THE YEAR IN HYPERTENSION 2001

THE YEAR IN HYPERTENSION

2001

HENRY L. ELLIOTT, JOHN M. C. CONNELL

and

GORDON T. McINNES

Department of Medicine and Therapeutics, University of Glasgow
Gardiner Institute, Western Infirmary, Glasgow

CLINICAL PUBLISHING SERVICES

OXFORD

Clinical Publishing Services Ltd

Oxford Centre for Innovation
Mill Street, Oxford OX2 0JX, UK

Tel: +44 1865 811116
Fax: +44 1865 251550
Web: www.clinicalpublishing.co.uk

Distributed by:

Plymbridge Distributors Ltd
Estover Road
Plymouth PL6 7PY, UK

Tel: +44 1752 202300
Fax: +44 1752 202333
E mail: orders@plymbridge.com

A catalogue record for this book is available from the British Library

ISBN 0 9537339 4 7

Project Manager: Rosemary Osmond
Typeset by Footnote Graphics, Warminster, Wiltshire
Printed in Spain by T G Hostench SA, Barcelona

Contents

Part III

Hypertension: emerging concepts

Part IV

Current practical issues

Contributors

STEPHEN CLELAND, BSc, MRCP, PhD, Lecturer in Clinical Medicine, Department of Medicine & Therapeutics, Gardiner Institute, Western Infirmary, University of Glasgow, Glasgow

JOHN CONNELL, MBChB, MD, FRCP, FMedSci, Professor of Endocrinology, Department of Medicine & Therapeutics, Gardiner Institute, Western Infirmary, University of Glasgow, Glasgow

HENRY ELLIOTT, MD, FRCP, Senior Lecturer in Medicine and Therapeutics, Department of Medicine & Therapeutics, Gardiner Institute, Western Infirmary, University of Glasgow, Glasgow

ANDREW KERNOHAN, BMedSci, MBChB, MRCP, Clinical Research Fellow, Department of Medicine & Therapeutics, Gardiner Institute, Western Infirmary, University of Glasgow, Glasgow

GORDON McINNES, BSc, MD, FRCP, FFPM, Senior Lecturer and Honorary Consultant Physician, Department of Medicine & Therapeutics, Gardiner Institute, Western Infirmary, University of Glasgow, Glasgow

Foreword

The authors' second annual review of the year in hypertension is timely in the light of many new trial outcomes which have recently been reported. As highlighted in the earlier volume, there remains considerable uncertainty as to whether 'newer' drugs, such as the angiotensin-converting enzyme inhibitors and calcium channel blocking drugs, confer advantages over older drugs in the treatment of hypertension in general and in important high-risk subgroups such as those with diabetes, existing vascular disease or renal impairment. To have waited almost 20 years without knowledge of the long-term outcomes of these drugs when used as hypertension treatment is a clear indictment of the profession whose responsibility surely should have been to demand that morbidity and mortality studies were set in place long before now.

It is against this background that the authors critically review many trials, the results of which have recently been published. They rightly emphasize the many shortcomings of trials such as INSIGHT, NORDIL and CAPPP, which were clearly underpowered to detect potential advantages of the newer drugs in protection against coronary heart disease. The discussion of the HOPE trial is important because of the remaining uncertainty as to whether the benefits observed were related to the drug ramipril, or to blood pressure differences between the groups.

Several new meta-analyses have been published this year and deserve mention. The reader is encouraged to be as critical in evaluation of these data as he or she might be in looking at the individual trials. As the Blood Pressure Trialists' Collaboration were at pains to point out, these are interim analyses and report end-point numbers that are still too small to allow definitive conclusions to be made on drug-drug comparisons.

Many on-going studies are cited and several will report in the next year, guaranteeing the wherewithal for future reviews!

The authors reiterate a summary of contemporary guidelines and it is likely that the various bodies will reconvene to review their recommendations in the light of new trial results.

The section on genetics and cardiovascular disease leads us through a particularly challenging and difficult field characterized by inconsistent and at times conflicting findings.

For the clinician, the book will come as an important and useful reference. Many issues, however, remain unresolved and one hopes that future editions of *The Year in Hypertension* will provide critical summaries of key outstanding studies aimed to establish the definitive evidence base upon which to establish optimal clinical practice and to reduce the prevailing and unacceptable burden of hypertension-related cardiovascular disease in contemporary society.

Peter S Sever, MA, MB, BChir, PhD, FRCP, FESC
Professor of Clinical Pharmacology & Therapeutics
Imperial College School of Medicine
London, UK

Preface

The task of keeping up to date with recent developments is becoming increasingly difficult, even for the specialist, on account of the exponential expansion in medical knowledge and the ever increasing numbers of journals and other publications. For the non-specialist, therefore, especially where time and the relevant resources are restricted, it may prove to be impossible to keep abreast of all recent developments. Accordingly, the principal aim of *The Year in Hypertension* is to distill and summarize the information contained in recent publications and to present to the reader an abbreviated version of any recent 'landmark' clinical trials and illustrative examples of smaller research studies that influence current therapeutic practice, or indicate likely future directions.

The Year in Hypertension cannot possibly be a comprehensive and extensive review of every recently published paper. While major studies, which are likely to influence clinical practice directly can readily be identified and commented upon, other smaller studies are selected on the pragmatic basis that they are illustrative of current lines of research. This does not mean that a chosen paper is necessarily definitive, or unique, or unexpected, but it has been selected because it provides the reader with ready access to current directions in terms of both clinical practice and ongoing research.

In addition to providing a distillate of the literature published within the last year or so, there is a necessary requirement to maintain a perspective on how these recent findings relate to existing knowledge. For this reason, specific comment and summarizing conclusions are made by the authors on the basis of their own personal experience and expertise. Additionally, in some instances, summarizing comments have been retained for influential studies that have been published within recent years.

Finally, the content of *The Year in Hypertension* is likely to evolve and alter as the relevance of different therapeutic areas changes with time. It is our intention to modify and adapt our chapters continuously in the light of these changes. Nevertheless, our primary aim is the presentation of up-to-date information in a readily accessible format.

Henry Elliott, John Connell and Gordon McInnes

Part I

Clinical trials and guidelines

1

Recent trial results

Introduction

In epidemiological studies, there is a close relationship between blood pressure (BP; systolic and diastolic) and risk of stroke, coronary heart disease (CHD) and other cardiovascular events |**1**|. The higher the BP, the greater is the risk. This relationship is consistent in different populations, in younger and older subjects, in men and women, and is independent of other cardiovascular risk factors. The relationship is continuous across the range of BP, indicating that there is no lower threshold or safe level of BP. The slope of the relationship between BP and stroke is about 50% steeper than that between BP and CHD. However, many more coronary events are experienced in Western populations, although strokes are the predominant events in individuals from South-East Asia.

Over the past four decades, numerous studies have examined the influence of drug treatment of hypertension on risk of cardiovascular events |**2**|. The usual aim was to achieve diastolic BP less than 90 mmHg. The average reduction in diastolic BP of 5–6 mmHg in these trials conferred a reduction of about 38% in stroke incidence, a 16% reduction in CHD events, a 21% reduction in all vascular events and a 12% reduction in all cause mortality, all highly significant. Effects on fatal and non-fatal events were similar. The proportional reductions were the same in high- and low-risk individuals, in the young and the elderly, and in mild, moderate and severe hypertension. At least equivalent benefits are associated with treatment of systolic hypertension |**3–7**|.

Benefits are likely to be greater with larger reductions of BP. Epidemiological data indicate no lower threshold for risk and observational findings suggest that patients with the lowest on-treatment BP have the best prognosis |**8**|. The Hypertension Optimal Treatment (HOT) Study |**9**| confirmed that rigorous control of BP is associated with a reduced risk of cardiovascular events. Attainment of low BP was achievable in a high proportion of patients |**10,11**| without unacceptable side-effects |**11**|, and was associated with an improved quality of life |**12**|. Concordance with therapy was high in all groups |**13**|. Failure to achieve target BP, therefore, cannot be attributed to side-effects or patient non-compliance.

Epidemiological data suggest that a difference in usual BP of the magnitude seen in the trials would result in a reduction in stroke incidence of 35–40% and of 20–25% for CHD events. Thus, treatment attains all that can be expected in stroke prevention but there appears to be a shortfall in protection against CHD events. As most of the trials used diuretics or beta-blockers, with potentially adverse metabolic effects, it has been suggested that newer agents might achieve greater cardiovascular protection for an equivalent reduction in BP. Early findings were inconclusive. The overall findings of the Captopril Prevention Project (CAPPP) |14| indicate that antihypertensive therapy based on an angiotensin-converting enzyme (ACE) inhibitor is no better than therapy based on diuretics and beta-blockers in the prevention of cardiovascular events and may be less effective in prevention of stroke although ACE inhibitors may confer an advantage in patients with diabetes mellitus. In the Swedish Trial of Old Patients with Hypertension-2 (STOP-2) study |15|, diuretics and beta-blockers and newer antihypertensive drugs (ACE inhibitors and calcium channel blockers) where equally useful in the management of elderly patients with hypertension. The hypothesis that some classes of drugs would have advantages was not substantiated. However, both trials had major shortcomings. In CAPPP |14|, the use of captopril once daily in half the patients randomized to this form of therapy was illogical in view of the short duration of action of this drug. The observed BP differences between the groups could not be explained by chance in such a large sample size and is almost certainly related to the use of envelopes for randomization |16|. The excess of stroke in captopril-treated patients is probably the consequence of the trial-long difference in BP; statistical adjustment cannot compensate for such an effect. The STOP-2 study |15| also had potential weaknesses and uncertainties. The newer drugs were used at low doses in a once daily regimen raising the possibility that 24-h control of BP might be less complete in these patients. Additional therapy was with older drugs regardless of the randomized group reducing the distinction between older and newer drugs. This is particularly relevant as about 50% of patients required older drugs and at least one-third of patients discontinued randomized therapy during the course of the trial.

The potential advantage of newer agents thus remains uncertain. The last year has seen the publication of several large outcome trials and meta-analyses that have addressed this question. In addition, a further overview has examined the risks associated with systolic BP in older patients with isolated systolic hypertension.

Influence of newer antihypertensive agents

The International Nifedipine GITS Study: Intervention as a Goal in Hypertension Treatment (INSIGHT)

 Morbidity and mortality in patients randomized to double-blind treatment with a long-acting calcium-channel blocker or diuretic in the International Nifedipine GITS Study: Intervention as a Goal in Hypertension Treatment (INSIGHT).
M J Brown, C R Palmer, A Castaigne, *et al. Lancet* 2000; **356**: 366–72.

BACKGROUND. The aim was to compare the effects of the calcium channel blocker nifedipine once daily with the diuretic combination co-amilozide on cardiovascular mortality and morbidity in high-risk patients with hypertension.

INTERPRETATION. Nifedipine once daily and co-amilozide were equally effective in preventing overall cardiovascular and cerebrovascular complications.

Comment

INSIGHT was a double-blind randomized trial of morbidity and mortality, in which the comparison was between older and newer classes of antihypertensive drugs in patients at high absolute risk of cardiovascular events. These patients are the main target for treatment in modern guidelines. The primary objective was to compare the efficacy in preventing the major complications from hypertension of nifedipine, a calcium channel blocker, administered in a long-acting gastro-intestinal therapeutic system (GITS) formulation and co-amilozide a common and effective combination of the diuretics hydrochlorothiazide and amiloride.

The study recruited 2929 men and 3392 women, aged 55–80 years, with BP during placebo run-in $\geq$ 150/95 mmHg or isolated systolic BP $\geq$ 160 mmHg, from nine countries (Israel, France, Italy, Spain, the Netherlands, UK, Norway, Sweden and Finland). To be eligible, patients had to have $\geq$ 1 other additional major cardiovascular risk factor. Treatment allocation to nifedipine GITS 30 mg daily (n = 3157) or co-amilozide (hydrochlorothiazide 25 mg/amiloride 5 mg) once daily (n = 3164) was performed by minimization rather than randomization to balance additional risk factors. Optimal increases in treatment by dose doubling and/or addition of atenolol or enalapril, and then by other antihypertensive drugs, excluding calcium channel blockers or diuretics, was allowed to achieve target BP $\leq$ 140/90 mmHg or a fall $\geq$ 20/10 mmHg.

The primary outcome variable was a composite of death from any cardiovascular or cerebrovascular cause, together with non-fatal stroke, myocardial infarction (MI) and heart failure. Three secondary variables were: (a) total mortality; (b) death from a vascular cause; and (c) non-fatal vascular events, including transient ischaemic attacks, angina (new or worsening), and renal failure.

Mean age of participants was 65 years. BP at randomization was 173/99 mmHg. The proportion of additional risk factors were: total cholesterol > 6.43 mmol/l, 52%; smoking > 10/day, 28%; diabetes mellitus, 21.6%; family history of premature MI or stroke, 21%; left ventricular hypertrophy 11%; previous MI, CHD and peripheral vascular disease, each 6%; proteinuria, 3%.

The main outcomes in INSIGHT are shown in Table 1.1. Primary outcomes occurred in 200 (6.3%) patients in the nifedipine group and in 182 (5.8%) in the co-amilozide group [18.2 vs 16.5 events per 1000 patient-years; relative risk (RR) 1.10 [95% confidence interval (CI) 0.91, 1.34], P = 0.35]. Overall mean BP fell from 173/99 mmHg to 138/82 mmHg. There was an 8% excess of withdrawals from the nifedipine group because of peripheral oedema (725 vs 518, P < 0.0001). Deaths were mainly non-vascular (nifedipine 176 vs co-amilozide 172; P = 0.81).

Table 1.1 Individual end-points in INSIGHT

	Nifedipine	Co-amilozide	Odds ratio (95% CI)	P
Primary outcomes				
Composite*	200 (6.3%)	182 (5.8%)	1.11 (0.90–1.36)	0.34
Myocardial infarction				
Non-fatal	61 (1.9%)	56 (1.8%)	1.09 (0.76–1.58)	0.52
Fatal	16 (0.5%)	5 (0.2%)	3.22 (1.18–8.80)	0.017
Sudden death	17 (0.5%)	23 (0.7%)	0.74 (0.39–1.39)	0.43
Stroke				
Non-fatal	55 (1.7%)	63 (2.0%)	0.87 (0.61–1.26)	0.52
Fatal	12 (0.3%)	11 (0.3%)	1.09 (0.48–2.48)	0.84
Heart failure				
Non-fatal	24 (0.8%)	11 (0.3%)	2.20 (1.07–4.49)	0.028
Fatal	2 (0.1%)	1 (<0.1%)	2.01 (0.18–22.13)	0.63
Other cardiovascular death	13 (0.4%)	12 (0.4%)	1.09 (0.50–2.38)	0.85
Secondary outcomes				
Composite†	383 (12.1%)	397 (12.5%)	0.96 (0.83–1.12)	0.62
Deaths				
All (first event)‡	153 (4.8%)	152 (4.8%)	1.01 (0.80–1.27)	0.95
Non-cardiovascular	71 (2.2%)	66 (2.1%)	1.08 (0.77–1.52)	0.67
Unknown cause	22 (0.7%)	34 (1.1%)	0.65 (0.38–1.11)	0.14
Cardiovascular	60 (1.9%)	52 (1.6%)	1.16 (0.80–1.69)	0.45
Non-fatal cardiovascular events	230 (7.3%)	245 (7.7%)	0.94 (0.78–1.13)	0.50
Primary events	140 (4.4%)	130 (4.1%)	1.08 (0.85–1.38)	0.53
Angina (worsening or new)	57 (1.8%)	77 (0.4%)	0.74 (0.52–1.04)	0.10
Transient ischaemic attacks	25 (0.8%)	25 (0.8%)	1.00 (0.57–1.75)	1.0
Renal failure	8 (0.3%)	13 (0.4%)	0.62 (0.26–1.49)	0.38

*MI, stroke, heart failure and cardiovascular death. †Primary outcomes plus non-cardiovascular deaths, renal failure, angina, and transient ischaemic attacks. ‡23 additional in nifedipine group and 20 in co-amilozide group occurred after a previous end-point.

Source: Brown *et al.* (2000).

Implications of INSIGHT

Overall, INSIGHT suggests no significant difference between nifedipine once daily and co-amilozide in patients with hypertension and additional cardiovascular risk factors. However, only 382 primary events were recorded, and 95% CIs for the composite end-point and cause-specific outcomes were wide. For the composite end-point, the findings do not exclude the possibilities that nifedipine is 10% better or 36% worse than diuretic-based therapy. For the cause-specific outcome of particular interest, MI, the 95% CI was even wider. Nifedipine might be 58% less effective than co-amilozide in preventing non-fatal heart attacks and indeed had a significant disadvantage for total heart attacks.

Of concern is the large loss of patients from randomized therapy. Some 2307 (almost 36%) patients were withdrawn from randomized therapy, the majority in the first year. Inclusion of such patients in the intention-to-treat analysis will tend to dilute the magnitude of any real cause-specific differences between individual therapies.

INSIGHT was simply too small. Alone, its findings contribute little to the debate about whether there are important differences between antihypertensive regimens. Thus INSIGHT provides little insight.

The Nordic Diltiazem (NORDIL) study

Randomized trial of effects of calcium antagonists compared with diuretics and β-blockers on cardiovascular morbidity and mortality in hypertension: the Nordic Diltiazem (NORDIL) study.
L Hansson, T Hedner, P Lund-Johansen, *et al.* for the NORDIL Study Group.
Lancet 2000; **356**: 339–65.

BACKGROUND. The effectiveness of diltiazem, a non-dihydropyridine calcium channel blocker, in reducing cardiovascular morbidity or mortality is unclear. NORDIL compared the effects of diltiazem with that of diuretics, beta-blockers, or both on cardiovascular morbidity and mortality in hypertensive patients.

INTERPRETATION. Diltiazem was as effective as treatment based on diuretics, beta-blockers, or both in preventing the combined primary end-point of all stroke, MI and other cardiovascular death.

Comment

Calcium channel blockers have been used extensively to treat hypertension for more than 15 years and are among the compounds listed as first-line treatment in the 1998 WHO/International Society of Hypertension guidelines for the management of mild hypertension (see Chapter 2). In addition, many observations on intermediary end-points, especially reversal of left ventricular hypertrophy (a powerful risk indicator in hypertension), show that a calcium channel blocker-based antihypertensive regimen is more effective than regimens based on diuretics, beta-blockers or both. Such findings suggest that calcium channel blockers ought to be at least as effective as diuretics or beta-blockers in lowering cardiovascular risks. Available trial data with calcium channel blockers are in elderly hypertensive patients |3,4,6,7,15| and mainly in patients with isolated systolic hypertension. Moreover, all those studies used dihydropyridine-derived calcium channel blockers.

In a prospective, randomized, open, blinded end-point study, 10 881 patients (5290 men and 5591 women), aged 50–74 years (mean 60 years) with diastolic BP $\geq$ 100 mmHg, were assigned diltiazem, or diuretics, beta-blockers, or both. All patients could receive additional antihypertensive treatment in several steps to lower diastolic BP to less than 90 mmHg.

In the diltiazem group, as step 1, patients were given 180–360 mg diltiazem daily. In step 2, ACE inhibitor was added, and in step 3, a diuretic or alpha-blocker was added to the ACE inhibitor. Any other antihypertensive compound could be added as step 4. In the diuretic and beta-blocker group, step 1 was a thiazide diuretic or a beta-blocker. In step 2, the two were combined. In step 3 an ACE inhibitor or alpha-blocker was added. In step 4, any other antihypertensive compound could be added except a calcium channel blocker. The mean follow-up was 4.5 years. The combined primary end-point was fatal and non-fatal stroke, MI and other cardiovascular death.

BP at baseline was similar in the treatment groups, 173.5/105.8 mmHg and 173.4/105.7 mmHg, in the diltiazem and diuretic/beta-blocker groups, respectively. Systolic and diastolic BP were lowered effectively in the diltiazem and diuretic and beta-blocker groups (reduction 20.3/18.7 vs 23.3/18.7 mmHg; difference in systolic reduction $P < 0.001$). A primary end-point occurred in 403 patients in the diltiazem group and in 400 in the diuretic and beta-blocker group [16.6 *vs* 16.2 events per 1000 patient-years; RR 1.00 (95% CI 0.87, 1.15), $P = 0.97$]. Fatal and non-fatal stroke occurred in 159 patients in the diltiazem group and in 196 in the diuretic and beta-blocker group [6.4 *vs* 7.9 events per 1000 patient-years; 0.80 (0.65, 0.99), $P = 0.04$] and fatal and non-fatal MI in 183 and 157 patients [7.4 *vs* 6.3 events per 1000 patient-years; 1.16 (0.94, 1.44), $P = 0.17$]. The main results are summarised in Fig. 1.1 and Table 1.2.

Antihypertensive treatment with a diltiazem-based regimen did not affect total mortality or the sum of major cardiovascular events differently from a thiazide diuretic and beta-blocker regimen. In prevention of the combined primary end-point of all stroke, MI and cardiovascular death, the two treatment approaches were almost indistinguishable. However, the diltiazem regimen was significantly more effective than the diuretic and beta-blocker regimen in lowering the rate of all stroke. This finding could be due to chance, in view of the many statistical comparisons conducted.

The reduction in diastolic BP was identical in the two groups, and for systolic BP was significantly greater (3 mmHg) in the diuretics and beta-blocker group than in

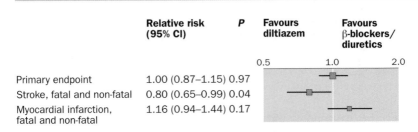

	Relative risk (95% CI)	P	Favours diltiazem	Favours β-blockers/diuretics
			0.5 1.0 2.0	
Primary endpoint	1.00 (0.87–1.15)	0.97		
Stroke, fatal and non-fatal	0.80 (0.65–0.99)	0.04		
Myocardial infarction, fatal and non-fatal	1.16 (0.94–1.44)	0.17		

Fig. 1.1 Relative risk of cardiovascular end-points in NORDIL. Source: Hansson *et al.* (2000).

Table 1.2 Relative risk and occurrence of end-points in NORDIL

	No. of patients with events		Event rate per 1000 patient-years		Relative risk (95% CI)*	P
	Diltiazem group	Diuretics and beta-blocker group	Diltiazem group	Diuretics and beta-blocker group		
Primary end-point	403	400	16.6	16.2	1.00 (0.87–1.15)	0.97
All stroke	159	196	6.4	7.9	0.80 (0.65–0.99)	0.04
Fatal stroke	21	22	0.8	0.9	0.96 (0.52–1.74)	0.89
All stroke plus TIA	200	236	8.1	9.5	0.84 (0.70–1.01)	0.07
All MI	183	157	7.4	6.3	1.16 (0.94–1.44)	0.17
Fatal MI	28	25	1.1	1.0	1.10 (0.64–1.88)	0.74
Cardiovascular death	131	115	5.2	4.5	1.11 (0.87–1.43)	0.41
Total mortality	231	228	9.2	9.0	1.00 (0.83–1.20)	0.99
All cardiac events	487	470	20.2	19.2	1.04 (0.91–1.18)	0.57
Diabetes mellitus	216	251	9.4	10.8	0.87 (0.73–1.04)	0.14
Atrial fibrillation	105	128	4.2	5.1	0.82 (0.64–1.07)	0.14
CHF	63	53	2.5	2.1	1.16 (0.81–1.67)	0.42

TIA, transient ischaemic attack; CHF, congestive heart failure. *Cox's regression model adjusted for age, sex, systolic pressure and baseline status of diabetes mellitus and smoking.

Source: Hansson *et al.* (2000).

the diltiazem group. A 3 mmHg difference in the reduction in BP should have a demonstrable effect on the frequency of stroke. The risk would have been 12% higher than that expected in the diltiazem group, and not the 20% lower frequency observed.

Implications of NORDIL

NORDIL suffered from a relative lack of patients who experienced end-points. Although the difference between diltiazem and conventional therapy for stroke events of 20% achieved borderline statistical significance, the 95% CI was wide and differences were not statistically significant for fatal strokes or when transient ischaemic attacks were included (Table 1.2). A detrimental effect of diltiazem on MI of similar magnitude (16%) was not statistically significant but the 95% CI does not exclude an adverse effect as great as 44%. For other cause-specific end-points, 95% CIs were also wide.

Although a high proportion of patients remained on randomized therapy throughout the trial (diltiazem group 71%, conventional therapy 93%), the study design ensured cross-contamination. Thus, in the diltiazem group, 916 patients (17%) received diuretics and 686 (13%) received beta-blockers; in the diuretic/beta-blocker group, 470 patients (9%) received a calcium channel blocker. As a consequence, any inferences concerning the influence of specific antihypertensive drug classes were diluted.

NORDIL provides the best evidence of the potential value of a non-dihydropyridine calcium channel blocker in hypertension. However, inequalities in BP control, the low event rate and the uncertainty arising from the use of supplementary drugs means that many questions remain unanswered.

The Antihypertensive and Lipid-Lowering Treatment to Prevent Heart Attack Trial (ALLHAT)

Major cardiovascular events in hypertensive patients randomized to doxazosin vs chlorthalidone. The Antihypertensive and Lipid-Lowering Treatment to Prevent Heart Attack Trial (ALLHAT).

The ALLHAT Officers and Coordinators for the ALLHAT Collaborative Research Group. *JAMA* 2000; **283**: 1967–75.

BACKGROUND. The objective was to compare the effect of doxazosin, an alpha-blocker, with chlorthalidone, a diuretic, on the incidence of cardiovascular disease in patients with hypertension as part of a study of four types of antihypertensive drugs: chlorthalidone, doxazosin, amlodipine and lisinopril.

INTERPRETATION. Compared with doxazosin, chlorthalidone yields essentially an equal risk of CHD death/non-fatal MI but significantly reduces the risk of combined cardiovascular disease events, particularly congestive heart failure, in high-risk hypertensive patients.

Comment

ALLHAT is a randomized, double-blind, active-controlled clinical trial, initiated in February 1994 (see Chapter 3). In January 2000, after an interim analysis, an independent data review committee recommended discontinuing the doxazosin treatment arm based on comparisons with chlorthalidone.

A total of 24 335 patients (aged $\geq$ 55 years) with hypertension and $\geq$ 1 other CHD risk factor were assigned randomly to receive chlorthalidone, 12.5–25 mg/day (n = 15268), or doxazosin, 2–8 mg/day (n = 9067), for a planned follow-up of 4–8 years. The primary outcome measure was fatal CHD or non-fatal MI; secondary outcome measures included all-cause mortality, stroke and combined cardiovascular disease (CHD, death, non-fatal MI, stroke, angina, coronary revascularization, congestive heart failure and peripheral arterial disease). Participants had a mean age of 67 years; 47% were women; 49% were white non-Hispanic, 35% black and 16% Hispanic; 36% were diabetic. The large sample size resulted in virtually identical distributions of baseline characteristics in the two treatment groups.

Median follow-up was 3.3 years. Mean seated BP was 145/83 mmHg in both groups and 135/76 mmHg and 137/76 mmHg at 4 years in the chlorthalidone and doxazosin group, respectively (Fig. 1.2). Outcome data that formed the basis for the decision to terminate the doxazosin arm are presented in Table 1.3.

A total of 365 patients in the doxazosin group and 608 in the chlorthalidone group had fatal or non-fatal MI, with no difference in risk between the groups (RR 1.03; 95% CI 0.90, 1.17; P = 0.71). Total mortality did not differ between the doxazosin and chlorthalidone arms (9.62% and 9.08%, respectively; RR 1.03; 95% CI 0.90, 1.15; P = 0.56). The doxazosin arm, compared with the chlorthalidone arm, had a higher risk of stroke (RR 1.19; 95% CI 1.01, 1.40; P = 0.04) and combined cardiovascular disease (25.45% vs 21.76%; RR 1.25; 95% CI 1.17, 1.33; $P <$ 0.001). Considered separately, heart failure risk was doubled (8.13% vs 4.45%; RR 2.04; 95% CI 1.79, 2.32; $P <$ 0.001).

While there were essentially no differences in the rates of the primary outcome or all-cause mortality between the two treatment groups, there was a statistically significant 25% higher incidence of major cardiovascular disease events in participants assigned to the doxazosin group compared with those assigned to the chlorthalidone group. In addition, the likelihood of observing a significant difference for the primary outcome by the scheduled end of the trial was very low. At the time of the decision to terminate the doxazosin vs chlorthalidone comparison, about 61% of the total number of expected CHD events had occurred in the chlorthalidone group. If the protocol-specific alternative hypothesis (16% reduction) was assumed for the remainder of the trial, there was only a 1% likelihood of finding a significant beneficial effect of doxazosin at the scheduled end of the trial.

Table 1.3 Outcomes in the BP component of ALLHAT by treatment group

Outcomes	4-year rate per 100 (SE)		No. of patients with outcomes		Relative risk (95% CI)	z Score†	P value†
	Chlorthalidone group (n = 15 268)	Doxazosin group (n = 9067)	Chlorthalidone group	Doxazosin group			
CHD‡	6.30 (0.38)	6.26 (0.30)	608	365	1.03 (0.90–1.17)	0.38	0.71
All-cause mortality	9.08 (0.35)	9.62 (0.49)	851	514	1.03 (0.90–1.15)	0.58	0.56
Combined CHD§	11.97 (0.38)	13.06 (0.53)	1211	775	1.10 (1.00–1.12)	2.00	0.05
Stroke	3.61 (0.22)	4.23 (0.32)	351	244	1.19 (1.01–1.40)	2.05	0.04
Combined cardiovascular disease¶	21.76 (0.49)	25.45 (0.68)	2245	1592	1.25 (1.17–1.33)	6.77	<.001
Congestive heart failure	4.45 (0.26)	8.13 (0.43)	420	491	2.04 (1.79–2.32)	10.95	<.001
Coronary revascularization	5.20 (0.27)	6.21 (0.39)	502	337	1.15 (1.00–1.32)	2.00	0.05
Angina	10.19 (0.35)	11.54 (0.48)	1082	725	1.16 (1.05–1.27)	3.01	<.001
Peripheral artery disease	2.87 (0.21)	2.89 (0.26)	264	165	1.07 (0.88–1.30)	0.67	0.05

The 4-year cumulative event rates were calculated using the Kaplan–Meier method. Other summary statistics are based on the entire trial experience.
†The z scores and two-sided P values were calculated using the log-rank test.
‡CHD is ALLHAT's primary outcome and consists of fatal CHD and non-fatal MI. The four secondary end-points are all-cause mortality, combined CHD, stroke and combined cardiovascular disease.
§Combined CHD consists of CHD death, non-fatal MI, coronary revascularization procedures and angina with hospitalization.
¶Combined cardiovascular disease consists of CHD death, non-fatal MI, stroke, coronary revascularization procedures, angina (treated in hospital or as outpatient), congestive heart failure (treated in hospital or as outpatient) and peripheral arterial disease (in-hospital or outpatient revascularization).
Source: The ALLHAT Officers and Coordinators for the ALLHAT Collaborative Research Group (2000).

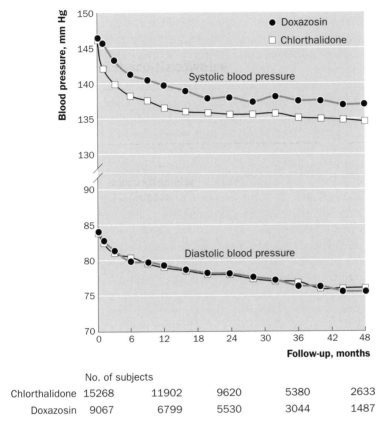

Fig. 1.2 Average systolic and diastolic BP during ALLHAT follow-up. Source: The ALLHAT Officers and Coordinators for the ALLHAT Collaborative Research Group (2000).

It was determined that participants assigned to the doxazosin group should be informed of their BP treatment assignment and that the major clinical findings regarding this treatment and its comparison agent, chlorthalidone, should be reported as soon as possible.

Implications of the comparisons of doxazosin and chlorthalidone in ALLHAT

The decision to discontinue the doxazosin arm was based on several factors. Foremost was a significantly higher incidence of combined cardiovascular events and, in particular, heart failure events, for the doxazosin group compared with the chlorthalidone group. In addition, with essentially equal rates in the two treatment groups for primary CHD outcome and total mortality, a beneficial effect of doxazosin at the scheduled trial termination was highly unlikely based on conditional power calculations. There was also a negative trend for stroke.

In ALLHAT, loss to follow-up and documentation of events were similar in the doxazosin and chlorthalidone groups. However, at 4 years, 86% of those assigned to chlorthalidone were still taking a diuretic, whereas only 75% of those assigned to doxazosin were still taking an alpha-blocker. Furthermore, although only 4% of patients randomized to chlorthalidone were taking an alpha-blocker, 24% of the doxazosin group were taking a diuretic. This lack of full adherence may have resulted in an underestimation of the true difference in cardiovascular rates between the two treatments.

Mean systolic BP in the doxazosin group was about 2–3 mmHg higher than in the chlorthalidone group; mean diastolic BP was the same. A 3 mmHg higher systolic BP could explain a 10–20% increase in heart failure, but not a doubling of the risk, a 15–20% increase in stroke risk and about a 12% increase in angina risk. Thus, the observed BP differential may explain much of the stroke and angina differences observed between chlorthalidone and doxazosin in ALLHAT.

These ALLHAT results demonstrate that chlorthalidone is superior to doxazosin as a first-line antihypertensive drug in a diverse group of older hypertensive patients with other cardiovascular risk factors. However, the use of doxazosin as part of a multidrug regimen for treating hypertension alone or hypertension with symptoms of benign prostatic hypertrophy was not tested in this trial. As ALLHAT was not a placebo-controlled trial but rather an active-controlled one, the study does not allow an assessment of whether doxazosin is better than placebo.

ALLHAT is continuing for participants in the remaining antihypertensive treatment arms and those in the lipid-lowering trial component. The trial is likely to provide important information about other pharmacological treatments of hypertension and the utility of lipid-lowering therapy in older, moderately hypercholesterolaemic persons with hypertension.

The Heart Outcomes Prevention Evaluation (HOPE) study

 Effects of an angiotensin-converting-enzyme inhibitor, ramipril, on cardiovascular events in high-risk patients.
The Heart Outcomes Prevention Evaluation Study Investigators.
N Engl J Med 2000; **342**: 145–53.

BACKGROUND. ACE inhibitors improve the outcome among patients with left ventricular dysfunction, whether or not they have heart failure. HOPE assessed the role of an ACE inhibitor, ramipril, in patients who were at high risk for cardiovascular events but who did not have left ventricular dysfunction or heart failure.

INTERPRETATION. Ramipril significantly reduced the rates of death, MI and stroke in a broad range of high-risk patients who are not known to have a low ejection fraction or heart failure.

Comment

A total of 9297 high-risk patients (55 years of age or older) who had evidence of vascular disease or diabetes plus one other cardiovascular risk factor and who were not known to have a low ejection fraction or heart failure were randomly assigned to receive ramipril (10 mg once daily) or matching placebo for a mean of 5 years. The primary outcome was a composite of MI, stroke or death from cardiovascular causes.

Some 10 576 eligible patients participated in a run-in phase in which they received ramipril 2.5 mg once daily for 7–10 days followed by matching placebo for 10–14 days. A total of 1035 patients were subsequently excluded from randomization because of non-compliance ($< 80\%$ of pills taken), side-effects, abnormal serum creatinine or potassium levels, or withdrawal of consent. Of the 9541 remaining patients, 4645 were assigned randomly to receive ramipril 10 mg, 4652 were assigned randomly to receive matching placebo, and 244 were assigned randomly to receive low-dose ramipril (2.5 mg daily). Treatment was scheduled to last 5 years.

Of the 9297 patients who underwent randomization, there were 2480 women, 5128 patients who were at least 65 years old, 8162 who had cardiovascular disease, 4355 who had hypertension, and 3577 who had diabetes. The mean BP at entry was 139/79 mmHg in both groups. The mean BP was 136/76 mmHg and 139/77 mmHg, respectively, at the end of the study.

A total of 651 patients who were assigned to receive ramipril (14.0%) reached the primary end-point, as compared with 826 patients who were assigned to receive placebo (17.8%) (RR 0.78; 95% CI 0.70, 0.86; $P < 0.001$) (Fig. 1.3). Treatment with ramipril reduced the rates of death from cardiovascular causes (6.1%, as compared with 8.1% in the placebo group; RR 0.74; $P < 0.001$), MI (9.9% vs 12.3%; RR 0.80; $P < 0.001$), stroke (3.4% vs 4.9%; RR 0.68; $P < 0.001$), death from any cause (10.4% vs 12.2%; RR 0.84; $P = 0.005$), revascularization procedures (16.0% vs 18.3%; RR 0.85; $P = 0.002$), cardiac arrest (0.8% vs 1.3%; RR 0.63; $P = 0.03$), heart failure (9.0% vs 11.5%; RR 0.77; $P < 0.001$) and complications related to diabetes (6.4% vs 7.6%; RR 0.84; $P = 0.03$). The beneficial effect of treatment with ramipril on the composite outcome was consistently observed among predefined subgroups (Fig. 1.4).

Implications of HOPE

An ACE inhibitor was beneficial in a broad range of patients without evidence of left ventricular dysfunction or heart failure who were at high risk of cardiovascular events. Treatment with ramipril reduced the rates of death, MI, stroke, coronary revascularization, cardiac arrest, and heart failure as well as risk of complications related to diabetes and of diabetes itself.

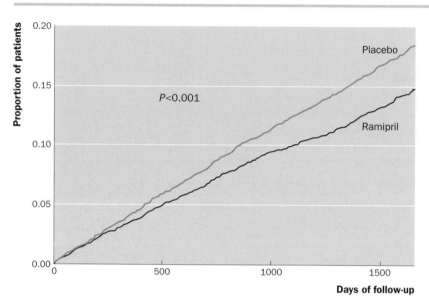

Fig. 1.3 Kaplan–Meier estimates of the composite outcome of MI, stroke or death from cardiovascular causes in the ramipril group and placebo group in HOPE. The relative risk of the composite outcome in the ramipril group as compared with the placebo group was 0.78 (95% CI 0.70, 0.86). Source: The Heart Outcomes Prevention Evaluation Study Investigators (2000).

The extent to which the beneficial effects of ramipril could be explained by BP reduction is controversial. The authors concluded that only a small part of the benefit could be attributed to a reduction in BP, as the majority of patients did not have hypertension at baseline (according to conventional definitions) and the mean reduction in BP with treatment was extremely small (3/2 mmHg). A reduction of 2 mmHg in diastolic BP might at best account for about 40% of the reduction the rate of stroke and about one-quarter of the reduction in the rate of MI |2|. However, the results of recent studies, such as the HOT study |9| suggest that for high-risk patients (e.g. those with diabetes), it may be beneficial to lower BP even if it is already within the 'normal' range (Table 1.4). In the absence of a positive control group with similar changes in BP, no definite conclusions can be reached about the benefits of ramipril beyond BP reduction.

HOPE observed a marked reduction in the incidence of complications related to diabetes and new cases of diabetes. The results are consistent with the results of CAPPP |14|, which indicated a lower rate of newly diagnosed diabetes in patients who were randomly assigned to receive captopril than in those who were assigned to receive a diuretic or beta-blocker, although the conduct of that study makes the results unreliable |16|.

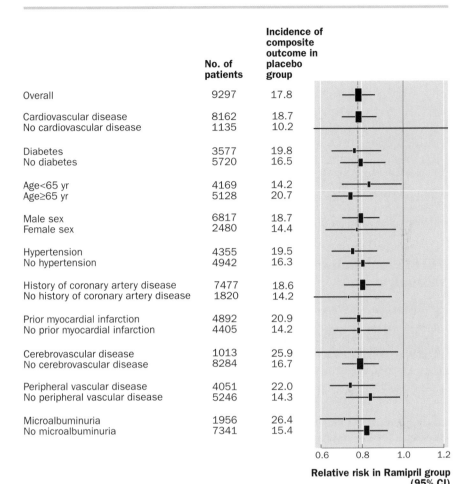

	No. of patients	Incidence of composite outcome in placebo group
Overall	9297	17.8
Cardiovascular disease	8162	18.7
No cardiovascular disease	1135	10.2
Diabetes	3577	19.8
No diabetes	5720	16.5
Age<65 yr	4169	14.2
Age≥65 yr	5128	20.7
Male sex	6817	18.7
Female sex	2480	14.4
Hypertension	4355	19.5
No hypertension	4942	16.3
History of coronary artery disease	7477	18.6
No history of coronary artery disease	1820	14.2
Prior myocardial infarction	4892	20.9
No prior myocardial infarction	4405	14.2
Cerebrovascular disease	1013	25.9
No cerebrovascular disease	8284	16.7
Peripheral vascular disease	4051	22.0
No peripheral vascular disease	5246	14.3
Microalbuminuria	1956	26.4
No microalbuminuria	7341	15.4

0.6   0.8   1.0   1.2

Relative risk in Ramipril group (95% CI)

Fig. 1.4 The beneficial effect of treatment with ramipril on the composite outcome of MI, stroke or death from cardiovascular causes overall and in various predefined subgroups in HOPE. Cerebrovascular disease was defined as stroke or transient ischaemic attacks. The size of each symbol is proportional to the number of patients in each group. The dashed line indicates overall relative risk. Source: The Heart Outcomes Prevention Evaluation Study Investigators (2000).

Table 1.4 Risk reduction for cardiovascular events. Comparison of findings in HOPE, MICRO-HOPE, SYST-EUR diabetic patients |19| and HOT diabetic patients |9|

Treatment	Risk Reduction			
	HOPE ACEI	MICRO HOPE ACEI	SYST-EUR DIABETES CCB ± others	HOT DIABETES CCB ± others
DBP (mmHg)	79	80	85	85
CV risk reduction (%)	22	25	69	51
Reduction DBP (mmHg)	2	1.4	3.3	4.1
CV risk reduction per mmHg (%)	11	17.9	20.9	12.4

ACEI, angiotensin converting enzyme inhibitor, CCB, calcium channel blocker, DBP, diastolic BP, CV, cardiovascular.

The Microalbuminuria and Renal Outcomes (MICRO) HOPE substudy

Effects of ramipril on cardiovascular and microvascular outcomes in people with diabetes mellitus: results of the HOPE study and MICRO-HOPE substudy.

Heart Outcomes Prevention Evaluation (HOPE) Study Investigators. *Lancet* 2000; **355**: 253–9.

BACKGROUND. Diabetes mellitus is a strong risk factor for cardiovascular and renal disease. HOPE investigated whether the ACE inhibitor ramipril can lower these risks in patients with diabetes.

INTERPRETATION. Ramipril was beneficial for cardiovascular events and overt nephropathy in people with diabetes. The cardiovascular benefit appeared greater than that attributable to the decrease in BP.

Comment

People with diabetes mellitus are at high risk of cardiovascular disease. Although studies suggest that ACE inhibitors may prevent or delay serious events in some subgroups, their role in a broader group of people with diabetes who are at high risk of cardiovascular events remains unknown. MICRO-HOPE substudy, the effect of this intervention on the risk of overt nephropathy was investigated.

Some 3577 people with diabetes included in HOPE, aged 55 years or older, who had a previous cardiovascular event or ≥ 1 other cardiovascular risk factor, no clinical proteinuria, heart failure or low ejection fraction, and who were not taking ACE inhibitors, were assigned randomly ramipril (10 mg daily) or placebo. The combined primary outcome was MI, stroke or cardiovascular death. Overt nephropathy was a main outcome in a substudy.

Eligible participants were included who completed a run-in period, during which they received ramipril 2.5 mg daily for 7–10 days, followed by matching placebo for 10–14 days, who were at least 80% compliant, tolerated the drug without side-effects, and maintained a serum creatinine concentration of 200 μmol/l or lower and potassium concentration of 5.5 mmol/l or lower. The mean age was 65.4 years, 1322 (37%) were women, and 1996 (56%) had a history of hypertension. Baseline characteristics of participants in the ramipril and placebo groups were similar.

The study was stopped 6 months early (after 4.5 years) by the independent data safety and monitoring board because of a consistent benefit of ramipril compared with placebo (Fig. 1.5). Ramipril lowered the risk of the combined primary outcome by 25% (95% CI 12, 36; $P = 0.0004$), MI by 22% (6, 36), stroke by 33% (10, 50), cardiovascular death by 37% (21, 51), total mortality by 24% (8, 37), revascularization by 17% (2, 30) and overt nephropathy by 24% (3, 40; $P = 0.027$).

BP decreased slightly more among participants on ramipril than among those on placebo. By the end of the study, systolic BP had fallen by 1.9 mmHg and risen by 0.6 mmHg in participants on ramipril and placebo, respectively ($P = 0.0002$); diastolic BP had fallen by 3.3 mmHg and 2.3 mmHg in the ramipril and placebo groups ($P = 0.008$). After adjustment for the changes in systolic (2.4 mmHg) and diastolic (1.0 mmHg) BPs, ramipril still lowered the risk of the combined primary outcome by 25% (12, 36; $P = 0.0004$).

Implications of MICRO-HOPE

Ramipril significantly lowered the risk of major cardiovascular outcomes by 25–30% in a broad range of high-risk middle-aged and elderly people with diabetes mellitus. The benefit was apparent irrespective of whether participants had a history of cardiovascular events, hypertension or microalbuminuria, were taking insulin or oral antihyperglycaemic agents, or had type 1 or type 2 diabetes mellitus. Ramipril also lowered the risk of overt nephropathy, renal failure or laser therapy. It had no long-term effect on glycaemic control.

Again the main controversy is to what extent the findings can be explained by BP reduction in the ramipril group. The authors propose that the risk reduction for cardiovascular events was greater than would be expected from the observed mean difference in BP between groups. For example, in the UK Prospective Diabetes Study (UKPDS) |17| mean differences between groups in systolic and diastolic BPs of 10 mmHg and 5 mmHg, respectively, lowered the risk of MI by 21% and stroke by 44%. Similarly, in participants with diabetes in the Systolic Hypertension in the Elderly (SHEP) study |18| a decrease in systolic and diastolic pressures of 10 mmHg and 2 mmHg, respectively (using a diuretic-based approach), reduced the risk of cardiovascular events by up to 34%. By contrast, in the HOPE study the differences in systolic and diastolic BPs were slight (2.2 mmHg and 1.4 mmHg), yet the decreases in risk of MI and stroke were similar to those seen in UKPDS. However,

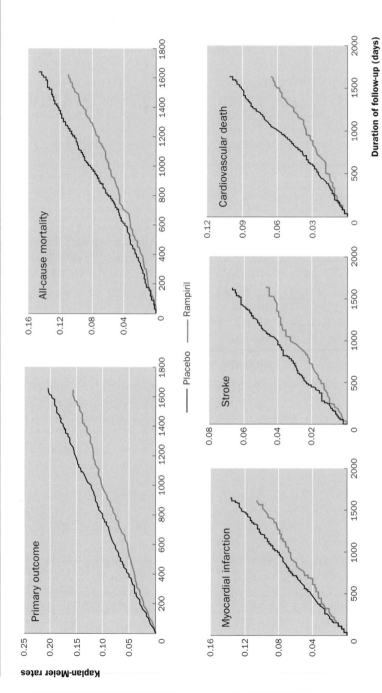

Fig. 1.5 Kaplan–Meier survival curves per patient with diabetes in MICRO-HOPE. Source: Heart Outcomes Prevention Evaluation (HOPE) Study Investigators (2000).

other studies in patients with type 2 diabetes |**9,19**| suggest much greater benefits from moderate reductions of diastolic BP following treatment with other classes of antihypertensive agents (Table 1.4). Thus, the findings of MICRO-HOPE (and HOPE) may merely confirm the value of small BP reductions within the 'normotensive' range in high-risk individuals.

Meta-analyses of trials of newer antihypertensive agents

Calcium antagonists compared with other first-line antihypertensive agents

Health outcomes associated with calcium antagonists compared with other first-line antihypertensive therapies: a meta-analysis of randomized controlled trials.
M Pahor, B M Psaty, M H Alderman, *et al. Lancet* 2000; **356**: 1949–54.

BACKGROUND. Several observational studies and individual randomized trials in hypertension have suggested that, compared with other drugs, calcium channel blockers may be associated with a higher risk of coronary events, despite similar blood-pressure control. The aim of this meta-analysis was to compare the effects of calcium channel blockers and other antihypertensive drugs on major cardiovascular events.

INTERPRETATION. In randomized controlled trials, the large available database suggests that calcium channel blockers are inferior to other types of antihypertensive drugs as first-line agents in reducing the risks of several major complications of hypertension. On the basis of these data, the longer-acting calcium channel blockers cannot be recommended as a first-line therapy for hypertension.

Comment

The main objective was to find out whether the intermediate-acting and long-acting calcium channel blockers used as first-line therapy are superior, equal or inferior to other treatments in reducing the frequency of cardiovascular complications. This was a meta-analysis of trials in hypertension that assessed cardiovascular events and included at least 100 patients, who were randomly assigned intermediate-acting or long-acting calcium channel blockers or other antihypertensive drugs and who were followed up for at least 2 years.

The nine trials included in the meta-analysis were Appropriate Blood Pressure Control in Diabetes (ABCD) |**20**|, the Cardiovascular Study in the Elderly (CASTEL) |**21**|, the Fosinopril *vs* Amlodipine Cardiovascular Events Trial (FACET) |**22**|, INSIGHT, the Multicenter Isradipine Diuretic Atherosclerosis Study (MIDAS)

|**23**|, the National Intervention Cooperative Study in Elderly Hypertensives study (NICS-EH) |**24**|, NORDIL, the STOP-2 study |**15**|, and Verapamil in Hypertension and Atherosclerosis Study (VHAS) |**25**|.

The nine eligible trials included 27 743 participants. Calcium channel blockers and other drugs achieved similar control of both systolic and diastolic BP. Compared with patients assigned diuretics, beta-blockers, ACE inhibitors or clonidine ($n = 15044$), those assigned calcium channel blockers ($n = 12699$) had a significantly higher risk of acute MI [odds ratio 1.26 (95% CI 1.11, 1.43), $P = 0.0003$], congestive heart failure [1.25 (95% CI 1.07, 1.46), $P = 0.005$], and major cardiovascular events [1.10 (95% CI 1.02, 1.18), $P = 0.018$]. The treatment differences were within the play of chance for the outcomes of stroke [0.90 (95% CI 0.80, 1.02), $P = 0.10$] and all-cause mortality [1.03 (95% CI 0.94, 1.13), $P = 0.54$].

The finding were quite similar when the analyses were restricted to double-blind trials (ABCD, INSIGHT, MIDAS, NICS-EH), to dihydropyridine (ABCD, CASTEL, FACET, INSIGHT, MIDAS, NICS-EH, STOP-2), and non-dihydropyridine (NORDIL, VHAS) calcium channel blockers , to shorter-acting (CASTEL, MIDAS, NORDIL) and longer-acting (ABCD, FACET, INSIGHT, NICS-EH, STOP-2, VHAS) calcium channel blockers, to patients with diabetes (ABCD, CASTEL, FACET, NORDIL), to large trials in which cardiovascular events were the primary outcome (INSIGHT, NORDIL, STOP-2), and when calcium channel blockers were compared with ACE inhibitors (ABCD, FACET, STOP-2) and with diuretics or beta-blockers (CASTEL, INSIGHT, MIDAS, NICS-EH, NORDIL, STOP-2, VHAS).

In comparative analyses of intermediate-acting or long-acting calcium channel blockers *vs* other antihypertensive therapies, the combined results of the nine trials that met the inclusion criteria showed that calcium channel blockers were associated with a significantly higher risk of major complications of hypertension, including acute MI, congestive heart failure and combined major cardiovascular events. No significant differences were found for the outcomes of stroke and all-cause mortality (Tables 1.5–1.10).

Table 1.5 Meta-analysis of direct comparisons between calcium channel blockers (CCB) and other drugs

Outcome	CCB versus other drugs All trials (n = 27,743)	
	OR	95% CI
MI (n = 1050)	1.26	1.11, 1.43
Stroke (n = 1227)	0.90	0.80, 1.02
MCE (n = 3409)	1.10	1.02, 1.18
CHF (n = 717)	1.25	1.07, 1.46
Mortality (n = 2078)	1.03	0.94, 1.13

OR, Odds ratio; MI, CHD events; MCE, major cardiovascular events; CHF, congestive heart failure.

Source: Pahor *et al.* (2000).

Table 1.6 Meta-analysis of direct comparisons between dihydropyrindine (DHP) and non-dihydropyridine (non-DHP) calcium channel blockers (CCB) and other drugs

Outcome	CCB versus other drugs			
	DHP (n = 15 448)		Non-DHP (12 295)	
	OR	95% CI	OR	95% CI
MI	1.31	1.12, 1.53	1.18	0.95, 1.46
Stroke	0.95	0.82, 1.10	0.81	0.66, 1.00
MCE	1.12	1.02, 1.23	1.05	0.92, 1.20
CHF	1.25	1.05, 1.48	1.24	0.86, 1.78
Mortality	1.03	0.93, 1.15	1.03	0.92, 1.20

OR, Odds ratio; MI, CHD events; MCE, major cardiovascular events; CHF, congestive heart failure.

Source: Pahor *et al.* (2000).

Table 1.7 Meta-analysis of direct comparisons between calcium channel blockers (CCB) and other drugs. Shorter and longer acting agents

Outcome	CCB versus other drugs			
	Shorter acting (n = 12 295)		Longer acting (n = 15 628)	
	OR	95% CI	OR	95% CI
MI	1.18	0.96, 1.46	1.41	1.12, 1.54
Stroke	0.85	0.69, 1.04	0.94	0.81, 1.08
MCE	1.09	0.96, 1.24	1.10	1.00, 1.21
CHF	1.46	1.05, 2.04	1.19	1.00, 1.42
Mortality	1.09	0.96, 1.24	0.99	0.90, 1.11

OR, Odds ratio; MI, CHD events; MCE, major cardiovascular events; CHF, congestive heart failure.

Source: Pahor *et al.* (2000).

However, the reviewed trials cannot provide evidence about whether calcium channel blockers have a harmful effect on CHD and congestive heart failure, or whether the other drugs have special benefits. In the Systolic Hypertension in Europe trial (SYST-EUR) trial, compared with placebo, nitrendipine had no significant effects on the risk of cardiac outcomes, but was associated with a lower risk of stroke |6|. In this meta-analysis, the effects of calcium channel blockers and their comparison therapies on the risk of stroke suggest that BP control may have an especially important role in preventing stroke.

The authors conclude that low-dose diuretics, which have proven efficacy and low cost, should continue to be the standard therapy for hypertension, and all new classes of drugs should be compared with diuretics. The use of long-acting calcium

Table 1.8 Meta-analysis of direct comparisons between calcium channel blockers (CCB) and other drugs in patients with diabetes mellitus

Outcome	CCB versus other drugs Diabetes mellitus (n = 1640)	
	OR	95% CI
MI	1.53	1.01, 2.31
Stroke	1.37	0.84, 2.20
MCE	1.44	1.09, 1.91
CHF	1.76	0.97, 3.21
Mortality	1.24	0.84, 1.83

OR, Odds ratio; MI, CHD events; MCE, major cardiovascular events; CHF, congestive heart failure.

Source: Pahor *et al.* (2000).

Table 1.9 Meta-analysis of direct comparisons between calcium channel blockers (CCB) and other drugs—ACE inhibitors

Outcome	CCB versus other drugs ACE inhibitors (n = 5251)	
	OR	95% CI
MI	1.43	1.15, 1.76
Stroke	1.01	0.84, 1.23
MCE	1.18	1.04, 1.33
CHF	1.24	1.00, 1.55
Mortality	0.97	0.83, 1.13

OR, Odds ratio; MI, CHD events; MCE, major cardiovascular events; CHF, congestive heart failure.

Source: Pahor *et al.* (2000).

channel blockers (and alpha-blockers) should be limited to patients who do not tolerate or do not respond to diuretics, beta-blockers and ACE inhibitors.

Blood Pressure Lowering Treatment Trialists' Collaboration

Effects of ACE inhibitors, calcium antagonists, and other blood-pressure-lowering drugs: results of prospectively designed overviews of randomized trials.
Blood Pressure Lowering Treatment Trialists' Collaboration. *Lancet* 2000; **355**: 1955–64.

BACKGROUND. This programme of overviews of randomized trials was established to investigate the effects of ACE inhibitors, calcium channel blockers, and other BP

Table 1.10 Meta-analysis of direct comparisons between calcium channel blockers (CCB) and other drugs—diuretics and beta-blockers

Outcome	CCB Versus Other Drugs Diuretics and beta-blockers (n = 24, 627)	
	Odds Ratio	95% CI
MI	1.20	1.04, 1.37
Stroke	0.86	0.76, 0.98
MCE	1.06	0.97, 1.15
CHF	1.22	1.03, 1.46
Mortality	1.04	0.94, 1.16

Odds ratios and 95% CI. MI, CHD events; MCE, major cardiovascular events; CHF, congestive heart failure.

Source: Pahor *et al.* (2000).

lowering drugs on mortality and major cardiovascular morbidity in several populations of patients. Separate overviews were made of trials comparing active treatment regimens with placebo, trials comparing more intensive and less intensive BP lowering strategies, and trials comparing treatment regimens based on different drug classes.

INTERPRETATION. Strong evidence of benefits of ACE inhibitors and calcium channel blockers is provided by the overviews of placebo-controlled trials. There is weaker evidence of differences between treatment regimens of differing intensities and of differences between treatment regimens based on different drug classes.

Comment

Over the past 5 years, a new series of trials has been completed, and several other trials started in efforts to elucidate further the effects of ACE inhibitors, calcium channel blockers, and other BP lowering drugs on mortality and major cardiovascular morbidity in several populations of patients, including those with hypertension, diabetes mellitus, CHD or renal disease. Before the results of any of these new trials were known, some studies were recognized as being too small individually to detect moderate, although potentially important, cause-specific effects of treatments or differences between treatment effects. Therefore, prospective overviews in which treatment effects and treatment differences would be estimated from the combined results of individual studies were planned (see Chapter 3). This report provides results from the first prospectively planned cycle of analyses by this collaborative group.

The hypotheses to be investigated, the trials to be included, and the outcomes to be studied were all selected before the results of any participating trial were known. Outcome data were available from 15 studies |6,9,14,15,17,20,24,26–32| along with HOPE, INSIGHT and NORDIL, that collectively included 74 696 individuals.

The overview of placebo-controlled trials of ACE inhibitors (four trials, 12 124 patients mostly with CHD) revealed reductions in stroke [30% (95% CI 15, 43)],

CHD [20% (95% CI 11, 28)] and major cardiovascular events [21% (95% CI 14, 27)]. Each study comparing ACE inhibitors with placebo was carried out in patients selected on the basis of a history of cardiovascular disease or diabetes mellitus rather than BP. One study provided most of the data: of the 1860 cardiovascular events and the 1165 deaths from all causes, 88% and 90%, respectively, were seen in the HOPE study.

The overview of placebo-controlled trials of calcium channel blockers (two trials, 5520 patients mostly with hypertension) showed reductions in stroke [39% (95% CI 15, 56)] and major cardiovascular events (28% (95% CI 13, 41)). The larger of these (SYST-EUR) |6| was carried out in patients with isolated systolic hypertension, and the smaller (Prospective Randomized Evaluation of the Vascular Effect of Norvasc Trial [PREVENT]) |28| was carried out in those selected on the basis of CHD. Of the 388 major cardiovascular events and 296 deaths from all causes, 86% and 95% respectively, were seen in SYST-EUR.

In the overview of trials comparing BP lowering strategies of different intensity (three trials, 20 408 patients with hypertension), there were reduced risks of stroke [20% (95% CI 2, 35)], CHD [19% (95% CI 2, 33)] and major cardiovascular events [15% (95% CI 4, 24)] with more intensive therapy. In the overviews comparing different antihypertensive regimens (eight trials, 37 872 patients with hypertension), several differences in cause-specific effects were seen between calcium-antagonist-based therapy and other regimens, but each was of borderline significance.

Overall, in the trials comparing ACE inhibitor-based regimens with diuretic-based or beta-blocker-based regimens, 2022 major cardiovascular events and 1257 deaths from all causes were seen (Table 1.11). There were no detectable differences between randomized groups in the risks of any of the outcomes studied (all $P > 0.1$), but for most of the comparisons, moderate differences in cause-specific outcome (e.g. 10% difference in the relative risk of CHD) were not excluded by the 95% CIs. There was borderline significant evidence of heterogeneity between the

Table 1.11 Meta-analysis of direct comparisons between ACE inhibitors (ACEI) and other drugs

Outcome	ACEI versus other drugs Patients (n = 16,061)	
	OR	95% CI
MI (n = 843)	1.00	0.88, 1.14
Stroke (n = 827)	1.05	0.92, 1.19
MCE (n = 2022)	1.00	0.93, 1.08
CHF (n = 473)	0.92	0.77, 1.09
Mortality (n = 1257)	1.03	0.93, 1.14

OR, Odds ratio; MI, CHD events; MCE, major cardiovascular events; CHF, congestive heart failure.

Source: Blood Pressure Lowering Treatment Trialists' Collaboration (2000).

results of individual studies for stroke ($P = 0.05$), because of an apparent excess of strokes among patients assigned ACE inhibitor-based treatment in CAPPP |24|—a difference that could be largely explained by the higher initial BP of patients assigned ACE-inhibitor-based therapy in this study. Exclusion of CAPPP from the overview analyses decreased the evidence of heterogeneity for this outcome, but did not materially alter the overall results for any outcome.

Among patients assigned calcium channel blockers based therapy, there was a significant 13% lower risk of stroke (95% CI 2, 23) than among those assigned diuretic-based or beta-blocker-based therapy. Additionally, there was a 12% greater risk of CHD events of borderline significance (95% CI 0, 26) among those assigned calcium channel blocker-based therapy. The results are summarized in Tables 1.12 and 1.13.

Table 1.12 Meta-analysis of direct comparisons between calcium channel blockers (CCB) and other drugs

Outcome	CCB versus other drugs Patients (n = 23 454)	
	OR	95% CI
MI (n = 1077)	1.12	1.00, 1.16
Stroke (n = 985)	0.87	0.77, 0.98
MCE (n = 2485)	1.02	0.95, 1.10
CHF (n = 528)	1.12	0.95, 1.33
Mortality (n = 1552)	1.01	0.92, 1.11

OR, Odds ratio; MI, CHD events; MCE, major cardiovascular events; CHF, congestive heart failure.

Source: Blood Pressure Lowering Treatment Trialists' Collaboration (2000).

Table 1.13 Meta-analysis of direct comparisons between dihydropyridine (DHP) and non-dihydropyridine (non-DHP) calcium channel blockers and other drugs

Outcome	CCB versus other drugs			
	DHP (n = 11 159)		Non-DHP (n = 12 295)	
	OR	95% CI	OR	95% CI
MI	1.11	0.96, 1.30	1.13	0.95, 1.35
Stroke	0.89	0.77, 1.04	0.83	0.68, 1.02
MCE	1.01	0.92, 1.10	1.04	0.92, 1.18
CHF	1.11	0.92, 1.34	1.18	0.82, 1.69
Mortality	1.00	0.89, 1.12	1.02	0.86, 1.22

OR, Odds ratio; MI, CHD events; MCE, major cardiovascular events; CHF, congestive heart failure.

Source: Blood Pressure Lowering Treatment Trialists' Collaboration (2000).

Only two trials compared directly ACE inhibitor-based regimens and calcium channel blocker-based regimens (Table 1.14), and most of the data were provided by one of these studies: of the 1178 major cardiovascular events and 774 deaths from all causes in these two trials, 93% and 96%, respectively, were observed in the STOP-2 study |**15**|. The combined analysis suggested a reduced risk of CHD events among the patients assigned ACE inhibitor-based therapy, but for this outcome and for major cardiovascular events, there was significant heterogeneity ($P = 0.01$ and 0.04, respectively) between the results of the two studies.

The results of the first cycle of analyses from this programme of prospectively designed overviews show that benefits of BP lowering drugs are not limited to regimens based on diuretics or beta-blockers. The overview of placebo-controlled trials of ACE inhibitors shows that, with only a modest reduction in BP, these agents decreased the risks of stroke, CHD, and major cardiovascular events by 20–30% among high-risk patients selected on the basis of a history of cardiovascular disease or diabetes mellitus.

The overview of placebo-controlled trials of calcium channel blockers shows that these agents reduced the risk of stroke and major cardiovascular events by about 30–40%; this was mainly among elderly patients with isolated systolic hypertension among whom study treatment reduced BP by about the same amount as that observed in earlier trials of diuretic-based or beta-blocker-based therapy. There was no clear evidence of reductions in CHD or heart failure.

The overview comparing the effects of more intensive and less intensive BP lowering strategies provided some evidence of potentially important differences between treatment regimens of differing intensity. In these trials of regimens based on ACE inhibitors, calcium channel blockers and beta-blockers, patients assigned the lowest BP targets (diastolic BP ≤ 75 to ≤ 85 mmHg) experienced lower risks of stroke, CHD and major cardiovascular events, although the exact sizes of all such differences remain uncertain because of the wide 95% CIs.

Table 1.14 Meta-analysis of direct comparisons between ACE inhibitors (ACEI) and calcium channel blockers (CCB)

Outcome	ACEI versus CCB Patients (n = 4871)	
	OR	95% CI
MI (n = 261)	0.81	0.68, 0.97
Stroke (n = 240)	1.02	0.85, 1.21
MCE (n = 1178)	0.92	0.83, 1.01
CHF (n = 353)	0.82	0.67, 1.00
Mortality (n = 774)	1.03	0.91, 1.18

OR, Odds ratio; MI, CHD events; MCE, major cardiovascular events; CHF, congestive heart failure.

Source: Blood Pressure Lowering Treatment Trialists' Collaboration (2000).

There may be moderate, although potentially important, differences between drug classes in their effects on cause-specific outcomes. In particular, the results of the overview comparing calcium channel blocker-based regimens with diuretic-based or beta-blocker-based regimens suggest a lower risk of stroke and a greater risk of CHD among patients assigned calcium channel blockers. As these trends were similar in trials of dihydropyridine and non-dihydropyridine calcium channel blockers, the results provide no clear support for the hypothesis that there may be qualitatively different effects of these agents on coronary risks. However, for stroke and CHD, the 95% CIs were wide and the size of any true differences between calcium channel blocker-based regimens and diuretic-based or beta-blocker-based regimens could not be determined reliably.

In comparisons of ACE inhibitor-based regimens with calcium channel blocker-based regimens, extreme reductions in the risk of CHD among patients assigned ACE inhibitor-based therapy were seen in one small trial with very few events [20], but no such difference was detected in the other much larger study with many more events [15]. The small trial was stopped early on the basis of an apparent difference in fatal or non-fatal MI, and so its results could provide an inflated estimate of any real treatment difference, which might explain the heterogeneity. For these reasons, the combined analysis of CHD events from these two trials does not provide reliable evidence of a difference between ACE inhibitor-based and calcium channel blocker-based regimens in their effects on this outcome.

In most of the trials included in these overviews, only about three-quarters of all randomized patients remained on assigned treatment at the end of follow-up. Such non-adherence makes it likely that analyses done by intention to treat, although keeping important biases to a minimum, will underestimate the effects of individual treatments and the differences between treatments that would be seen had there been full adherence to the randomized regimens.

Although the results of these prospectively planned overviews provide answers to some of the questions they were designed to address, uncertainty remains. For example, although there is clear evidence from the placebo-controlled trials that, with only modest reductions in BP, ACE inhibitors confer marked beneficial effects on the risks of major cardiovascular events in high-risk patients, there is no clear evidence from other trials in hypertensive patients that the benefits of ACE inhibitor-based therapy are any greater than those of diuretic-based or beta-blocker-based regimens. Additionally, although there is clear evidence of benefits of calcium channel blocker-based regimens for stroke and major cardiovascular events in older hypertensive patients, the evidence suggestive of greater benefits for stroke and lesser benefits for CHD with calcium channel blocker-based regimens than with diuretic-based or beta-blocker-based regimens is not sufficiently reliable to allow precise assessments of the differing balance of benefits and risks that might be experienced by patients at varying risks of stroke or coronary disease.

Implications of the meta-analyses of trials of newer anti-hypertensive agents

The study done by the Blood Pressure Lowering Treatment (BPLT) Trialists' Collaboration has several methodological strengths. Its prospective design reduces the potential for bias due to selection of studies. In addition, the availability of data from individual trial participants enabled use of the same criteria for defining study outcomes. Because of differences in selection criteria, Pahor and colleagues' analysis was based on experience in 27 743 participants from nine trials, whereas the corresponding analysis conducted by the BPLT Trialists' Collaboration was based on experience in 26 129 participants from six of the nine trials.

One limitation of the effect of ACE inhibitor therapy on cardiovascular disease as found by the BPLT trialists was that it was heavily dependent on results from one trial (HOPE). Furthermore, there is reason to be concerned about the generalizability of the findings because all the study participants were selected on the basis of a history of cardiovascular disease or diabetes rather than the level of their BP before randomization.

Although published simultaneously, these meta-analyses were very different in numbers of individuals, trials included and in method of counting events. Despite these differences in scope and overall conclusions the results were in fact very similar (Tables 1.15–1.18). The main dispute reflects the arbitrary nature of statistical significance ($P < 0.05$). The trends were very similar. Thus, calcium channel blockers, regardless of type, may have an advantage over other drugs, except ACE inhibitors, in prevention of stroke and disadvantage compared with other drugs in prevention of heart attacks. For all-cause-specific outcomes, 95% CIs were wide, emphasizing that much uncertainty remains.

Table 1.15 Meta-analyses of direct comparisons between calcium channel blockers (CCB) and other drugs

Outcome	CCB versus other drugs			
	Pahor (n = 27 743)		Trialists (n = 23 454)	
	OR	95% CI	OR	95% CI
MI	1.26	1.11, 1.43	1.12	1.00, 1.16
Stroke	0.90	0.80, 1.02	0.87	0.77, 0.98
MCE	1.10	1.02, 1.18	1.02	0.95, 1.10
CHF	1.25	1.07, 1.46	1.12	0.95, 1.33
Mortality	1.03	0.94, 1.13	1.01	0.92, 1.11

OR, Odds ratio; MI, CHD events; MCE, major cardiovascular events; CHF, congestive heart failure.

Source: Blood Pressure Lowering Treatment Trialists' Collaboration. Pahor *et al.* (2000).

Table 1.16 Meta-analyses of direct comparisons between dihydropridine calcium channel blockers (DHP CCB) and other drugs

Outcome	DHP CCB versus other drugs				
	Pahor (n = 15 448)		Trialists (n = 11 159)	
	OR	95% CI	OR	95% CI
MI	1.31	1.12, 1.53	1.11	0.96, 1.30
Stroke	0.95	0.82, 1.10	0.89	0.77, 1.04
MCE	1.12	1.02, 1.23	1.01	0.92, 1.10
CHF	1.25	1.05, 1.48	1.11	0.92, 1.34
Mortality	1.03	0.93, 1.15	1.00	0.89, 1.12

OR, Odds ratio; MI, CHD events; MCE, major cardiovascular events; CHF, congestive heart failure.

Source: Blood Pressure Lowering Treatment Trialists' Collaboration. Pahor *et al.* (2000).

Table 1.17 Meta-analyses of direct comparisons between non-dihydropyridine calcium channel blockers (non-DHP CCB) and other drugs

Outcome	Non-DHP CCB versus other drugs				
	Pahor (n = 12 295)		Trialists (n = 12 295)	
	OR	95% CI	OR	95% CI
MI	1.18	0.95, 1.46	1.13	0.95, 1.35
Stroke	0.81	0.66, 1.00	0.83	0.68, 1.02
MCE	1.05	0.92, 1.20	1.04	0.92, 1.18
CHF	1.24	0.85, 1.78	1.18	0.82, 1.69
Mortality	1.03	0.92, 1.20	1.02	0.86, 1.22

OR, Odds ratio; MI, CHD events; MCE, major cardiovascular events; CHF, congestive heart failure.

Source: Blood Pressure Lowering Treatment Trialists' Collaboration. Pahor *et al.* (2000).

Table 1.18 Meta-analyses of direct comparisons between calcium channel blockers (CCB) and ACE inhibitors (ACEI)

Outcome	CCB versus ACEI				
	Pahor (n = 5251)		Trialists (n = 4871)	
	OR	95% CI	OR	95% CI
MI	1.43	1.15, 1.76	1.23	1.03, 1.47
Stroke	1.01	0.84, 1.23	0.98	0.83, 1.18
MCE	1.18	1.04, 1.33	1.07	0.99, 1.20
CHF	1.24	1.00, 1.55	1.22	1.00, 1.49
Mortality	0.97	0.83, 1.13	0.97	0.85, 1.10

OR, Odds ratio; MI, CHD events; MCE, major cardiovascular events; CHF, congestive heart failure.

Source: Blood Pressure Lowering Treatment Trialists' Collaboration. Pahor *et al.* (2000).

Meta-analysis of outcome trials of isolated systolic hypertension in the elderly

Risks of untreated and treated isolated systolic hypertension in the elderly: meta-analysis of outcome trials.

A Staessen, J Gasowski, J G Wang, *et al. Lancet* 2000; **355**: 865–72.

BACKGROUND. Previous meta-analysis of outcome trials in hypertension have not specifically focused on isolated systolic hypertension or have explained treatment benefit mainly in function of the achieved diastolic BP reduction. A quantitative overview of the trials was undertaken to evaluate further the risks associated with systolic BP in treated and untreated older patients with isolated systolic hypertension.

INTERPRETATION. Drug treatment is justified in older patients with isolated systolic hypertension whose systolic BP is 160 mmHg or higher. Absolute benefit is larger in men, in patients aged 70 or more and in those with previous cardiovascular complications or wider pulse pressure. Treatment prevented stroke more effectively than coronary events. However, the absence of a relation between coronary events and systolic BP in untreated patients suggests that the coronary protection may have been underestimated.

Comment

Three trials exclusively involved older patients with isolated systolic hypertension: SHEP |**5**|, the SYST-EUR |**6**| and the Systolic Hypertension in China trial (SYST-CHINA) |**4**|. Also included were elderly patients with isolated systolic hypertension enrolled in five other trials: the study conducted by the European Working Party on High Blood Pressure in the Elderly (EWPHE) |**33**| the trial on Hypertension in Elderly Patients in Primary Care (HEP) |**34**| the Swedish Trial in Old Patients with Hypertension (STOP) |**35**| and the Medical Research Council trials in mild hypertension (MRC1) |**36**|, and in older adults (MRC2) |**37**|.

In the eight trials 15 693 patients with isolated systolic hypertension were followed up for 3.8 years (median). Patients were 60 years old or more. Systolic BP was 160 mmHg or greater and diastolic BP was less than 95 mmHg. BP at enrolment averaged 174 mmHg systolic and 83 mmHg diastolic. The mean baseline-corrected differences in systolic and diastolic BP between patients assigned control of active treatment were 10.4 (95% CI 9.8, 11.0) mmHg and 4.1 (95% CI 3.8, 4.4) mmHg.

After correction for regression dilution bias, sex, age and diastolic BP, the relative hazard rates associated with a 10 mmHg higher initial systolic BP were 1.26 ($P = 0.0001$) for total mortality, 1.22 ($P = 0.02$) for stroke, but only 1.07 ($P = 0.37$) for coronary events. Independent of systolic BP, diastolic BP was inversely correlated with total mortality, highlighting the role of pulse pressure as a risk factor.

Active treatment reduced total mortality by 13% (95% CI 2, 22, $P = 0.02$), cardiovascular mortality by 18%, all cardiovascular complications by 26%, stroke by 30%, and coronary events by 23% (Fig. 1.6). Furthermore, if only the three trials that focused specifically on isolated systolic hypertension were considered, active treatment decreased total mortality by 17% (95% CI 5, 28; $P = 0.008$), cardiovascular mortality by 25% (95% CI 8, 39; $P = 0.005$), all cardiovascular complications by 32% (95% CI 13, 41; $P < 0.001$), stroke by 37% (95% CI 24, 48; $P < 0.001$) and coronary events by 25% (95% CI 9, 39; $P < 0.001$). The number of patients to treat for 5 years to prevent one major cardiovascular event was lower in men (18 vs 38), at or above age 70 (19 vs 39), and in patients with previous cardiovascular complications (16 vs 37).

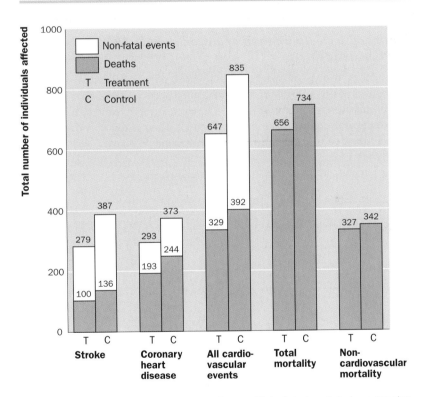

Fig. 1.6 Summarized results in older patients with isolated systolic hypertension enrolled in eight trails of antihypertensive drug treatment. Analysis included 15 693 patients. BP at entry averaged 174 mmHg systolic and 83 mmHg diastolic. During follow-up (median 3.8 years), mean difference in BP between treated and control patients was 10.4 mmHg systolic and 4.1 mmHg diastolic. Source: Staessen et al. (2000).

In untreated patients systolic BP was a more accurate than diastolic BP as a predictor of mortality and cardiovascular complications. After correction of regression dilution bias, a 10 mmHg increase in systolic BP was significantly and independently correlated with increases by nearly 10% in the risk of all fatal and non-fatal complications, except for coronary events. Diastolic BP, on the other hand, was inversely correlated with total and cardiovascular mortality. At any given level of systolic BP, the risk of death rose with lower diastolic BP and therefore also with greater pulse pressure.

The findings on the role of systolic BP as a risk factor may have important clinical implications. The target level of BP to be reached by antihypertensive drug treatment should, in older patients, be based on systolic rather than on diastolic BP. In terms of the number of patients to treat to prevent one event, antihypertensive therapy was particularly effective in men and in patients with previous cardiovascular complications and in patients aged ≥ 70 years.

Implications of the meta-analysis of outcome trials of isolated systolic hypertension in the elderly

Drug treatment is justified in older patients whose systolic BP is 160 mmHg or higher. Absolute benefit is greater in men, in older patients, and in those with previous cardiovascular complications or greater pulse pressure. In relative and absolute terms, treatment prevented stroke more effectively than it did coronary events. However, the absence of a relation between coronary events and systolic BP in untreated patients suggests that the coronary protection achievable in elderly hypertensive patients might have been underestimated.

Lessons from the recent trials of antihypertensive therapy

Introduction

The evidence base in support of the drug treatment of hypertension is among the strongest in medicine. Prospective, randomized clinical trials in 50 000 individuals have demonstrated conclusively that pharmacological reduction of BP reduces the risk of cardiovascular events and all-cause mortality [2].

The magnitude of reduction in stroke events in the trials is exactly that predicted from long-term epidemiological studies for the differences in systolic and diastolic BP achieved [1]. However, reduction in CHD events, the predominant complication of hypertension in Western populations, while significant, is rather less than that expected. The shortfall in CHD prevention might be explained by deleterious effects of diuretics or beta-blockers, which formed the basis of therapy in almost all the trials. Other antihypertension agents should avoid these unwanted actions and could have advantages in cardioprotection.

Stroke events appear to be prevented to the extent predicted by BP reduction regardless of how this is achieved. The question of interest is whether newer drugs are superior to earlier agents in the prevention of CHD events for the same reduction in BP, i.e. have benefits beyond BP control.

At usual doses, all antihypertensive agents produce reductions in BP of similar magnitude. Hence any difference in CHD risk between regimens based on diuretics and other drugs would have to be due to properties of the drugs that are independent of BP lowering effect.

It is unknown whether these influences augment the benefits of lowering BP and any independent effect is unlikely to be large. Detection of feasible and worthwhile differences in relative risk (10–15%) between various antihypertensive regimens requires evidence from randomized trials involving thousands of patients and yielding a rich harvest of CHD events.

Recent trials

Selective alpha-blockers, ACE inhibitors and calcium channel blockers have potential advantages over diuretics and beta-blockers in the prevention of CHD events and advantages for surrogate end-points have been claimed. These agents avoid the metabolic complications of the older drugs (and in the case of alpha-blockers may improve the metabolic profile), have possible vascular protective properties and advantages for surrogate end-points have been claimed.

Results of large outcome trials did not appear until 20 years after their introduction. The wait was hardly worthwhile. Although none detected a significant difference in CHD events between therapy based on newer drugs and that based on conventional agents, the precision of comparisons in individual trials was weak with wide 95% CIs for differences. As clinically useful differences between therapies in CHD events could not be excluded in any of the trials, individually the trials were not informative.

Individual trials had other shortcomings that cloud their interpretation. In CAPPP, BP at randomization and persistently throughout the trial was higher in patients treated with captopril compared with those given conventional therapy |14|. It is almost certain that there was failure in the randomization procedure |16| rendering the results unreliable. This extends to the findings in the subset with diabetes mellitus where there appeared to be an advantage of ACE inhibition |14|. In STOP-2 (ACE inhibitors or calcium channel blockers *vs* beta-blockers or diuretic) |15| and INSIGHT (calcium channel blockers *vs* diuretics), withdrawal rates from randomized therapy were unacceptably high (34–39% and 33–40%, respectively). Where less than 70% of all randomized patients remained on assigned therapy at the end of follow-up, intention-to-treat analysis will underestimate differences in treatment that would have been seen had there been full adherence to the randomized regimens. Significantly fewer fatal and non-fatal events were observed in the ACE inhibitor-treated patients than in calcium channel blockers treated patients in STOP-2 |15|. However, this was only one of 48 statistical comparisons and interpretation must be treated with caution.

The only information on the relative value of alpha-blockade in CHD prevention comes from the prematurely discontinued arm of ALLHAT. The primary reason was an apparent excess risk of heart failure in doxazosin-treated patients compared with those randomized to chlorthalidone. However, several factors make interpretation difficult. The diagnostic criteria for heart failure were unconvincing, on-treatment systolic BP was higher in doxazosin-treated subjects and the discontinuation rate was almost twice as high in patients randomized to alpha-blockers. The other reason for early discontinuation was futility—even if continued, the chance of detecting an advantage of doxazosin- over chlorthalidone-based therapy for CHD outcomes was less than 1%. We are left, probably for ever, with the unsatisfactory finding that alpha-blocker therapy might be 10% better or 17% worse than diuretic therapy for this outcome. Thus ALLHAT has also been uninformative. ALLHAT is the only study with sufficient statistical power to assess the impact on CHD separately; however, if the rest of the trial is conducted similarly to the doxazosin arm, ALLHAT may end in disappointment.

The HOPE study merits particular mention. Although not a comparison of a new drug against conventional therapy in hypertensive patients, it has been interpreted as showing an advantage of ACE inhibition beyond BP control. That active therapy (ramipril) was better than inactive therapy (placebo) in reducing heart attacks is hardly surprising but the magnitude of the reduction was greater than that predicted from epidemiological data for the small difference in BP observed. However, the reduction in cardiovascular events per mmHg difference in BP was no greater than that seen in other high-risk populations, such as diabetes, treated with other forms of antihypertensive therapy. In the absence of a positive control group, treated with another agent providing equivalent BP control, no definitive conclusions can be reached. A better acronym for HOPE might be 'HYPE'.

The recent trials of newer drugs against older drugs have failed us because they were too small, the event rate was low and almost 50% of the deaths were not cardiovascular. Insufficient power and the large proportion of non-vascular mortality make it difficult to detect differences between treatments for the outcome of interest—CHD (Table 1.19). The wide 95% CIs indicate that individual trials were uninformative.

Meta-analyses

In the face of uncertainty from individual trials it has become fashionable to resort to meta-analysis. The BPLT Trialists' Collaboration, which is collecting data from over 30 trials, should provide adequate power to compare more reliably different antihypertensive regimens with respect to particular events. However, the recently published preliminary analysis has not taken the matter of differential protection against CHD much further forward.

Differences in cause-specific effects between active therapies were of borderline significance. No differences were detected in comparisons of ACE inhibitors and conventional therapy but this analysis was heavily dependent on the unreliable CAPPP |14| and STOP-2 |15|. Compared with conventional therapy, calcium channel blocker-based therapy was associated with a 13% reduction in strokes and an increase of similar magnitude (12%) in CHD events, with no difference between

Table 1.19 Relative risk of MI and 95% CI in comparisons of newer drugs and conventional drugs (diuretics and beta-blockers)

Trial	Myocardial infarction New drugs versus conventional drugs		
	Drug	Relative risk	95% CI
CAPPP	ACEI	0.96	0.77, 1.19
STOP-2	ACEI	0.90	0.72, 1.13
	CCB	1.18	0.96, 1.47
NORDIL	CCB	1.16	0.94, 1.44
INSIGHT	CCB	1.09	0.76, 1.58
ALLHAT	AB	1.03	0.90, 1.17

ACEI, ACE inhibitor; CCB, calcium channel blocker; AB, alpha blocker. CAPP, Captopril Prevention Project |14|; STOP-2, Swedish Trial in Old Patients with Hypertension 2 |15|; NORDIL, Nordic Diltiazem Study; INSIGHT, International Nifedipine GITS study: Intervention as a Goal in Hypertension Treatment; ALLHAT = Antihypertension and Lipid-Lowering Treatment to Prevent Heart Attack Trial.

calcium channel blocker types. For both outcomes, 95% CIs were wide and the sizes of any true differences could not be determined reliably. Direct comparison of ACE inhibitor and calcium channel blocker-based therapies depended on only two trials, between which there was significant heterogeneity and with over 90% of events from STOP-2 |15|; it does not provide reliable evidence of a difference between ACE inhibitor and calcium channel blocker-based regimens.

The Pahor *et al.* meta-analysis suggested a highly significant 26% excess risk of CHD events with calcium channel blocker-based therapy compared with other treatments. This retrospective analysis used data on 27 743 patients from nine trials while the BPLT Trialist' review was based on 23 454 patients from six of these trials. The Pahor analysis had fewer CHD events and more strokes than the BPLT Trialists' (ratio 0.86 *vs* 1.09), emphasizing differences in the populations included. Nevertheless, there was no real difference between the meta-analyses—the clinically relevant message is that there remains uncertainty.

Both meta-analyses had limited statistical power to detect differences in cause-specific outcomes. There are insufficient data to suggest that ACE inhibitors are superior to diuretic and beta-blockers and insufficient power to provide a definitive comparison of the efficacy of calcium channel blockers against that of diuretics, beta-blockers and ACE inhibitors for CHD events. The quality of a meta-analysis depends on the quality of the studies included; in both of these examples, the studies included had major shortcomings.

Other concerns

The pattern of events in recent trials (relatively low proportion of cardiovascular deaths and high rate of stroke events) is not anticipated from epidemiological data or from trials comparing active therapy against placebo where cardiovascular

Table 1.20 CHD and stroke events in recent outcome trials

Trial	Events in Outcome Trials Recent trials		
	CHD	Stroke	Ratio
CAPPP	343	337	1.02
STOP-2	614	659	0.93
INSIGHT	191	163	1.17
NORDIL	443	355	1.25
Overall	1591	1514	1.05

CAPPP, Captopril Prevention Project |14|; STOP-2, Swedish Trial in Old Patients with Hypertension 2 |15|; INSIGHT; International Nifedipine GITS study: Intervention as a Goal in Hypertension Treatment; NORDIL, Nordic Diltiazem study.

deaths and CHD predominate |1,2|. In early trials |2|, the ratio of CHD to stroke events was 3:2 while in the recent trials the ratio is 1:1 (Table 1.20). Therefore, the newer drugs appear to have been tested in an environment very different from that where older drugs were evaluated and the hypothesis of a shortfall in CHD prevention was generated.

Uncertainties remain about the application of experience based upon the relative reduction in risk in individual populations with varying absolute risk for cause-specific outcomes. The generalization of results is only appropriate if the population to be treated is similar to that studied. Data from populations in which stroke outcomes are as common as CHD events may not be readily extrapolated to Western societies where CHD predominates. For this outcome, there appears to be little to choose between therapies.

The short duration of trials might have contributed to failure to detect differential effects on CHD events. It is conceivable that BP lowering *per se* may have a particularly important role in preventing stroke that is manifest rapidly while the influence of drug therapy on CHD may take longer to appear. Clinical trials provide short-term answers to long-term problems and are in effect surrogates for real life where treatment is often given for a lifetime.

Conclusion

The recent trials of hypertension treatment have provided few practical lessons and leave many questions unanswered. It appears that, for equivalent changes in BP, newer drugs are equivalent to earlier agents in preventing cardiovascular complications. Over the years since new drugs were introduced, expectations appear to have waned. Whereas, in the beginning, the new drugs were promoted as being superior to older drugs, now the objective seems to be to suggest equivalence with diuretics and beta-blockers. In the absence of any clear overall advantage, diuretics and beta-blockers should remain first-step drug therapies with newer agents added as necessary to achieve the target BP control that is clearly desirable.

Recent trials have demonstrated the critical importance of rigorous control of BP in reducing the risk of cardiovascular disease. Compared with less intensive control, tight control reduces CHD by 19% and underreporting of events in the largest individual trial may have led to an underestimate of the benefit. In the majority of patients, rigorous BP control necessitates the use of two or more anti-hypertensive agents in combination. The beneficial effects of additional BP lowering far outweighs any postulated differential effect between drugs.

References

1. MacMahon S, Peto R, Cutler J, Collins R, Sorlie P, Neaton J, Abbot R, Godwin J, Dyer A, Stamler J. Blood pressure stroke and coronary heart disease. Part 1, Prolonged differences in blood pressure: prospective observational studies corrected for the regression dilution bias. *Lancet* 1990; **335**: 765–74.

2. Collins R, MacMahon S. Blood pressure, antihypertensive drug treatment and the risks of stroke and of coronary heart disease. *Br Med Bull* 1994; **50**: 272–98.

3. He J, Whelton PK. Elevated systolic blood pressure as a risk factor for cardiovascular and renal disease. *J Hypertens* 1999; **17** (Suppl. 2): S7–S13.

4. Liu L, Wang JG, Gong L, Liu G, Staessen JA. Comparison of active treatment and placebo for older patients with isolated systolic hypertension. *J Hypertens* 1998; **16**: 1823–9.

5. SHEP Co-operative Research Group. Prevention of stroke by antihypertensive drug treatment in older persons with isolated systolic hypertension: Final results of the Systolic Hypertension in the Elderly Program (SHEP). *JAMA* 1991; **265**: 3255–64.

6. Staessen JA, Fagard R, Thijs L, Celis H, Arabidze GG, Birkenhager WH, Bulpitt CJ, de Leeuw PW, Dollery CT, Fletcher AE, Forette F, Leonetti G, Nachev C, O'Brien ET, Rosenfield J, Rodicio JL, Tuomilehto J, Zanchetti A. Randomised double-blind comparison of placebo and active treatment for older patients with isolated systolic hypertension. *Lancet* 1997; **350**: 757–64.

7. Staessen JA, Wang JG, Thijs L, Fargard R. Overview of the outcome trials in older patients with isolated systolic hypertension. *J Hum Hypertens* 1999; **13**: 859–63.

8. Isles CG, Walker LM, Beevers DG, Brown I, Cameron HL, Clarke J, Hawthorne V, Hole D, Lever AF, Robertson JWK, Wapshaw JA. Mortality in patients of the Glasgow Blood Pressure clinic. *J Hypertens* 1986; **4**: 141–56.

9. Hansson L, Zanchetti A, Carruthers SG, Dahlöf B, Elmfeldt D, Julius S, Ménard J, Rahn KH, Wedel H, Westerling S, for the HOT study group. Effects of intensive blood pressure lowering and low-dose aspirin in patients with hypertension: principal results of the Hypertension Optimal Treatment (HOT) randomised trial. *Lancet* 1998; **351**: 1755–62.

10. Hansson L, Zanchetti A. The Hypertension Optimal Treatment (HOT) Study–patient characteristics: randomization, risk profiles and early blood pressure results. *Blood Press* 1994; **3**: 322–7.

11. Hansson L, Zanchetti A for the HOT Study Group. The Hypertension Optimal Treatment (HOT) Study: 24-month data on blood pressure and tolerability. *Blood Pressure* 1997; **6**: 313–17.

12. Wiklund I, Halling K, Rydén-Bergsten T, Fletcher A. Does lowering of blood pressure improve mood? Quality of life results from the Hypertension Optimal Treatment (HOT) Study. *Blood Press* 1997; **6**: 357–64.

13. Waeber B, Leonetti G, Kolloch R, McInnes GT. Compliance with aspirin or placebo in the hypertension optimal treatment (HOT) Study. *J Hypertens* 1999; **17**: 1041–5.

14. Hansson L, Lindholm LH, Niskanen L, Lanke J, Hedner T, Niklason A, Luomanmäki K, Dählöf B, de Faire U, Mörlin C, Karlberg BE, Wester PO, Björck J-E, for the Captopril Prevention Project (CAPPP) study group. Effect of angiotensin-converting enzyme inhibition compared with conventional therapy on cardiovascular morbidity and mortality in hypertension: the Captopril Prevention Project (CAPPP) randomised trial. *Lancet* 1999; **353**: 611–16.

15. Hansson L, Lindholm LH, Ekbom T, Dahlöf B, Lanke J, Scherston B, Wester PO, Hedner T, de Faire U. Randomised trial of old and new antihypertensive drugs in elderly patients: cardiovascular mortality and morbidity the Swedish Trial in Old Patients with Hypertension-2 Study. *Lancet* 1999; **354**: 1751–6.

16. Peto R. Failure of randomisation by 'sealed' envelope. *Lancet* 1999; **354**: 73.

17. UK Prospective Diabetes Study Group. Tight blood pressure control and risk of macrovascular and microvascular complications in type 2 diabetes: UKPDS 38. *BMJ* 1998; **317**: 703–13.

18. Curb JD, Pressel SL, Cutler JA, Savage PJ, Appelgate WB, Black H, Camel G, Davis BR, Frost PH, Gonzalez N, Guthrie G, Oberman A, Rutan GH, Stamler J. Effect of diuretic-based antihypertensive treatment on cardiovascular disease risk in older diabetic patients with isolated systolic hypertension. *JAMA* 1996; **276**: 1886–92.

19. Tuomilehto J, Rastenyte D, Birkenhager WH, Thijs L, Antikainen R, Bulpitt CJ, Fletcher AE, Forette F, Goldhaber A, Palatini P, Sarti C, Fagard R, Staessen JA, for the Systolic Hypertension in Europe Trial Investigators. Effects of calcium channel blockers in older patients with diabetes and systolic hypertension. *N Engl J Med* 1999; **340**: 677–784.

20. Estacio RO, Jeffers BW, Hiatt WR, Biggi SL, Gifford N, Schrier RW. The effect of nisoldipine as compared with enalapril on cardiovascular events in patients with non-insulin-dependent diabetes and hypertension. *N Engl J Med* 1998; **388**: 645–52.

21. Casiglia E, Spolaore P, Mazz A. Effect of two different therapeutic approaches on total and cardiovascular mortality in a Cardiovascular Study in the Elderly (CASTEL). *Jpn Heart J* 1994; **35**: 589–600.

22. Tatti P, Pahor M, Byington RP, Di Mauro P, Guarisco R, Strollo G, Strollo F. Outcome results of the Fosinopril versus Amlodipine Cardiovascular Events randomized trial in patients with hypertension and NIDDM. *Diabetes Care* 1998; **21**: 597–603.

23. Borhani NO, Mercuri M, Borhani PA, Buckalew VM, Canossa-Terris M, Carr AA, Kappagoda T, Rocco MV, Schnaper HW, Sowers JR, Bond MG. Final outcome results of

the Multicenter Isradipine Diuretic Atherosclerosis Study (MIDAS): a randomized controlled trial. *JAMA* 1996; **276**: 785–91.

24. National Intervention Cooperative Study in Elderly Hypertensives Study Group. Randomized double-blind comparison of a calcium antagonist and a diuretic in elderly hypertensives. *Hypertension* 1999; **34**: 1129–33.

25. Rosei EA, Dal Palu C, Leonetti G, Magnani B, Pessina A, Zanchetti A. Clinical results of the Verapamil in Hypertension and Atherosclerosis Study. *J Hypertens* 1997; **15**: 1337–44.

26. UK Prospective Diabetes Study Group. Efficacy of atenolol and captopril in reducing risk of macrovascular and microvascular complications in type 2 diabetes: UKPDS 39. *BMJ* 1998; **317**: 713–20.

27. MacMahon S, Sharpe N, Gamble G, Clague A, Ni Mhurchu C, Clark T, Hart H, Scott J, White H and PART-2 Collaborative Research Group. Randomized, placebo-controlled trial of the angiotensin converting enzyme inhibitor, ramipril, in patients with coronary and other exclusive vascular disease. *J Am Coll Cardiol* 2000; **36**: 438–43.

28. Pitt B, Byington R, Farberg CD, Hunninghake DB, Mancini GBJ, Miller ME, Riley W, for the PREVENT Investigators. Effect of amlodipine on the progression of atherosclerosis and the occurrence of clinical events. *Circulation* 2000; **102**: 1503–10.

29. Cashin-Hemphill L, Holmvang G, Chan R, Pitt B, Dunsmore R, Lees R. Angiotensin converting enzyme inhibition as antiatherosclerotic therapy: no answer yet. *Am J Cardiol* 1999; **83**: 43–7.

30. Teo KK, Burton JR, Buller CE, Plant S, Catellier D, Tymchak W, Dzavik V, Taylor D, Yokoyama S, Montague TJ, for the SCAT Investigators. Long-term effects of cholesterol lowering and angiotensin-converting enzyme inhibition on coronary atherosclerosis: the Simvastatin/enalapril Coronary Atherosclerosis Trial (SCAT). *Circulation* 2000; **102**: 1749–54.

31. Agabiti-Rosei E, Dal Palu C, Leonetti G, Magnani B, Pessina A, Zanchetti A, on behalf of the VHAS Investigators. Clinical results of the Verapamil in Hypertension in Atherosclerosis Study. *J Hypertens* 1997; **15**: 1337–44.

32. Zanchetti A, Agabiti-Rosei E, Dal Palu C, Leonetti G, Magnani B, Pessina A. The Verapamil in Hypertension and Atherosclerosis Study (VHAS): results of long-term randomized treatment with either verapamil or chlorthalidone on intima-media thickness. *J Hypertens* 2000; **12**: 1667–76.

33. Amery A, Birkenhager W, Brixko P, Bulpitt C, Clement D, Deruyttere M, DeSchaepdryver A, Dollery C, Fagard R, Forette F, Forte J, Hamdy R, Henry JF, Joossens JV, Leonetti G, Lund-Johansen P, O'Malley K, Petrie J, Strasser T, Tuomilehto J, Williams B. Mortality and morbidity results from the European Working Party on High Blood Pressure in the Elderly trial. *Lancet* 1985; **i**: 1349–54.

34. Coope J, Warrender TS. Randomised trial of treatment of hypertension in elderly patients in primary care. *BMJ* 1986; **293**: 1145–51.

35. Dahlöf B, Lindholm LH, Hansson L, Schersten B, Ekbom T, Wester P-O. Morbidity and mortality in the Swedish Trial in Old Patients with Hypertension (STOP-Hypertension). *Lancet* 1991; **338**: 1281–5.

36. Medical Research Council Working Party. MRC trial of treatment of mild hypertension: principal results. *Br Med J* 1985; **291**: 97–104.

37. MRC Working Party. Medical Research Council trial of treatment of hypertension in older adults: principal results. *BMJ* 1992; **304:** 405–12.

2

Current guidelines

Introduction

The conclusive evidence for the benefits of treating hypertension has encouraged the treatment of patients at risk. Unfortunately, the standards of care are extremely variable, ranging from total neglect to over-intensive use of drugs in individuals who stand to gain little if anything from treatment. These considerations have stimulated the publication of guidelines to assist practitioners in the management of hypertension.

Various national and international guidelines have endeavoured to distil the plethora of available information into practical recommendations. The guidelines range from lengthy and extremely detailed reports to relatively succinct advice. Each guideline is a consensus, a compromise among different views, and therefore subject to change which is not always evidence-based.

The guidelines essentially address three questions: when to treat; how to treat; and the target blood pressure. Despite a general consensus, health care practices in different countries can dictate various interpretations of the evidence. Earlier guidelines differed in their views of the optimal threshold for treatment, the choice of first-line drugs and the goals of treatment. Recent guidelines have come closer together in these respects. Those reviewed in this chapter are united in their recognition of the need to include other risk factors for cardiovascular disease in determining the threshold for intervention, the role of other cardioprotective drugs and the optimal target blood pressure.

The sixth report of the Joint National Committee on Prevention, Detection, Evaluation, and Treatment of High Blood Pressure (JNC VI) [1]

This comprehensive and lengthy document embraces many aspects of the epidemiology and management of hypertension. It follows the pattern of earlier reports and expands on advice, sometimes on the basis of new evidence. JNC VI places more emphasis on absolute risk and benefit, and uses risk stratification as part of the treatment strategy.

Table 2.1 Trends in awareness, treatment and control of high blood pressure in adults in the United States, 1978–1994

	Adults 18–74 years		
	1976–80	**1988–91**	**1991–94**
Awareness (%)	51	73	68
Treatment (%)	31	55	53
Control (%)	10	29	27

Threshold blood pressure 140/90 mmHg.

Source: NHANES II, III.

Hypertension awareness, treatment and control rates have increased during the last three decades. However, the rates of increase have lessened since the publication of the JNC V report in 1993 |2| (National Heart and Nutrition Examination Surveys: NHANES II, III: Table 2.1). Age-adjusted mortality rates for stroke and coronary heart disease (CHD) declined during this time, but thereafter were levelling. The incidence of end-stage renal disease and the prevalence of heart failure were increasing.

In considering the evidence to formulate clinical policy, absolute rather than relative changes were used, because the absolute benefit derived from treating hypertension depends on the absolute risk, i.e. those with the greatest risk achieve the greatest benefit (Fig. 2.1). Despite limitations, evidence from randomized clinical trials was given emphasis.

Blood pressure measurement and clinical evaluation

Although classification of adult blood pressure (BP) is somewhat arbitrary, it is useful for clinicians who must make treatment decisions based on a constellation of factors including the actual level of BP (Table 2.2). When systolic BP (SBP) and diastolic BP (DBP) fall into separate categories, the higher category should be selected to classify the individuals BP.

Table 2.2 JNC VI guidelines classification of blood pressure for adults aged 18 years and older

	Systolic (mmHg)		Diastolic (mmHg)
Optimal	< 120	and	< 80
Normal	< 130	and	< 85
High–normal	130–139	or	85–89

Hypertension (≥ 2 readings at ≥ 2 visits after screening)

	Systolic (mmHg)		Diastolic (mmHg)
Stage 1	140–159	or	90–99
Stage 2	160–179	or	100–109
Stage 3	≥ 180	or	≥ 110

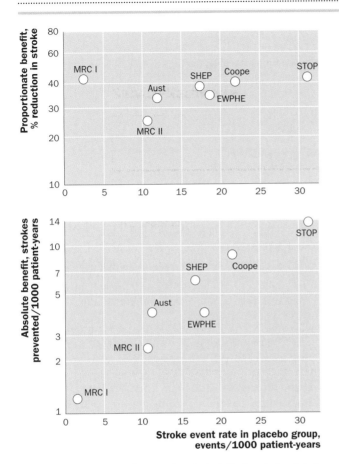

Fig. 2.1 Comparison of proportionate (relative) and absolute benefit from reduction in the incidence of stroke.
MRC I = Medical Research Council trial I; MRC II = MRC trial II; Aust = Australian study; SHEP = Systolic Hypertension in the Elderly Program; EWPHE = European Working Party on High Blood Pressure in the Elderly trial; Coope = Coope and Warrender |3|; STOP = Swedish Trial in Old Patients with Hypertension.

Recommendations for detection, confirmation and evaluation of high BP remain consistent with those in the JNC V report |2|. Two or more readings should be carried out on each occasion, and periodic re-measurement is essential (Table 2.3).

Measurement of BP outside the clinician's office—self-measurement or ambulatory blood pressure monitoring (ABPM)—may have a role in some patients. However, these procedures should not be used indiscriminately in the routine evaluation of patients with suspected hypertension. Since BP tends to be higher when measured in the clinic than when measured outside, new definitions of

Table 2.3 JNC VI guidelines recommendations for follow-up based on initial BP measurement in adults

Systolic (mmHg)	Diastolic (mmHg)	Follow-up
< 130	< 85	2 years
130–139	85–89	1 year
140–159	90–99	≤ 2 months
160–179	100–109	≤ 1 month
≥ 180	≥ 110	≤ 1 week

hypertension are proposed: ≥ 135/85 mmHg for self-measured and mean daytime BP (ABPM) and ≥ 120/75 mmHg for mean night-time BP (ABPM).

Evaluation of patients with documented hypertension has three objectives:

- to identify known causes of hypertension;
- to assess the presence or absence and extent of target organ damage (TOD) and cardiovascular disease; and
- to identify other cardiovascular risk factors (RFs) and concomitant disorders that may define prognosis and guide treatment.

Data for evaluation are acquired through medical history, physical examination, laboratory tests and other diagnostic procedures.

Laboratory tests recommended before initiation of therapy are tests to determine the presence of TOD and other RFs—urinalysis, complete blood cell count, blood chemistry (potassium, sodium, creatinine, fasting glucose, total cholesterol, high density lipoprotein cholesterol) and 12-lead electrocardiogram (ECG). Optional tests include microalbuminuria, blood calcium and uric acid, and echocardiography.

Risk stratification

This depends not only on the level of BP but also on the presence or absence of other RFs (Table 2.4a) and TOD (Table 2.4b). Three stages of BP and three levels of risk form a matrix against which physicians can determine therapy (Table 2.5). In

Table 2.4a Components of cardiovascular risk stratification in patients with hypertension–1

Major risk factors

- Smoking
- Dyslipidaemia
- Diabetes mellitus
- Age > 60 years
- Male/post-menopausal female
- Family history

Source: JNC VI (1997).

Table 2.4b Components of cardiovascular risk stratification in patients with hypertension–2

Target organ damage

- Left ventricular hypertrophy
- Clinical ischaemic heart disease
- Heart failure
- Stroke/TIA
- Nephropathy
- Peripheral vascular disease
- Retinopathy

TIA = transient ischaemic attack.

Source: JNC VI (1997).

Table 2.5 Risk stratification and treatment

BP (mmHg)	Risk group A No RF/TOD	Risk group B ≥ 1 RF*/No TOD	Risk group C TOD ± RF+
130–139/85–89	Lifestyle	Lifestyle	Drugs++
140–159/90–99	Lifestyle (1 yr)	Lifestyle (6 m)	Drugs
≥ 160/≥ 100	Drugs	Drugs	Drugs

*Not DM ++HF, RI, DM +Including DM

RF = risk factor; TOD = target organ damage; DM = diabetes mellitus; HF = heart failure; RI = renal insufficiency.

Source: JNC VI (1997).

patients with stage 1 hypertension, drug therapy should be instituted if lifestyle modification does not achieve goal BP. In risk group B, clinicians should consider antihypertensive drugs as initial therapy if multiple RFs are present.

Treatment of high blood pressure

The goal of treatment is to achieve and maintain SBP < 140 mmHg and DBP < 90 mmHg, and lower if tolerated. Goals based on out-of-office measurements should be lower than those based on office readings.

The first step in hypertension management is lifestyle modification (Table 2.6). This can also reduce other cardiovascular RFs at little cost and minimal risk. Even when lifestyle modifications alone are not adequate to control hypertension, these measures may reduce the number and dosage of antihypertensive medications needed for management. Implementation of lifestyle modification should not delay the start of effective antihypertensive drug regimens in those at higher risk.

A diuretic or beta-blocker should be used as initial therapy unless there are compelling or specific indications for another drug. For most drugs, a low dose should be used, slowly titrating upwards according to response. Formulations that provide 24-hour control are recommended, although no advice is given on how such agents

Table 2.6 Lifestyle modifications for hypertension prevention and management

- Lose weight if overweight
- Limit alcohol intake
- Increase aerobic exercise
- Reduce sodium intake (≤ 100 mmol/day)
- Maintain potassium intake (90 mmol/day)
- Maintain calcium and magnesium intake
- Stop smoking and reduce saturated fats

Source: JNC VI (1997).

should be selected. Examples of compelling and specific indications for and contraindications to individual drugs are shown in Table 2.7(a,b,c). An algorithm for the treatment of hypertension is given in Fig. 2.2. The use of immediate-release nifedipine is not recommended, because of the risk of precipitating ischaemic events.

If the response to the initial drug advice is inadequate after reaching the full

Table 2.7a Considerations for individualizing antihypertensive drug therapy–1

Compelling indications for drugs

• DM (type 1) with proteinuria	ACE inhibitor (ARB)
• Heart failure	ACE inhibitor (ARB)
	Diuretic
• ISH in elderly	Diuretic
	Long-acting DHP
• MI	Beta-blocker
—systolic dysfunction	ACE inhibitor (ARB)

DM = diabetes mellitus; ACE = angiotensin-converting enzyme; ARB = angiotensin receptor blocker; ISH = isolated systolic hypertension; DHP = dihydropyridine; MI = myocardial infarction.

Source: JNC VI (1997).

Table 2.7b Considerations for individualizing antihypertensive drug therapy–2

Specific indications for drugs

• Angina	Beta-blocker
	Calcium antagonist
• DM (types 1 and 2)	ACE inhibitor (ARB)
with proteinuria	Calcium antagonist
• DM (type 2)	Diuretic
• Dislipidaemia	Alpha-blocker
• Renal insufficiency	ACE inhibitor (ARB)

DM = diabetes mellitus; ACE = angiotensin-converting enzyme; ARB = angiotensin receptor blocker.

Source: JNC VI (1997).

Table 2.7c Considerations for individualizing antihypertensive drug therapy–3

Contraindications for drugs

● Bronchospasm	Beta-blocker
● Depression	Reserpine
● Gout	Diuretic
● Heart block (second or third degree)	Beta-blocker
	Rate-limiting calcium antagonist
	ACE inhibitor (ARB)

ACE = angiotensin-converting enzyme; ARB = angiotensin receptor blocker.

Source: JNC VI (1997).

dose, two options for subsequent therapy should be considered—combination or substitution (Fig. 2.2). Treatment decisions should be made after at least 4 weeks of a particular therapy. The control of BP, avoiding side-effects, may take several months. A diuretic should be selected as first- or second-step therapy, because addition will enhance the effect of other agents.

Before proceeding to each successive treatment step, clinicians should consider possible reasons for lack of responsiveness (Table 2.8). Stepwise decrease of dosage and number of antihypertensive drugs should be considered after hypertension has been controlled effectively for at least 1 year, with careful follow-up arrangements.

Resistant hypertension is defined as SBP $\geq$ 140 mmHg ($\geq$ 160 mmHg in older patients with isolated systolic hypertension) or DBP $\geq$ 90 mmHg despite adequate adherence to triple therapy including a diuretic, with all drugs at near-maximal dose. Management strategies can improve concordance (adherence) with therapy (Table 2.9). Strategies for management of hypertensive emergencies and urgencies are described.

Special population and situations

Coexisting cardiovascular disease

In patients with *coronary artery disease*, a goal BP even lower than the usual target is desirable if angina persists. Beta-blockers and calcium antagonists may be specifically useful, but short-acting calcium antagonists should not be used. After

Table 2.8 Reasons for lack of responsiveness to therapy

- Pseudotolerance, e.g. white-coat hypertension
- Non-adherence to therapy
- Volume overload, e.g. excess salt intake or inadequate diuretic therapy
- Drug interactions, e.g. non-steroidal anti-inflammatory drugs
- Associated conditions, e.g. smoking, chronic pain
- Secondary hypertension

Source: JNC VI (1997).

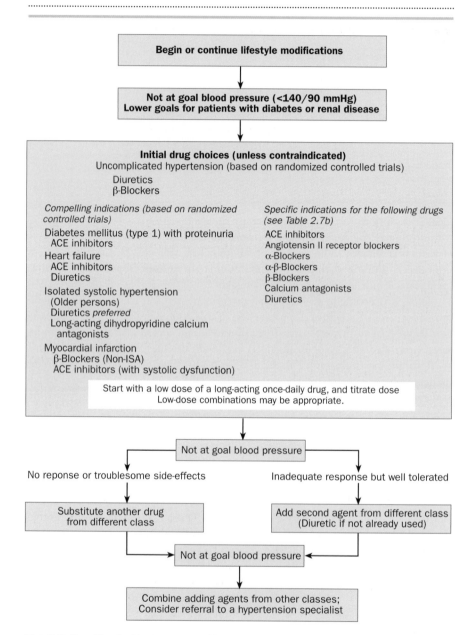

Fig. 2.2 Algorithm for the treatment of hypertension. ISA = intrinsic sympathomimetic activity.

Table 2.9 General guidelines to improve patient adherence to antihypertensive therapy

- Consider non-adherence
- Establish goals with patient
- Educate patients/families
- Maintain contact
- Avoid expensive management
- Respond to patient needs/concerns
- Avoid adverse drug effects
- Consider nurse care management

Source: JNC VI (1997).

myocardial infarction, beta-blockers without intrinsic sympathomimetic activity should be given, and ACE inhibitors are also useful if there is left ventricular systolic dysfunction. If beta-blockers are ineffective or contraindicated, verapamil or diltiazem may be used. Identification of patients with *left ventricular hypertrophy* should be based on the ECG, with echocardiography reserved for patients with untreated stage 1 hypertension, no cardiovascular RFs, no evidence of clinical cardiovascular disease and no TOD. Lifestyle modification and all antihypertensive drugs (except direct vasodilators such as hydralazine and minoxidil) reduce left ventricular mass. Patients with *cardiac failure* should receive an ACE inhibitor; addition of carvedilol has been shown to be beneficial. When an ACE inhibitor is contraindicated or not tolerated, the combination of hydralazine and isosorbide dinitrate is also effective, and an angiotensin receptor blocker (ARB) should be considered. Amlodipine and felodipine appear relatively safe in treating patients with chronic heart failure when used in addition to an ACE inhibitor, a diuretic and digoxin; other calcium antagonists are not recommended.

Renal insufficiency

Reversible causes of renal failure should always be sought. Those patients with proteinuria > 1 g/day should be treated to a goal BP of 125/75 mmHg; if proteinuria is less, the target BP is 130/85 mmHg. The most important action to slow progressive renal failure is to lower BP to goal. All classes of antihypertensive drugs are effective and, in most cases, multiple drugs are necessary. ACE inhibitors appear to have additional renal protective effects and should be included in the regimen (in most cases along with a diuretic) unless contraindicated. In patients with serum creatinine ≥ 265.2 μmol/l (3 mg/dl), ACE inhibitors should be used with caution. If serum creatinine rises by ≥ 88.4 μmol/l (1 mg/dl) and persists on re-checking, the diagnosis of renal artery stenosis should be considered and any ACE inhibitor (or ARB) discontinued. Thiazide diuretics are not effective at serum creatinine ≥ 221 μmol/l (2.5 mg/dl) and loop diuretics (often at high doses) are needed. Potassium-sparing diuretics should be avoided.

Diabetes mellitus

The goal of antihypertensive therapy is a BP < 130/85 mmHg. Drugs from all of the main classes can be used, and combinations are usually necessary. ACE inhibitors (or ARBs if these are not tolerated) are preferred as the first step in diabetic nephropathy.

Comment

JNC VI provides comprehensive advice on the prevention, evaluation and treatment of hypertension. It emphasizes risk factor stratification and multiple risk factor intervention. The new targets for therapy are rigorous. JNC VI represents a major effort that should help clinicians to appreciate the importance of treating hypertension. However, it has uncertain relevance to health care systems outside the United States.

1999 World Health Organization–International Society of Hypertension Guidelines for the Management of Hypertension |4|

The second half of the twentieth century saw a progressive decline in cardiovascular mortality in North America, Western Europe, Japan and Australasia. At the same time, the control of hypertension in these regions improved considerably, although most hypertensive subjects have imperfect control (or no treatment at all). Moreover, given the ageing population structure of most developed countries, the total numbers of strokes and CHD events are increasing or remaining static. Even more worrying is the rapid development of the 'second wave' epidemic of cardiovascular disease (CVD) that is flowing through developing countries and the former socialist republics.

Scope and purpose

These guidelines concentrate on the practical clinical management of mild hypertension. The primary aim is to offer balanced information to guide clinicians who

Table 2.10 Cardiovascular disease risk factors–1: the relative contribution of blood pressure and selected other factors

BP (mmHg)	Age (yrs)	DM	TIA	Risk
140/90	40	No	No	1
170/105	40	No	No	×2–3
145/90	65	Yes	Yes	×20

BP = blood pressure; DM = diabetes mellitus; TIA = transient ischaemic attack. Otherwise healthy male.

Source: WHO–ISH Guidelines (1999).

Table 2.11 Cardiovascular disease risk factors–2: factors other than blood pressure

- Age
- Male sex
- Prior event
- Renal disease
- IGT
- Cigarettes
- Lipids

- Obesity
- Fibrinogen
- Alcohol
- Physical activity
- Socio-economic status
- Ethnicity
- Geographical region

IGT = impaired glucose tolerance.

Source: WHO–ISH Guidelines (1999).

manage patients from a wide range of ethnic and cultural backgrounds with very different health systems and varying availabilities of resources.

Contribution of blood pressure and other risk factors to cardiovascular risk

Differences in risk of CVD are determined not only by the level of BP, but also by the presence or levels of other RFs (Table 2.10). Thus differences in the absolute level of cardiovascular risk between patients with hypertension will often be determined to a greater extent by other RFs than by the level of BP. Examples of other cardiovascular RFs are shown in Table 2.11.

Clinical evaluation

The aims of the clinical and laboratory evaluation of hypertensive patients are summarized in Table 2.12. A comprehensive clinical history and full physical examination are essential. Because BP is characterized by large spontaneous variations, the diagnosis of hypertension should be based on multiple BP measurements taken on several occasions.

Home and ABPM provide useful additional clinical information and have a limited place in the management of hypertensive patients (Table 2.13). The information from these methods must be regarded as supplementary to conventional measurements, and not a substitute. Average 24-hour BP values of around 125/80

Table 2.12 Aims of clinical evaluation of the hypertensive patient

- Sustained blood pressure level
- Target organ damage
- Other cardiovascular risk factors
- Conditions that may influence treatment
- Secondary hypertension

Source: WHO–ISH Guidelines (1999).

Table 2.13 Circumstances in which ambulatory blood pressure monitoring should be considered

- Variability in blood pressure
- Low cardiovascular risk
- Symptoms suggesting hypotension
- Resistant hypertension

Source: WHO–ISH Guidelines (1999).

mmHg correspond to a clinic BP of 140/90 mmHg. Home devices that measure BP in the fingers or the arm below the elbow should be avoided.

In a few patients, office BP is persistently elevated, whereas daytime BP outside the office environment is not ('white-coat' or better 'isolated office' hypertension). Physicians should aim at its identification (by use of home BP or ABPM) whenever clinical suspicion is raised. The decision to treat or not should be based on the overall risk profile and the presence or absence of TOD. Close follow-up is essential for subjects with isolated office hypertension when the physician chooses not to treat.

Routine investigations should include urinalysis for blood, protein and glucose, microscopic examination of urine, blood potassium, creatinine, fasting glucose and total cholesterol, and ECG. Optional investigations are guided by the findings from history, examination and routine investigations. Echocardiography should be performed whenever the clinical assessment reveals the presence of TOD or suggests the possibility of left ventricular hypertrophy or other cardiac disease. Vascular ultrasonography should be performed whenever the presence of arterial disease is suspected in the aorta or the carotid or peripheral arteries. Renal ultrasonography should be performed if renal disease is suspected. Whether such expensive high-technology investigations are appropriate in all health care systems is not discussed.

Definition and classification of hypertension

To reduce confusion and provide more consistent advice to clinicians, the WHO–ISH guidelines adopt in principle the definition and classification provided by JNC VI |1|. However, the term 'grade' rather than 'stage' has been chosen to avoid implying progression. The guidelines emphasize that the decision to lower BP in particular patients is not based on the level of BP alone but on assessment of the total cardiovascular risk.

Stratification of patients by absolute level of cardiovascular risk

These guidelines provide a simple method by which to estimate the combined effect of several RFs and conditions on the future absolute risk of cardiovascular events. The estimates in Table 2.14 are based on the RFs, TOD and associated clinical conditions (ACC) listed in Table 2.15(a,b,c). Among individuals in the low-risk group, the risk of a major cardiovascular event in the next 10 years is typically < 15%; in the medium-risk group 15–20%; and in the high-risk group 20–30%.

Table 2.14 Stratifying risk to quantify prognosis

Other risk factors and disease history	Blood pressure (mmHg)		
	Grade 1 (mild hypertension) SBP 140–159 or DBP 90–99	**Grade 2** (moderate hypertension) SBP 160–179 or DBP 100–109	**Grade 3** (severe hypertension) SBP ≥ 180 or DBP ≥ 110
I. no other risk factors	Low risk	Medium risk	High risk
II. 1–2 risk factors	Medium risk	Medium risk	Very high risk
III. 3 or more risk factors or TOD or diabetes	High risk	High risk	Very high risk
IV. ACC	Very high risk	Very high risk	Very high risk

TOD = target organ damage; ACC = associated clinical conditions, including clinical cardiovascular disease or renal disease. The typical 10-year risk of stroke or myocardial infarction is shown, where 'low risk' corresponds to below 15%, 'medium risk' to 15–20%, 'high risk' to 20–30%, and 'very high risk' to 30% or higher.

Table 2.15a Factors influencing prognosis. A: risk factors

- Men > 55 years
- Women > 65 years
- Cigarette smoking
- Total cholesterol > 6.5 mmol/l
- Diabetes mellitus
- FH of premature CVD

FH = family history; CVD = cardiovascular disease.

Source: WHO–ISH Guidelines (1999).

Table 2.15b Factors influencing prognosis. B: target organ damage

- LVH (ECG/echo/CXR)
- Proteinuria/slight elevation ser Cr
- Atherosclerotic plaque (US/X-ray)
- Retinopathy (grade II)

LVH = left ventricular hypertrophy; ECG = electrocardiogram; CXR = chest X-ray; ser Cr = serum creatinine; US = ultrasound.

Source: WHO–ISH Guidelines (1999).

Table 2.15c Factors influencing prognosis. C: associated clinical conditions

- Cerebrovascular disease
- Heart disease
- Renal disease
- Vascular disease
- Advanced retinopathy

Source: WHO–ISH Guidelines (1999).

Patients with grade 3 hypertension and one or more RFs and all patients with CVD or renal disease carry the very highest risk of cardiovascular events (around 30% over 10 years) and qualify for the most intensive and rapidly instituted therapeutic regimens.

Goals of treatment

Effective treatment requires management of all reversible RFs and ACCs as well as of raised BP. BP targets are < 130/85 mmHg in young, middle-aged and diabetic subjects; and < 140/90 mmHg in the elderly. When home or ABP measurements are used, targets should be lower: 10–15 mmHg for SBP and 5–10 mmHg for DBP.

Management strategy

Lifestyle measures

Lifestyle measures should be instituted wherever appropriate in all patients including those who require drug therapy:

- to lower BP;
- to reduce the need for antihypertensive drugs and maximize their efficacy; and
- to address other RFs present.

Lifestyle measures that are widely agreed to lower BP and that should be considered in all patients are weight reduction, reduction of excessive alcohol consumption, reduction of high salt intake and increase in physical activity. Particular emphasis should be placed on cessation of smoking and on healthy eating patterns that contribute to the treatment of associated RFs and CVD.

Drug treatment

- Begin with the lowest dose to minimize adverse effects. If there is a good response and treatment is well tolerated but BP control remains inadequate, it is reasonable to increase the dose.
- Use appropriate drug combinations (Table 2.16). Using both drugs at low doses minimizes side-effects. Fixed low-dose combinations may be advantageous. Most patients are likely to require more than one drug.

Table 2.16 Effective drug combinations

- Diuretic + beta-blocker
- Diuretic + ACE inhibitor (or ARB)
- Calcium antagonist (dihydropyridine) + beta-blocker
- Calcium antagonist + ACE inhibitor
- Alpha-blocker + beta-blocker

ACE = angiotensin-converting enzyme; ARB = angiotensin receptor blocker.
Source: WHO–ISH Guidelines (1999).

- Change to a different drug class if there is little response or poor tolerability to the first drug choice.

- Use long-acting drugs providing 24-hour efficacy on a once-daily basis to improve compliance with therapy and to minimize BP variability.

For patients in the high- and very high-risk groups, drug treatment should be instituted within a few days, as soon as repeated measurements have confirmed the patient's BP. For patients in the medium-risk groups, lifestyle measures with re-inforcement should be continued for 3–6 months before initiating drug treatment if goal BP is not achieved. For patients in the low-risk group, drug treatment should be initiated after 6 months to 1 year of assiduous lifestyle modification; in the border-line subgroup (DBP 90–94 mmHg and SBP 140–149 mmHg), lifestyle measures alone may be continued in the long-term. In contrast, in patients with high normal BP (130–139/85–95 mmHg) who also have diabetes mellitus and/or renal insuffi-ciency, early antihypertensive drug therapy should be considered to reduce the risk of loss of renal function. A practical framework for the management of patients with grade 1 or 2 hypertension is shown in Fig. 2.3.

All available drugs are suitable for the initiation and maintenance of anti-hypertensive therapy, but the choice of drugs will be influenced by many factors (Table 2.17). The absolute effect of treatment on cardiovascular risk depends on absolute risk and BP reduction (Table 2.18).

Hypertension is termed refractory when a therapeutic plan that has included attention to lifestyle measures and the prescription of combination therapy at adequate doses has failed to lower BP to below 140/90 mmHg. Common causes of refractory hypertension are listed in Table 2.19.

Since the aim of treatment is the reduction of total cardiovascular risk, it is at least as important to treat the other RFs and ACCs in the individual hypertensive patient. It is reasonable to recommend, where BP has been rigorously controlled, the use of low-dose aspirin in hypertensive patients who are at high risk of CHD and who are not particularly at risk of bleeding from the gastrointestinal tract or from other sites. The use of cholesterol-lowering therapy can be recommended for hypertensive patients who have elevated serum cholesterol and who, for other reasons, are at high risk of CHD.

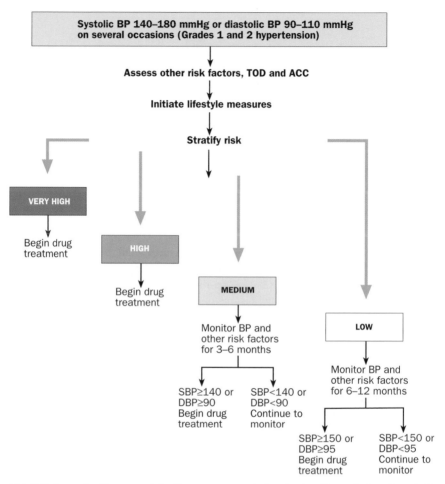

Fig. 2.3 A practical framework for the management of patients with grade 1 and grade 2 hypertension. TOD = target organ damage; ACC = associated clinical conditions; (S/D) BP = (systolic/diastolic) blood pressures.

Follow-up

The frequency of visits will depend on the overall risk category as well as the level of BP (Fig. 2.4). After prolonged BP control it may be possible to attempt careful progressive reduction in the dose and number of drugs used under careful supervision.

Implementation

These guidelines are accompanied by a briefer companion set of 'Practice Guidelines' intended for translation into many languages and distribution to medical

Table 2.17 Guidelines for selecting drug treatment of hypertension

Class of drug	Compelling indications	Possible indications	Compelling contraindications	Possible contraindications
Diuretics	Heart failure Elderly patients Systolic hypertension	Diabetes	Gout	Dyslipidaemias Sexually active males
Beta-blockers	Angina After myocardial infarction	Heart failure Pregnancy	Asthma and COPD Heart block (a)	Dyslipidaemias Athletes and physically active patients Peripheral vascular disease
ACE inhibitors	Heart failure Left ventricular dysfunction After myocardial infarction Diabetic nephropathy		Pregnancy Hyperkalaemia Bilateral renal artery stenosis	
Calcium antagonists	Angina Elderly patients Systolic hypertension	Peripheral vascular disease	Heart block (b)	Congestive heart failure (c)
Alpha-blockers	Prostatic hypertrophy	Glucose intolerance Dyslipidaemias		Orthostatic hypotension
Angiotensin II antagonists	ACE inhibitor cough	Heart failure	Pregnancy Bilateral renal artery stenosis Hyperkalaemia	

(a) Grade 2 or 3 atrioventricular block; (b) Grade 2 or 3 atrioventricular block with verapamil or diltiazem; (c) verapamil or diltiazem
COPD = chronic obstructive pulmonary disease.

Source: WHO–ISH Guidelines (1999).

Table 2.18 Absolute effects of treatment on cardiovascular risk

Patient group	Absolute risk (CVD events/ 10 years)	Absolute treatment effect (CVD events prevented/ 1000 pt-years)	
		10/5 mmHg	20/10 mmHg
Low risk	< 15%	< 5	< 9
Medium risk	15–20%	5–7	8–11
High risk	20–30%	7–10	11–17
Very high risk	> 30%	> 10	> 17

CVD = cardiovascular disease; pt-years = patient treatment years.

Source: WHO–ISH Guidelines (1999).

Table 2.19 Causes of refractory hypertension

- Secondary hypertension
- Poor concordance
- Drug interaction, e.g. NSAID
- Lifestyle, e.g. weight/alcohol
- Volume overload, e.g. inadequate diuretic
- Spurious, e.g. white-coat hypertension

NSAID = non-steroidal anti-inflammatory drug.

Source: WHO–ISH Guidelines (1999).

practitioners in many countries. The WHO–ISH guidelines can act as a model and a stimulus for the development of national recommendations adopted to suit the local culture and economic and social realities. It is hoped that such modified recommendations could be embedded in an implementation plan that reaches local medical practitioners and local communities alike.

Comment

The WHO–ISH guidelines provide recommendations that are based on the collective expert interpretation of the available evidence from epidemiological studies and clinical trials. The primary aim is to offer balanced information to guide clinicians rather than rigid rules that would constrain their judgement about the management of individual patients who will differ in their personal, medical, social, economic, ethnic and cultural characteristics.

These are both strengths and weaknesses. The guidelines are more a consensus statement than evidence-based recommendations, and there is a lack of clear practical advice. The WHO–ISH guidelines are written for a global audience of communities that vary widely in the nature of their health systems and the availability of resources. This challenge may have been beyond the capabilities of the authors.

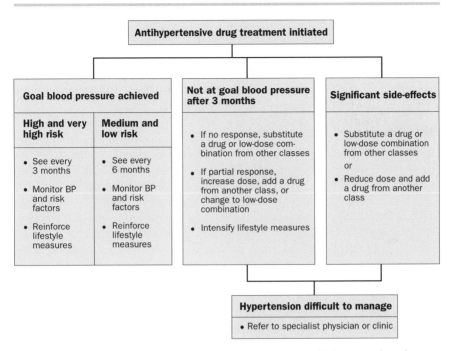

Fig. 2.4 Stabilization, maintenance and follow-up of patients with hypertension after initiation of drug therapy.

Guidelines for management of hypertension: report of the third working party of the British Hypertension Society |5,6|

These guidelines update previous reports in 1989 |7| and 1993 |8|. Since the 1993 guidelines, much more evidence has emerged, notably on optimal BP targets during antihypertensive therapy, management of hypertension in diabetic patients and treatment of isolated systolic hypertension in the elderly. These important additions to an already formidable body of evidence provide the basis for the new recommendations. The guidelines embrace the concept that effective management of hypertension requires the identification of those at highest cardiovascular risk and the adoption of multifactorial intervention, targeting not only BP levels, but also associated cardiovascular RFs.

The guidelines recommend formal estimation of 10-year CHD risk using a computer program or risk chart. CHD risk is a good predictor of CVD risk (the proper focus of hypertension management), which can be approximated by multiplying the estimated 10-year CHD risk level by 4/3 (i.e. 30% CHD risk approximates to 40% CVD risk).

These guidelines are intended for general practitioners, practice nurses and generalists in hospital practice, and aim to present as clearly as possible the best currently available evidence on hypertension management. The guidelines should be applied with due regard to local circumstances and policies, and with appropriate clinical judgement with regard to the needs of individual patients.

Blood pressure measurement

All adults should have BP measured routinely every 5 years until the age of 80 years. Those with high–normal values (135–139/85–89 mmHg) should have BP measured annually. Measurement should follow standard recommendations (Table 2.20).

In uncomplicated mild hypertension, measurements at monthly intervals over 4–6 months should be used to guide the decision to treat. In more severe hypertension prolonged observation before treatment is not necessary or warranted. Formal assessment of CHD/CVD risk needs to take account of age, sex, smoking habit, diabetes, total high-density lipoprotein (HDL) cholesterol ratio and family history in addition to BP.

ABPM may be indicated in the circumstances shown in Table 2.21. Normal BP values by ABPM may alter management when there are no TOD or cardiovascular complications, the estimated CHD risk is < 15%, and elevated clinic BP (average ≥ 160/100 mmHg) is the only indication of high risk. The average daytime BP

Table 2.20 Blood pressure measurement

- Well-validated and maintained device
- Patient seated, arm at level of heart
- Bladder size appropriate
- Cuff deflated 2 mmHg/sec
- Measure ± 2 mmHg
- Phase V diastolic
- Two measurements per visit
- Repeated visits

Source: BHS Guidelines (1999).

Table 2.21 Circumstances where ambulatory blood pressure monitoring may be indicated

- Unusual variability in blood pressure
- Resistant hypertension
- Symptoms suggestive of hypotension
- White-coat hypertension

Resistant hypertension is defined as blood pressure > 150/90 mmHg on a regimen of three or more anti-hypertensive drugs.

Source: BHS Guidelines (1999).

should be used for treatment decisions. Since ABP measurements are systematically lower than clinic measurements, treatment thresholds and targets must be adjusted downwards by about 12/7 mmHg when making decisions based on ABPM: i.e. an ABPM average daytime BP of 148/83 mmHg is approximately equivalent to a clinic BP of 160/90 mmHg, and may require treatment in some patients. Furthermore, a normal value from ABPM should be confirmed by a second ABPM record, because of within-patient variability and limited reproducibility. Also, patients left untreated on the basis of ABPM need reassessment of BP (perhaps repeated ABPM) and cardio-vascular risk at least once a year. The same considerations apply to self-measurement of BP at home.

Non-pharmacological measures

Measures that lower blood pressure:

- weight reduction by calorie restriction
- reduced salt intake
- moderation of alcohol consumption
- physical exercise
- increased fruit and vegetable consumption
- reduced total and saturated fat intake

Measures to reduce cardiovascular risk:

- stop cigarette smoking
- increase polyunsaturated and monounsaturated fats
- increase oily fish consumption
- reduce total and saturated fat

Evaluation of hypertensive patients

All hypertensive patients should have a thorough history and physical examination (Table 2.22) but need only a limited number of routine investigations (Table 2.23). An echocardiogram is valuable to confirm or refute the presence of left ventricular hypertrophy when the ECG shows 'high' left ventricular voltage without T-wave abnormalities, as is often the case in young people. When the clinical evaluation or

Table 2.22 Aims of clinical evaluation of the hypertensive patient

- Causes of hypertension
- Contributory factors
- Complications of hypertension
- Cardiovascular risk factors
- Contraindications to specific drugs

Source: BHS Guidelines (1999).

Table 2.23 Routine investigations in the hypertensive patient

- Urine strip test
- U and E
- BS
- TC:HDL-C
- ECG

U and E = serum urea and electrolytes; BS = blood sugar; TC:HDL-C = serum total cholesterol: HDL cholesterol; ECG = electrocardiogram.

Source: BHS Guidelines (1999).

Table 2.24 Indications for referral for specialist advice or treatment

- Urgent treatment
- Suspicion of secondary hypertension
- Therapeutic problem
- ABPM
- Pregnancy

ABPM = ambulatory blood pressure monitoring.

Source: BHS Guidelines (1999).

the results of these simple investigations suggest a need for further investigation, it is usually best to refer for specialist advice. Indications for referral for specialist advice or treatment are summarized in Table 2.24.

Thresholds for antihypertensive therapy

Drug therapy should be started in all patients with sustained SBP ≥ 160 mmHg or DBP ≥ 100 mmHg despite non-pharmacological measures (Fig. 2.5). Drug treatment is also indicated in patients with a sustained SBP of 140–159 mmHg or DBP of 90–99 mmHg if TOD or diabetes is present, or if the 10-year CHD risk is $\geq 15\%$ (Fig. 2.6). The preferred method for estimation of risk is a computer program; but, where this is not practicable, a 'coronary risk chart' is recommended (Fig. 2.7a,b). Thresholds for intervention and times to intervention are summarized in Fig. 2.6 and Table 2.25.

When a decision is reached not to treat a patient with mild hypertension, it is essential to continue observation and monitoring of BP and CHD risk at least once per year. These patients should be encouraged to continue with non-pharmacological measures to lower BP and cardiovascular risk.

Treatment goals

Recommendations for target BP during treatment are shown in Table 2.26(a,b). Systolic and diastolic targets should both be attained. The audit standard reflects the minimum recommended level of BP control.

BHS Guidelines

Threshold blood pressure (mmHg)

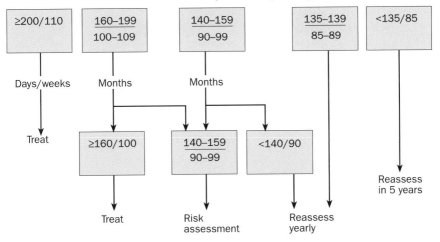

Fig. 2.5 Thresholds for antihypertensive drug therapy.

BHS Guidelines

Risk assessment

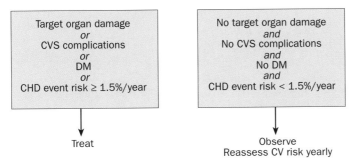

Fig. 2.6 Risk assessment in hypertensive patients. CVS = cardiovascular system; DM = diabetes mellitus; CHD = coronary heart disease; CV risk = cardiovascular risk.

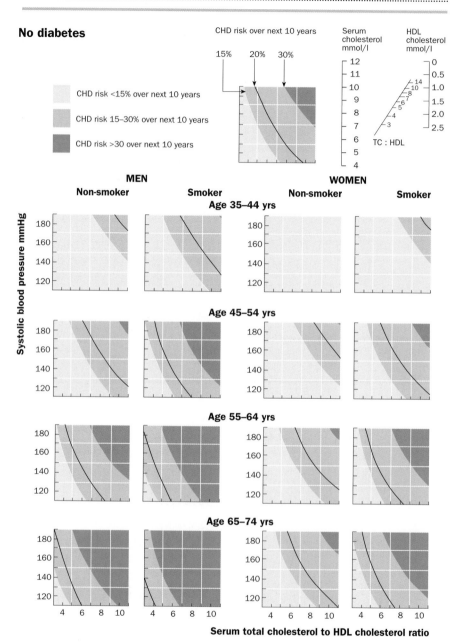

Fig. 2.7a Joint British Societies Coronary Risk Prediction Chart: without diabetes. CHD = coronary heart disease; HDL = high-density lipoprotein; TC = total serum cholesterol.

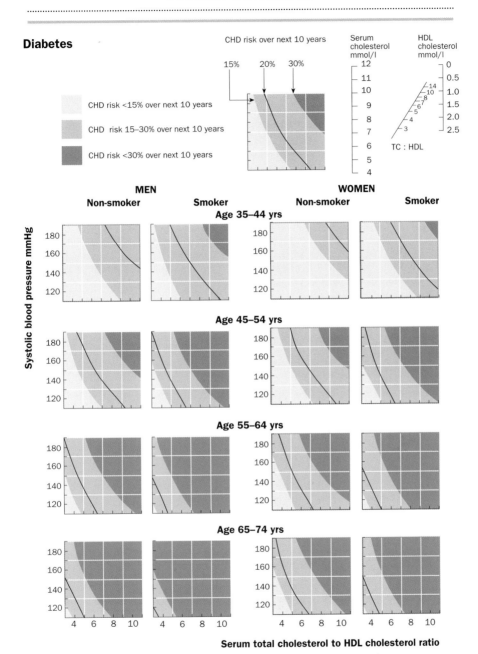

Fig. 2.7b Joint British Societies Coronary Risk Prediction Chart: with diabetes.
CHD = coronary heart disease; HDL = high-density lipoprotein; TC = total serum
cholesterol.

How to use the coronary risk prediction chart for primary prevention (Fig. 2.7)

These charts are for estimating coronary heart disease (CHD) risk (non-fatal myocardial infarction and coronary death) for individuals who have not developed symptomatic CHD or other major atherosclerotic disease.

The use of these charts is not appropriate for patients who have existing disease which already puts them at high risk. Such diseases are:
- CHD or other major atherosclerotic disease
- Familial hypercholesterolaemia or other inherited dyslipidaemia
- Established hypertension (SBP >160 mmHg and/or DBP >100 mmHg) or associated target organ damage (TOD)
- Diabetes mellitus with associated TOD
- Renal dysfunction

- To estimate an individual's absolute 10-year risk of developing CHD, find the table for their gender, diabetes (yes/no), smoking status (smoker/non-smoker) and age. Within this square define the level of risk according to SBP and the ratio of total cholesterol to HDL cholesterol. If there is no HDL cholesterol result, then assume this is 1.0 mmol/l and then the lipid scale can be used for total cholesterol alone.

- High-risk individuals are defined as those whose 10-year CHD risk exceeds 15% (equivalent to a cardiovascular risk of 20% over the same period). As a minimum, those at highest risk (30%) should be targeted and treated now, and as resources allow, others with a risk of >15% should be progressively targeted.

- Smoking status should reflect lifetime exposure to tobacco and not simply tobacco use at the time of risk assessment.

- The initial BP and the first random (non-fasting) total cholesterol and HDL cholesterol can be used to estimate an individual's risk. However, the decision on using drug therapies should be based on repeat risk factor measurements over a period of time. The chart should not be used to estimate risk after treatment of hyperlipidaemia or BP has been initiated.

- CHD risk is higher than indicated in the charts for:
  - Those with a family history of premature CHD (men <55 years and women <65 years), which increases the risk by a factor of approximately 1.5
  - Those with raised triglyceride levels
  - Those who are not diabetic but have impaired glucose tolerance
  - Women with premature menopause
  - Persons approaching the next age category. As risk increases exponentially with age the risk will be closer to the higher decennium for the last 4 years of each decade

- In ethnic minorities the risk chart should be used with caution, as it has not been validated for these populations.

- The estimates of CHD risk from the chart are based on groups of people, and in managing an *individual* the physician also has to use clinical judgement in deciding how intensively to intervene on lifestyle and whether or not to use drug therapies.

- An individual can be shown on the chart the direction in which the risk of CHD can be reduced by changing smoking status, BP, or cholesterol.

Table 2.25 Time to intervention in hypertension

- Immediate—malignant phase/emergencies
- 1–2 weeks—BP ≥ 200/110
- 3–4 weeks—BP ≥ 160/100 + complications/TOD/DM
- 4–12 weeks—BP ≥ 160/100
- 12 weeks—BP ≥ 140/90 + complications/TOD/DM
- 6 months—BP ≥ 140/90 + 10-year CHD risk ≥ 15%

BP = blood pressure; TOD = target organ damage; DM = diabetes mellitus; CHD = coronary heart disease.
Source: BHS Guidelines (1999).

Table 2.26a Treatment targets for antihypertensive drug therapy–1: office blood pressure (mmHg)

	No diabetes	Diabetes
Optimal	< 140/85	< 140/80
Audit standard	< 150/90	< 140/85

Source: BHS Guidelines (1999).

Table 2.26b Treatment targets for antihypertensive drug therapy–2: ambulatory blood pressure monitoring (mmHg)

	No diabetes	Diabetes
Optimal	< 130/80	< 130/75
Audit standard	< 140/85	< 140/80

Source: BHS Guidelines (1999).

Choice of antihypertensive drug treatment

A low dose of thiazide is the first-line treatment unless there is a contraindication or a compelling indication for another drug. A long-acting dihydropyridine calcium antagonist is a suitable alternative for isolated systolic hypertension in the elderly when a low-dose thiazide is not tolerated or is contraindicated. The choice of drug will depend on relative indications and contraindications in individual patients (Table 2.27).

The drug or formulation used should ideally be effective when taken as a single daily dose. An interval of 4 weeks should be allowed to observe the full response, unless it is necessary to lower BP more urgently. The dose of thiazide diuretic should not be titrated upwards, whereas other drugs should be titrated according to the manufacturers' instructions. When the first drug is well tolerated but the

Table 2.27 Compelling and possible indications, contraindications and cautions for the major classes of antihypertensive drugs

Class of drug	Indications		Contraindications	
	Compelling	Possible	Possible	Compelling
α-blockers	Prostatism	Dyslipidaemia	Postural hypotension	Urinary continence
ACE inhibitors	Heart failure Left ventricular dysfunction Type I diabetic	Chronic renal disease Type II diabetic nephropathy	Renal impairment Peripheral vascular disease	Pregnancy Renovascular disease
Angiotensin II receptor antagonists	Cough induced by ACE inhibitor	Heart failure Intolerance of other antihypertensive drugs	Peripheral vascular disease	Pregnancy Renovascular disease
β-blockers	Myocardial infarction Angina	Heart failure	Heart failure Dyslipidaemia Peripheral vascular disease	Asthma or chronic obstructive pulmonary disease Heart block
Calcium antagonists (dihydropyridine)	Isolated systolic hypertension in elderly patients	Angina Elderly patients	—	—
Calcium antagonists (rate-limiting)	Angina	Myocardial infarction	Combination with β-blockade	Heart block Heart failure
Thiazides	Elderly patients	—	Dyslipidaemia	Heart failure

ACE = angiotensin-converting enzyme.

Source: BHS Guidelines (1999).

response is insufficient, the options are to substitute another drug or add a second drug. Substitution is appropriate when hypertension is mild and uncomplicated, and the response to the initial drug is small. In more severe or complicated hypertension, it is safer to add drugs stepwise until BP control is attained. Treatment can be stepped down later if the BP falls substantially below the optimal level.

Drugs from the major classes have additive antihypertensive effects, but certain drugs should not be co-presented. These include beta-blockers with diltiazem or verapamil, ACE inhibitors with ARBs and potassium-sparing diuretics with ACE inhibitors.

Other measures to reduce cardiovascular risk

Patients with established CVD or at high risk should be considered for aspirin and statin therapy.

- For *primary prevention*, aspirin 75 mg is recommended for hypertensive patients aged ≥ 50 years who have satisfactory control of BP ($< 150/90$ mmHg) and TOD, diabetes or a 10-year CHD risk $\geq 15\%$; statin therapy is indicated when serum total cholesterol is $\geq 5\%$ mmol/l and the 10-year CHD risk is $\geq 30\%$ in patients aged ≤ 70 years.

- For *secondary prevention*, aspirin should be prescribed unless contraindicated; statin therapy is indicated when the serum total cholesterol is ≥ 5.0 mmol/l in patients aged ≤ 75 years.

Follow-up

The frequency of follow-up for treated patients after adequate BP control is attained is variable. A review every three months is sufficient when treatment and BP are stable, and the interval should not exceed 6 months.

Special patient groups

Elderly

Once started, antihypertensive therapy should be continued after patients reach the age of 80 years. Patients with newly diagnosed hypertension after the age of 80 years should be considered for treatment provided they are generally fit and have reasonable life expectancy, particularly if there are hypertensive complications or TOD. Similarly, doctors should consider the anticipated benefits and resource implications when reaching treatment decisions about patients aged > 60 years with borderline isolated systolic hypertension (140–159/< 90 mmHg).

Diabetes

In type I and type II diabetes, the threshold for starting antihypertensive therapy is $\geq 140/90$ mmHg and the target BP is $< 140/80$ mmHg. In type I diabetes with nephropathy, the target BP is $< 130/80$ mmHg, or lower ($< 125/75$ mmHg) when proteinuria is ≥ 1 g/24 hours; an ACE inhibitor titrated to the maximum dose recommended and tolerated is the preferred first-line therapy. In both forms of diabetes, rigorous control of BP invariably necessitates the use of combinations of antihypertensive drugs. As well as ACE inhibitors, low-dose diuretics, calcium antagonists, beta-blockers and alpha-blockers are all suitable.

Renal disease

In patients with chronic renal impairment, good BP control is essential to retard this process. Thresholds and targets are the same as for hypertensive patients with type I diabetes complicated by nephropathy. Multiple drugs, including a diuretic, are usually required. Since thiazide diuretics may be ineffective in patients with renal impairment, loop doses, frequently in high doses, are often required. Patients with renal failure have a very high risk of cardiovascular complications, and may need aspirin or statin in addition to antihypertensive management to reduce the burden of risk.

Oral contraceptives

BP should be measured before starting oral contraceptives and 6-monthly there-after. In hypertensive women, other non-hormonal forms of contraception should be sought, particularly if other RFs for CVD coexist. If other methods of contraception are unacceptable, changing to a progestogen-only pill is recommended. If BP does not fall to < 160/100 mmHg, antihypertensive medication should be instituted.

Hormone replacement therapy

Hormone replacement therapy is not contraindicated for women with hypertension provided BP can be controlled by antihypertensive medication. It is prudent to monitor BP 2–3 times in the first 6 months and then 6-monthly. Hormone replacement therapy should be discontinued temporarily in women with resistant hypertension to assess its contribution to BP.

Implementation

All practices and primary care groups should develop protocols for hypertension management, including methods for identifying and recalling patients who drop out of follow-up. Written information should be available for patients. The practice policy should detail those aspects of management that are in the province of the practice nurse and the doctor, and the indications and procedures for passing management decisions from nurse to doctor and vice versa. It is recommended that implementation of the practice policy should be audited periodically.

Comment

The British Hypertension Society guidelines are a natural progression from earlier reports. However, the new recommendations introduce the concept of formal risk assessment incorporating all cardiovascular risk factors, advocate much more rigorous treatment targets, formalize advice on other cardioprotective strategies, and promote greater efforts in implementations. The guidelines are supported by information material for patients and doctors prepared by and available from the Society.

In contrast to the JNC VI and WHO–ISH guidelines, the brevity of the British Hypertension Society guidelines will make them especially useful for clinicians. Perhaps the most controversial issue is the recommendation to initiate treatment on the basis of level of risk rather than level of BP in patients with the mildest hypertension. This algorithm represents an important new direction that will require evaluation, since it alters fundamentally the way in which doctors are encouraged to think about treatment of hypertension.

Joint British recommendations on prevention of coronary heart disease in clinical practice [9]

The British Cardiac Society, the British Hyperlipidaemia Association and the British Hypertension Society cooperated in preparing national recommendations, which have been endorsed by the British Diabetic Association. Previously, each society had worked independently, publishing independent guidelines. This professional isolation is mirrored in clinical practice, where major determinants of cardio-vascular risk can be overlooked.

It is hoped that collaboration among professional societies will result in a more unified and hence more effective approach to the prevention of CHD. To achieve this, it is necessary to include all cardiovascular RFs, rather than focusing on treat-ing a single RF. The authors concede that the recommendations are based on evidence rather than strictly 'evidence-based'.

Priorities and objectives

Individuals who present to doctors vary enormously in their risk of CHD. Priority should depend on risk, and the following is proposed:

- patients with established CHD or other major atherosclerotic disease; and
- individuals with hypertension, or other RFs, or combinations of RFs that put them at high risk of CHD.

The specific objectives are:

- in patients with established CHD or other major atherosclerotic disease, to pre-vent the risk of further major cardiac events and to reduce overall mortality; and
- in high-risk individuals in the general population, to reduce the risk of CHD or other major atherosclerotic disease.

Coronary heart disease risk

Patients with established CHD identify themselves to medical services, are at high risk and gain considerable benefit from treatment. Therefore, in these cases it is not necessary to calculate absolute coronary risk before deciding on intervention.

In the general 'healthy' population, individuals may be at high or low but unknown risk. Since benefit depends on risk, it is necessary to calculate absolute risk before taking treatment decisions.

A staged approach is recommended (Table 2.28). Those at highest risk should be targeted first, and, as a minimum, healthy individuals with $\geq 30\%$ CHD risk over 10 years should be identified and treated. This is consistent with advice from the Standing Medical Advisory Committee (SMAC) and the Scottish Intercollegiate Guidelines Network (SIGN). Patients with DBP ≥ 100 mmHg, familial hyper-lipidaemia and diabetes mellitus with TOD should be included in the priority group. As a next step, it is appropriate to expand RF intervention down to indi-viduals with a 15% CHD risk over 10 years, provided those at higher levels of risk have already received effective preventive care.

To calculate risk, the computer program or coronary risk chart (Fig. 2.7a,b) subsequently adopted by the British Hypertension Society is recommended. The RFs used to calculate CHD risk are listed in Table 2.29.

Table 2.28 Priorities for coronary heart disease (CHD) prevention

- Stage 1   Established vascular disease
- Stage 2   CHD risk ≥ 30%*
              plus
              SBP ≥ 160 mmHg
              DBP ≥ 100 mmHg
              Familial hypercholesterolaemia
              DM + TOD
- Stage 3   CHD ≥ 15%

* As recommended by the Standing Medical Advisory Committee (1998) and the Scottish Intercollegiate Guidelines Network (1999).
SBP = systolic blood pressure; DBP = diastolic blood pressure; DM = diabetes mellitus; TOD = target organ damage.

Source: Joint British Recommendations (1998).

Secondary prevention

The interventions recommended are listed in Table 2.30. Lifestyle changes (Table 2.31) are the starting point, but only one component of management. Treatment of hypertension follows the British Hypertension Society guidelines (Table 2.32). Recommendations concerning serum lipids (≤ age 75 years), patients with diabetes mellitus, and the use of cardioprotective drugs are summarized in Tables 2.33–2.35.

Table 2.29 Risk factors used to calculate coronary heart disease (CHD) risk

- Smoking (current or recent)
- Blood pressure (repeated measures)
- Total cholesterol (repeated measures)
- HDL cholesterol (repeated measures)
- Diabetes
- FH of premature CHD
- ECG evidence of LVH

HDL = high-density lipoprotein; FH = family history; ECG = electrocardiogram; LVH = left ventricular hypertrophy.

Source: Joint British Recommendations (1998).

Table 2.30 Management of risk factors in secondary prevention of coronary heart disease

- Lifestyle
- Blood pressure
- Serum lipids
- Glucose
- Cardioprotective drugs

Source: Joint British Recommendations (1998).

Table 2.31 Lifestyle modifications to prevent coronary heart disease

- Stop smoking
- Avoid obesity
- Reduce saturated fat intake
- Increase intake of poly(mono)unsaturated fat
- Increase fruit/vegetables/fish
- Moderate alcohol
- Increase physical activity

Source: Joint British Recommendations (1998).

Table 2.32 Treatment of blood pressure for secondary prevention of coronary heart disease

- Beta-blocker-based therapy
- Rate-limiting calcium antagonist
  —intolerant of beta-blocker
  —no LV dysfunction
- ACE inhibitor
  —LV dysfunction or failure
- Rigorous control
  —target SBP < 140 mmHg < 130 (DM)
           DBP < 85 mmHg < 80 (DM)
  —combination therapy often required

LV = left ventricular; ACE = angiotensin-converting enzyme; SBP = systolic blood pressure;
DBP = diastolic blood pressure; DM = diabetes mellitus.

Source: Joint British Recommendations (1998).

Table 2.33 Treatment of serum lipids for secondary prevention of coronary heart disease

- Dietary advice
- Statin if TC ≥ 5.0 mmol/l after diet
  or TC ≥ 6.0 mmol/l without diet
  (post-MI or unstable angina)
- Target TC < 5.0 mmol/l
  AND ≥ 33% reduction

TC = serum total cholesterol; MI = myocardial infarction.

Source: Joint British Recommendations (1998).

Table 2.34 Management of diabetes mellitus for secondary prevention of coronary heart disease

- Lifestyle
- Blood pressure
- Serum lipids
- Glycaemic control

Source: Joint British Recommendations (1998).

Table 2.35 Cardioprotective drugs for secondary prevention of coronary heart disease

- Aspirin*
- Beta-blockers*
- Rate-limiting calcium antagonists+
- ACE inhibitors+
- Cholesterol-lowering drugs+
- Anticoagulants+

* Unless contraindicated. + Selected patients. ACE = angiotensin-converting enzyme.

Source: Joint British Recommendations (1998).

Primary prevention

For patients without clinical atherosclerotic disease, the absolute risk of developing CHD or other atherosclerotic disease during the next 10 years should strongly influence the intensity of lifestyle and therapeutic intervention. The decision not to introduce a particular therapy for a particular individual should be reviewed regularly since risk increases with age, and may in the course of time become sufficient to justify intervention.

It is recommended that intervention is initiated at the absolute risk levels indicated in Table 2.28. For individuals with an absolute CHD risk < 15% over the next 10 years, drug therapy is not usually recommended.

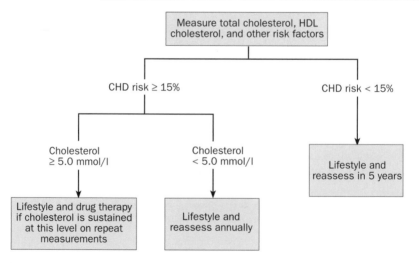

Fig. 2.8 Absolute coronary heart disease (CHD) risk and management of blood lipids in primary prevention of CHD and other atherosclerotic disease. HDL = high-density lipoprotein.

Lifestyle measures (Table 2.31) should be given priority, and will be the only approach offered to those with a CHD risk insufficient to justify pharmacotherapy. BP should be managed according to British Hypertension Society guidelines. The strategy for management of blood lipids in patients aged ≤69 years is shown in Fig. 2.8. In patients with type I and type II diabetes mellitus, efforts should be made to achieve not only tight glycaemic control, but also rigorous control of BP. The strategy for management of hypertension in diabetes is given in Table 2.36. Low-dose aspirin is recommended in selected high-risk patients using the criteria adopted in the British Hypertension Society guidelines. The management of patients with chronic renal failure is summarized in Table 2.37.

Table 2.36 Strategy for management of hypertension in a diabetic patient

- **Threshold**
  Type I   SBP ≥ 160   DBP ≥ 80 mmHg
  Type II   SBP ≥ 160   DBP ≥ 90 mmHg
                  SBP ≥ 140 mmHg (TOD)
- **Treatment**
  Type I   ACE inhibitor (ARB)
                  + others
  Type II   ACE inhibitor (ARB)
                  or beta-blocker
                  + thiazide/DHP calcium antagonist
- **Target**
  Type I/II   SBP < 130   DBP < 80 mmHg
                  SBP < 125   DBP <75 (proteinuria)

SBP = systolic blood pressure; DBP = diastolic blood pressure; TOD = target organ damage;
ACE = angiotensin-converting enzyme; DHP = dihydropyridine; ARB = angiotensin receptor blocker.

Source: Joint British Recommendations (1998).

Table 2.37 Strategy for management of hypertension in a patient with chronic renal failure

- **Blood pressure**
  —threshold   SBP ≥ 140   DBP ≥ 90 mmHg
  —treatment   ACE inhibitor (ARB)
                  loop diuretic
                  others
  —target   SBP ≥ 130   DBP ≥ 80 mmHg
- **Serum lipids**
  —statin
  —high risk

SBP = systolic blood pressure; DBP = diastolic blood pressure; ACE = angiotensin-converting enzyme;
ARB = angiotensin receptor blocker.

Source: Joint British Recommendations (1998).

Other recommendations

Screening of first-degree blood relatives (principally siblings and offspring aged ≥ 18 years) of patients with premature CHD or other atherosclerotic disease (men < 55 years and women < 65 years) is encouraged, and is essential in the context of familial hyperlipidaemia.

Auditing of the impact of common clinical protocols for hospital and general practice in the management of patients with CHD and other atherosclerotic diseases, and for the identification and management of high-risk individuals, is strongly recommended.

Comment

The Joint British Recommendations on Prevention of Coronary Heart Disease emphasize the need for practitioners to prioritize patients on the basis of risk, and advocate a staged approach to management. Patients with established CHD or other atherosclerotic diseases have the highest priority; therapeutic attention should be paid to individuals with hypertension and other risk predictors. The highest-priority patients should be treated appropriately and effectively. There is a need to calculate cardiovascular risk accurately in those without overt CVD.

Implementation requires an integrated care plan involving doctors and nurses in the primary and secondary care settings, and the patient. All RFs should be addressed by appropriate lifestyle measures and drug therapy. Regular audit of care protocols is essential.

Recommendations of the Second Joint Task Force of European and other Societies on Coronary Prevention |10|

These are similar in concept and objectives to the Joint British Recommendations (Fig. 2.9). The main differences relate to the threshold of absolute CHD risk at which drug treatment is recommended and the target BP. The Joint Task Force suggests an absolute CHD risk of ≥ 20% over 10 years or ≥ 20% if projected to the age of 60 years. A different risk chart is also recommended (Fig. 2.10a,b). Optimal target BP is defined as < 140/90 mmHg in both primary and secondary prevention. Treatment algorithms for BP and blood lipids are shown in Figs. 2.11 and 2.12.

Comment

The differences from the British guidelines reflect national prejudices. The most controversial recommendation is the option to project an individual's predicted CHD risk to the age of 60 years. The accuracy of this approach is untested. An inevitable consequence will be a large number of individuals at currently low risk committed to long-term drug therapy. The advantages and disadvantages of this policy require careful scrutiny.

Lifestyle and therapeutic goals for patients with CHD, or other atherosclerotic disease, and for healthy high-risk individuals

Patients with CHD or other atherosclerotic disease	Healthy high-risk individuals Absolute CHD risk ≥ 20% over 10 years, or will exceed 20% if projected to age 60

Lifestyle

Stop smoking, make healthy food choices, be physically active and achieve ideal weight

Other risk factors

Blood pressure <140/90 mmHg, total cholesterol <5.0 mmol/l (190 mg/dl) LDL cholesterol <3.0 mmol/(115 mg/dl) When these risk factor goals are not achieved by lifestyle changes, blood pressure and cholesterol-lowering drug therapies should be used.

Other prophylatic drug therapies

Aspirin (at least 75mg) for all coronary patients, those with cerebral atherosclerosis and peripheral atherosclerotic disease. β-blockers in patients following myocardial infarction. ACE inhibitors in those with symptoms or signs of heart failure at the time of myocardial infarction, or with chronic LV systolic dysfunction (ejection fraction <40%). Anticoagulants in selected coronary patients.	Aspirin (75mg) in treated hypertensive patients, and in men at particularly high CHD risk.

Screen close relatives

Screen close relatives of patients with premature (men <55 yrs, women <65 yrs) CHD	Screen close relatives if familial hypercholesterolaemia or other inherited dyslipidaemia is suspected.

Fig. 2.9 Framework for prevention of coronary heart disease (CHD) in clinical practice. LDL = low-density lipoprotein; ACE = angiotensin-converting enzyme; LV = left ventricular.

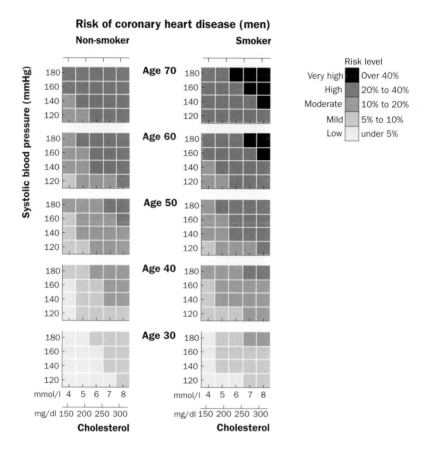

Fig. 2.10a Coronary risk chart: men.

How to use the coronary risk chart for primary prevention (Fig. 2.10)

- **To estimate a person's absolute 10-year risk of a CHD event**, find the table for their gender, smoking status, and age. Within the table, find the cell nearest to their systolic blood pressure (mmHg) and total cholesterol (mmol/l or mg/dl).

- **The effect of lifetime exposure to risk factors** can be seen by following the table upwards. This can be used when advising younger people.

- **High-risk individuals are defined as those whose 10-year CHD risk exceeds 20% or will exceed 20% if projected to age 60.**

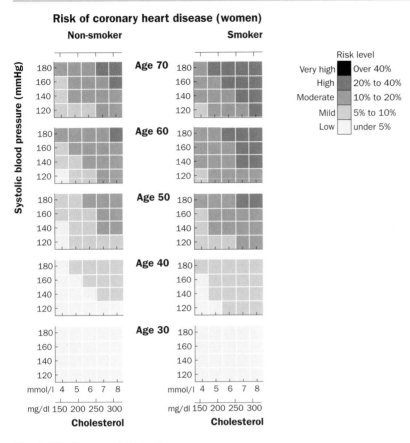

Fig. 2.10b Coronary risk chart: women.

- **CHD risk is higher than indicated** in the chart for those with:
  - Familial hyperlipidaemia (diabetes risk is approximately doubled in men and more than doubled in women);
  - Those with a family history of premature cardiovascular disease;
  - Those with low HDL cholesterol. These tables assume HDL cholesterol to be 1.0 mmol/l (39 mg/dl) in men and 1.1 (43) in women;
  - Those with raised triglyceride levels >2.0 mmol/l (>180 mg/dl);
  - As the person approaches the next age category.
- **To find a person's relative risk**, compare his/her risk category with that for other people of the same age. The absolute risk shown here may not apply to all populations, especially those with a low CHD incidence. Relative risk is likely to apply to most populations.
- **The effect of changing** cholesterol, smoking status, or BP can be read from the chart.

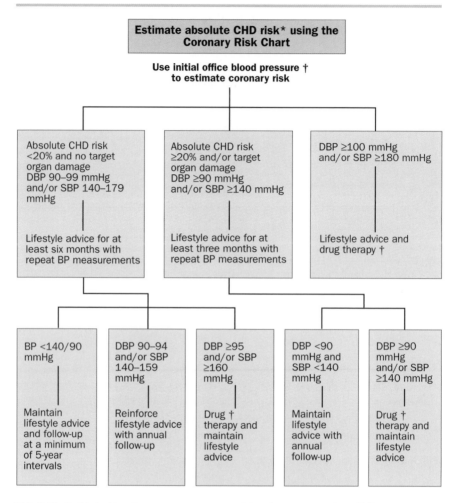

Fig. 2.11 Guide to blood pressure management in primary prevention. CHD = coronary heart disease; (S/D)BP = (systolic/diastolic) blood pressures.

* Ten-year CHD risk ≥ 20% or will exceed 20% if projected to age 60 years.

† Consider causes of secondary hypertension. If appropriate, refer to a specialist.

American Heart Association/American College of Cardiology statement on risk assessment |11|

This joint statement endorses the concept of calculating CHD risk. Absolute risk should be estimated from the major RFs. Thereafter, consideration can be given

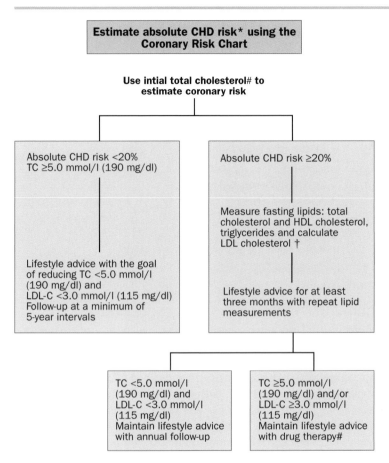

Fig. 2.12 Guide to lipid management in primary prevention. CHD = coronary heart disease; TC = total cholesterol; LDL(-C) = low-density lipoprotein (cholesterol); HDL = high-density lipoprotein.

* Ten-year CHD risk ≥ 20% or will exceed 20% if projected to age 60 years.

† HDL cholesterol < 1.0 mmol/l (40 mg/dl) and fasting triglycerides > 2.0 mmol/l (180 mg/dl) are markers for increased coronary risk.

\# Consider genetically determined hyperlipidaemias (total cholesterol usually > 8.0 mmol/l (above 300 mg/dl) with stigmata of hyperlipidaemia such as obesity, diabetes, alcohol, liver and renal diseases. If appropriate, refer to a specialist.

to modifying the estimate in the presence of other RFs (Table 2.38). Clinical judgement is required to estimate the incremental risk incurred by these RFs.

Detection of patients at high risk with the aid of global risk assessment should be an important aim of routine medical evaluation of all patients. The reader is referred

Table 2.38 Other cardiovascular risk factors after consideration of major independent risk factors

Predisposing

- Obesity (Body Mass Index)
- Abdominal obesity
- Physical inactivity
- Family history of premature CHD
- Ethnic characteristics
- Psychosocial factors

Conditional

- Elevated serum triglycerides
- Small LDL particles
- Elevated serum homocysteine
- Elevated serum lipoprotein (a)
- Prothrombotic factors (e.g. fibrinogen)
- Inflammatory markers (e.g. C-reactive protein)

CHD = coronary heart disease; LDL = low-density lipoprotein.

Source: AHA/ACC Statement (1999).

to JNC VI for specific therapy of hypertensive patients. Once appropriate therapies are selected, global risk scores can also be used to help instruct patients and to improve compliance with preventive interventions.

Global risk assessment is particularly useful in young and middle-aged adults for assessing both absolute and relative risk. Even though short-term risk may not be high in younger patients who have multiple RFs of only moderate severity, long-term risk can be unacceptably high. Risk assessment in those patients will highlight the need for early and prolonged intervention on RFs. In young adults, relative risk ratios help to reveal long-term risk of CHD, i.e. those within a particular age cohort who are most likely to suffer events. Although long-term prevention may not call for the use of risk-reducing drugs, it requires the introduction of lifestyle modification. Appropriate intervention, guided by risk assessment that is performed periodically in early adulthood and early middle age, has the potential to bring about a significant reduction in long-term risk.

Comment

This statement for health care professionals is long on rhetoric but short on practical advice. The method of calculating relative risk is complex and would be difficult to apply in most clinical settings. Furthermore, clear recommendations based on relative risk are not provided. Much of the advice depends on 'clinical judgement', and consistent implementation is unlikely. Again, risk projection is implicit in this statement.

Simple blood pressure guidelines for primary health care |12|

Professor Peter Sever has published a counterblast to the current epidemic of complex guidelines. He suggests four simple rules.

- **Rule 1** Abandon DBP measurement and rely on SBP values for decisions on treatment thresholds and goals.

- **Rule 2** Assess overall cardiovascular risk by history, physical examination and simple investigations (urine dipsticks, serum creatinine, glucose, lipids and ECG).

- **Rule 3** Apply a systolic threshold of 150 mmHg for the introduction of drug treatment when repeated measures of BP, following a trial of non-pharmaco-logical treatment, remain persistently above this level. This threshold may be reduced to 140 mmHg for high-risk patients (e.g. those with TOD or diabetes) or raised to 160 mmHg for low-risk patients and the elderly.

- **Rule 4** Modify treatment if initial drug treatment is ineffective, partially effect-ive or poorly tolerated. If BP does not fall below the pretreatment threshold, drug dosage should be increased (except that of diuretics), treatment should be changed or combinations should be used to achieve goal BP.

Comment

At first sight, these rules appear practical and refreshing, but, on closer inspection, problems appear. Apart from the elimination of DBP from the assessment, these simple guidelines are little different from a summary of the 1993 British Hypertension Society guidelines (lead author, Professor Sever). Reliance on SBP is unlikely to alter the individuals offered treatment, since very few will have DBP ≥ 100 mmHg (the 1993 guidelines threshold) and SBP < 150 mmHg.

Perhaps more importantly, it is left to the practitioner to identify high-risk patients from clinical clues. Sadly, doctors are very poor at this, as can be seen from the continued failure to identify and treat patients who are at high risk by any criteria, almost a decade after publication of the 1993 guidelines.

The goals of treatment are conservative. A target BP of 'below the treatment threshold' means that someone with a threshold SBP of 150 mmHg would be con-sidered to have achieved satisfactory control if, on treatment, SBP was 149 mmHg. Intuitively, this makes no sense. Furthermore, the distribution of BP in the com-munity dictates that the majority of patients who qualify for treatment will cluster around levels just above the threshold. Thus these guidelines will ensure only marginal improvement in BP in most treated patients. These guidelines may be simple, but are unlikely to result in great benefit for the individual.

Conclusion

The current guidelines all emphasize the importance of risk assessment in identifying individuals who merit treatment. Intuitive or informal assessment of risk by doctors is highly inaccurate. Without formal risk assessment, prescribing policies are very inconsistent, and are also prejudiced against certain high-risk groups such as smokers and older people. Some method of formal assessment is clearly necessary for rational prescribing.

Guidelines based on simple counting of RFs are distinctly less accurate than methods that count and weight RFs for CVD. These fail to treat individuals with high or even extremely high risk, while identifying for treatment many with a CHD risk of $< 0.6\%$ per year. Provided the method of formal risk assessment is simple, it is easy to classify individuals.

Cardiovascular risk assessment has tremendous potential, but the future cannot be predicted with any real certainty for the presymptomatic individual. For 1000 adults with a 20% CVD risk, neither the 200 potential losers nor the 800 potential winners can be identified. Nevertheless, multi-variable risk equations can forecast accurately the absolute risk of future events and predict the benefit of intervention.

The challenge is to 'operationalize' the information so that patients and physicians can make informed decisions. Reaching a consensus about the threshold of absolute risk for intervention is difficult. Also, there are limitations of short-term risk assessment, which favours treatment of older individuals in whom the immediate absolute risk of disease is high. However, older individuals without symptomatic disease can be classified among the winners, since they have tolerated RFs over years. Younger patients with RFs may have short-term absolute risk below a prespecified threshold, yet gain the most benefit over the long term, and are at increased risk of premature disease.

Nonetheless, cardiovascular risk assessment is an important addition to the doctor's diagnostic and prognostic black bag. If nothing else, it provides a framework to help inform otherwise healthy individuals of increased risk and help them to make informed decisions. The poor compliance with cardioprotective drug therapy suggests that patients who start treatment are not convinced of its benefit.

Professional compliance is also poor. Despite many national and international guidelines offering evidence-based recommendations on the management of hypertension, there is little evidence that clinical practice has improved. Guidelines are widely acknowledged but largely ignored.

It appears to be assumed that recommendations will filter down to the local level; but the flow is unlikely to be successful without efforts to improve implementation. Implementation depends on availability, accessibility, audit and education. For education to be successful it must be authoritative, simple, short, practical, attractive and repeated.

Practitioners value management guidelines, but consider those available to be too scientific, excessively demanding of resources, and of impractical complexity, of limited local applicability, and also to have a short shelf-life. Guidelines appear to be updated every few years to follow current fashion rather than to respond to important new evidence. Useful guidelines would be simple, practical, consider local resources and priorities, and incorporate local experience, opinion and judgement. Guidelines are likely to be implemented if they are clear and evidence-based, but not if they are vague, controversial, or demand change in practice or practice routines.

Interventions to promote implementation have met with varied success. The most consistently successful approaches include educational outreach with an interactive component and repeated reminders of key priorities. A multifactorial targeted approach involving audit, reminders and consensus is often particularly useful. The techniques usually employed, such as dissemination of summary guidelines, have no effect.

If management of hypertension is to improve, a much more practical approach is needed. Evidence and evidence-based guidelines are still necessary, but more attention must be paid to generation, dissemination and implementation. Only then can professional non-compliance with recommendations on best practice be corrected.

References

1. Joint National Committee on Prevention, Detection, Evaluation and Treatment of High Blood Pressure. The sixth report of the Joint National Committee on Prevention, Detection, Evaluation and Treatment of High Blood Pressure. *Arch Intern Med* 1997; **157**: 2413–46.

2. Joint National Committee on Detection, Evaluation and Treatment of High Blood Pressure. Fifth report of the Joint National Committee on Detection, Evaluation and Treatment of High Blood Pressure. *Arch Intern Med* 1993; **153**: 154–83.

3. Coope JN, Warrender TS. Randomised trial of hypertension in elderly patients in primary care. *BMJ* 1986; **293**: 1148–51.

4. Guidelines Subcommittee. 1999 World Health Organisation–International Society of Hypertension guidelines for the management of hypertension. *J Hypertens* 1999; **17**: 151–83.

5. Ramsay LE, Williams B, Johnston GD, MacGregor GA, Poston L, Potter JF, Poulter NR, Russell G. Guidelines for management of hypertension: report of the third working party of the British Hypertension Society. *J Hum Hypertens* 1999; **13**: 569–92.

6. Ramsay LE, Williams B, Johnston GD, MacGregor GA, Poston L, Potter JF, Poulter NR, Russell G. British Hypertension Society guidelines for hypertension management 1999: summary. *BMJ* 1999; **319**: 630–5.

7. Swales JD, Ramsay LE, Coope JR, *et al*. Treating mild hypertension. Report of the British Hypertension Society working party. *BMJ* 1989; **298**: 694–8.

8. Sever P, Beevers G, Bulpitt C, Lever A, Ramsay L, Reid J, Swales J. Management guidelines in essential hypertension. Report of the second working party of the British Hypertension Society. *BMJ* 1993; **306**: 983–7.

9. Wood D, Durrington P, McInnes G, Poulter N, Rees A, Wray A. Joint British recommendations on prevention of coronary heart disease in clinical practice. *Heart* 1998; **80** Suppl 2: S1–S29.

10. Wood D, De Backer G, Faergeman O, Graham I, Mancia G, Pyörälä K. Prevention of coronary heart disease in clinical practice. Summary of recommendations of the Second Joint Task Force of European and other Societies on Coronary Prevention. *J Hypertens* 1998; **16**: 1407–14.

11. Grundy SM, Pasternak R, Greenland P, Smith S, Fuster V. Assessment of cardiovascular risk by use of multiple-risk-factor assessment equations. A statement for healthcare professionals from the American Heart Association and the American College of Cardiology. *Circulation* 1999; **100**: 1481–92.

12. Sever PS. Simple blood pressure guidelines for primary health care. *J Hum Hypertens* 1999; **13**: 725–7.

3

Ongoing trials

Introduction

The combined results of previous randomized controlled trials, involving a total of about 47 000 patients with hypertension, have demonstrated that diuretic- and beta-blocker-based regimens produce much of the epidemiologically expected benefit of the blood pressure (BP) reduction achieved |1|. The proportional reduction in the risk of stroke and coronary heart disease (CHD) events appeared to be broadly similar for patients with mild, moderate and more severe hypertension, for older and younger patients, and for patients with and without a history of cerebrovascular disease. Thus, the magnitude of the absolute benefit of treatment varied in direct proportion to the background level of risk (i.e. patients with the highest absolute risk of stroke or CHD experienced the largest absolute reduction of risk).

Data from four direct randomized comparisons of diuretic- and beta-blocker-based regimens collectively demonstrated no evidence of a difference between these treatments on stroke or CHD outcomes. However, although a total of 24 000 patients was studied, even in combination these studies lacked adequate statistical power to determine reliably modest but potentially important treatment differences (e.g. a 10–15% difference in the relative risk of CHD).

Even less information is available concerning the effects of newer classes of antihypertensive agents. The Systolic Hypertension in Europe (SYST-EUR) trial |2| and the Shanghai Trial of Nifedipine in the Elderly (STONE) |3| indicated a significant reduction in stroke risk of about 40–50% compared with placebo in patients treated with nitrendipine and nifedipine, respectively. In comparison with conventional therapy (diuretics, beta-blockers), long-acting calcium antagonists showed no advantage in elderly hypertensive patients |4|. Likewise, angiotensin-converting enzyme (ACE) inhibitors and conventional agents had similar effects in Swedish Trial of Old Patients with Hypertension-2 (STOP-2) |4| and in the Captopril Prevention Project (CAPPP) |5|, although advantages of captopril were reported in the diabetic subset of CAPPP |5|. Unfortunately, deficiencies in the conduct of CAPPP make its results unreliable. Results of more recent trials, e.g. Heart Outcomes Prevention Evaluation (HOPE), Intervention as a Goal in Hypertension Treatment (INSIGHT), Nordic Diltiazem (NORDIL), have not defined clearly the role of newer agents (see Chapter 1).

Ongoing randomized controlled trials have been designed primarily to provide more reliable data about the effects of newer drug classes on cardiovascular mortality and morbidity in various patient populations. The trials fall into two categories

- comparison of newer and older drug classes for the treatment of patients with high BP, and
- evaluation of newer drugs in patients with high risk (e.g. established cardiac disease, cerebrovascular disease, diabetes, renal disease, the elderly).

At usual doses, most of the newer agents produce reductions in BP of similar magnitude to that produced by diuretics and beta-blockers |6|. Hence, any differences between the effects on stroke risk and CHD risk of regimens based on older and newer agents would have to be due to properties of the drugs that are independent of BP-lowering effects. Many such properties have been postulated. However, it is unknown whether these influences augment the benefits of lowering BP and any independent effects are not likely to be large. Detection of plausible differences in relative risk (of 15% or less) between various antihypertensive regimens on stroke and CHD will require evidence from randomized trials involving many thousands of patients and a thousand or more outcome events. Fewer events are required to detect the effect of the same treatment compared with placebo as the likely effects of treatment will be larger, but such studies are ethically acceptable in only a few clinical circumstances.

This chapter reviews the design and current status of a selection of the more important ongoing trials. Examples from both the main categories of outcome trials will be discussed. However, a clear distinction between comparisons of newer drugs and older drugs in hypertensive patients and those of newer drugs in patients with a high risk of cardiovascular events is not always easy since patients with multiple risk factors are targeted in most trials to increase the probability of achieving the necessary event rate. In addition, in many studies, the influence of other cardioprotective strategies (such as lipid lowering therapy) is often incorporated.

Comparison of older and newer drug classes

Antihypertensive therapy and Lipid Lowering Heart Attack prevention Trial (ALLHAT)

 Rationale and design for the Antihypertensive and Lipid Lowering to prevent Heart Attack Trial (ALLHAT).
B R Davis, J A Cutler, D J Gordon, *et al. Am J Hypertens* 1996; **9**: 342–60.

BACKGROUND. ALLHAT is a randomized double-blind trial in high-risk hypertensive patients. It compares a calcium channel blocker (amlodipine), an ACE inhibitor (lisinopril), and an alpha-blocker (doxazosin) with the thiazide diuretic

(chlorthalidone). The main eligibility criteria are systolic and diastolic hypertension in patients aged ≥ 55 years, who have at least one further CHD risk factor, e.g. left ventricular hypertrophy (LVH), known atherosclerotic cardiovascular disease, cigarette smoking or type 2 diabetes mellitus.

INTERPRETATION. ALLHAT is the only clinical trial of this nature with sufficient statistical power to assess the impact on CHD events separately from other cardiovascular events. It is designed to assess whether or not newer antihypertensive drugs can provide greater reductions in cardiovascular events relative to treatment with thiazide diuretics.

Outline

Patients: 42 448
Planned follow-up: 6 years
Randomized treatment: Diuretic, ACE inhibitor, alpha blocker, dihydropyridine calcium antagonist
Factorial assignment: Lipid lowering therapy, usual care
Completion date: 2002
Entry criteria: Hypertension + cardiovascular disease risk
Age: ≥ 55 years
Diastolic BP: 90–109 mmHg
Systolic BP: 140–179 mmHg
Projected events:
   CHD: 2580
   Strokes: 2790

ALLHAT is the largest hypertension outcome trial ever undertaken. It is a randomized, double-blind study in men and women aged ≥ 55 years. Representatives of four major classes of antihypertensive agents are compared: a diuretic (chlorthalidone), a calcium channel blocker (amlodipine), an ACE inhibitor (lisinopril) and an alpha-blocker (doxazosin). The treatment goal is diastolic BP < 90 mmHg and systolic BP < 140 mmHg. The study duration is 6–8 years.

The principal questions addressed by ALLHAT is whether different antihypertensive agents differ in the prevention of CHD mortality and morbidity, independent of BP lowering, particularly newer agents compared with a diuretic. ALLHAT also examines the question of whether lowering low-density lipoprotein (LDL) cholesterol with an HMG CoA reductase inhibitor (pravastatin) prevents cardiovascular disease and all cause mortality compared with usual care (diet alone).

The primary end-point is CHD death or non-fatal myocardial infarction (MI). Secondary end-points include all-cause mortality, combined cardiovascular disease, stroke and LVH. Recruitment at 625 community centres and Veterans Administration sites throughout the USA, Canada, Puerto Rica and the US Virgin Islands was completed in 1998 and results are expected in 2002. Projected follow-up is 4–8 years (average 6 years).

Participants are high-risk patients with BP ≥ 140/90 mmHg and ≥ 1 of the following risk factors: MI (not recent), stroke, coronary artery bypass graft or angioplasty, major ST segment depression or T wave inversion on electrocardiogram (ECG), known atherosclerotic cardiovascular disease, type 2 diabetes, high-density lipoprotein (HDL) cholesterol ≤ 35 mg/dl, LVH and cigarette smoking. Exclusion criteria include symptomatic ischaemic heart disease (angina), left ventricular systolic dysfunction (injection fraction < 35%) and renal impairment (serum creatinine > 2 g/dl).

Preliminary data on patient characteristics indicate that 53% are men, 35% are Afro-Americans, 16% are Hispanic and 36% have type 2 diabetes mellitus. ECG evidence of LVH was present at randomization in > 15% of participants. Average age is about 70 years and around 20% are cigarette smokers. About 25% of patients (n = 10337) are enrolled in the lipid lowering area of the trial, which involves patients with mild to moderately elevated total cholesterol. Patient characteristics are evenly distributed between the treatment groups.

It is projected that ALLHAT will accumulate to 2580 CHD events and 2790 strokes. This makes it the only trial of this nature with sufficient statistical power to assess the impact on CHD events separately from all other cardiovascular events.

One part of ALLHAT was stopped prematurely in early 2000 (Chapter 1). In summary, users of doxazosin had 25% more cardiovascular events and were twice as likely to be hospitalized for congestive heart failure as users of chlorthalidone (Table 3.1). The drugs were similarly effective in preventing heart attacks and in reducing the risk of death from all causes. Those in the doxazosin group had systolic BP slightly higher than those in the chlorthalidone group, although diastolic BP was the same (137/76 mmHg *vs* 135/76 mmHg, respectively) in each group. The doxazosin group also had poorer compliance with therapy; only 75% were still taking the drug or another alpha-blocker after 4 years, compared with 86% still taking chlorthalidone or another diuretic. Another reason for discontinuation was futility—the study had < 1% chance of detecting an advantage of doxazosin over chlorthalidone for CHD events.

Table 3.1 Cardiovascular events in ALLHAT

	RR	95% CI	*P*-value
Combined cardiovascular disease events	1.25	1.17, 1.35	< 0.001
Congestive heart failure	2.04	1.75, 2.32	< 0.001
Combined cardiovascular disease events (excluding congestive heart failure)	1.13	1.06, 1.21	< 0.001
Stroke	1.19	1.01, 1.40	0.04
CHD events	1.03	0.90, 1.17	0.71

Relative risk (RR) doxazosin *vs* chlorthalidone. 95% CI, 95% confidence interval.

Source: The ALLHAT Officers and Coordinators for the ALLHAT Collaborative Research Group (2000).

It was advised that patients taking an alpha-blocker should consult their doctor about alternative therapy. An alpha-blocker may not be the best choice for initial therapy. It cannot be concluded that doxazosin is harmful but it is less effective than chlorthalidone in reducing cardiovascular disease.

Comment

ALLHAT is a formidable scientific and logistical undertaking. Its findings will have far reaching consequences. However, ALLHAT has limitations that may cloud interpretation. Many patients are likely to require more than one antihypertensive agent in combination and many will have established cardiovascular disease. As beta-blockers, with known secondary protective properties, are likely to be added as second step agent, interpretation of the results may be complex. Also, findings in high-risk patients may not be easy to extrapolate to the majority of hypertensive patients with a much lower cardiovascular risk.

Early findings suggest that not all antihypertensive agents are created equal and that BP reduction alone cannot be considered as a valid surrogate end-point that reflects real outcomes (MI, stroke and death). That the reassuring concept of the primacy of BP reduction has been shattered by the discovery that doxazosin is associated with poorer outcome than chlorthalidone is ironic as alpha-blockers have been widely advocated on the basis that their metabolic influence afford advantages over diuretics. Thus, there has been much hope (or hype) that doxazosin would have benefits (over diuretics) beyond BP reduction by improving the hypertensive metabolic syndrome (surrogate marker). The outcome of the doxazosin arm of ALLHAT is a warning to those who advocate management decisions based on surrogate (or intermediate) end-points. Such optimism should not have been allowed to distract from the lack of outcome data with this drug class and its relatively moderate antihypertensive efficacy certainly in the supine posture (where we spend one-third of our lives) and relatively poor tolerability leading to poor compliance.

The Anglo Scandinavian Cardiac Outcomes Trial (ASCOT)

Rationale, design, methods and baseline demography of participants of the Anglo-Scandinavian Cardiac Outcomes Trial.

P S Sever, B Dahlöf, N R Poulter, *et al.* for the ASCOT investigators.
J Hypertens 2001; **19**: 1139–47.

BACKGROUND. ASCOT tests directly two important practical hypotheses as its primary aims:

- that a newer antihypertensive treatment regimen (calcium channel blocker ± an ACE inhibitor) is more effective than an older regimen (beta-blocker ± a diuretic) in the primary prevention of CHD.

- **that a statin compared with placebo will further protect against CHD end-points in hypertensive subjects with a total cholesterol ≤ 6.5 mmol/l.**

INTERPRETATION. The primary end-points in ASCOT are reductions in fatal and non-fatal CHD; secondary end-points include other cardiovascular events and total mortality. The factorial study design allows the benefits of BP reduction and cholesterol reduction to be analysed separately.

Outline

Patients: 19 342
Planned follow-up: 5 years
Randomized treatment: Dihydropyridine calcium antagonist ± ACE inhibitor, beta-blocker ± diuretic
Factorial assignment: Atorvastatin, placebo
Completion: 2003
Entry criteria: Hypertension + cardiovascular disease risk
Age: 40–79 years
Diastolic BP: ≥ 90 mmHg
Systolic BP: ≥ 140 mmHg
Projected events:
  CHD: 1150
  Strokes: 400

ASCOT is a prospective, randomized, open, blinded end-point (PROBE) trial with a double-blinded 2 × 2 factorial design with an antihypertensive and lipid lowering wing. In the antihypertensive limb, standard therapy based on atenolol (50/100 mg) ± bendrofluazide (1.25/2.5 mg) + potassium is compared with contemporary therapy based on amlodipine (5/10 mg) ± perindopril (4/8 mg). Supplementary therapy in both regimens is with doxazosin (GITS, Gastro Intestinal Therapeutic System) ± moxonidine ± free choice but avoiding drug classes in the comparator regimens. The lipid lowering arm consists of a double-blind comparison of atorvastatin 10 mg daily and placebo in participants with a serum total cholesterol ≤ 6.5 mmol/l (Fig. 3.1). In those subjects with higher serum total cholesterol levels, lipid lowering management is according to local guidelines.

Some 19 342 eligible subjects have been recruited mainly from general practices in the UK, Ireland, Denmark, Finland, Iceland, Norway and Sweden. All participants were randomized to standard or contemporary antihypertensive regimens and 10 297 subjects eligible for the lipid lowering arm were secondarily randomized to atorvastatin or placebo. Patient recruitment was completed in 2000 and the study should end in 2003. Average planned follow-up is 5 years or until 1150 primary events have occurred.

The primary objectives of ASCOT are to compare the effects of the two antihypertensive regimens on non-fatal acute MI plus total CHD events, and to compare the effects of atorvastatin and placebo on the same outcomes. There are 16

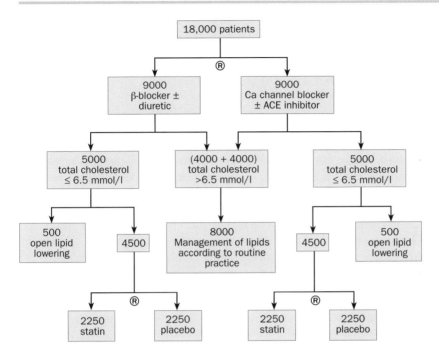

® Randomization

Fig. 3.1 Target numbers for study treatment comparisons in ASCOT. Source: Sever *et al.* (2001).

further secondary and tertiary objectives, including effects on total (fatal and non-fatal) stroke, all-cause mortality and heart failure. It will enable an evaluation of whether greater than additive effects on the study end-points or on all cardiovascular events and procedures are observed between the different antihypertensive regimens and the cholesterol lowering regimen. It will enable comparisons of the effects of the antihypertensive and lipid-lowering regimens on health care costs, and on all major study end-points among specific subgroups of patients (e.g. diabetics, smokers, the obese [body mass index (BMI) > 30 kg/m²], those with LVH, older/younger (≤ 60/> 60 years), male/female, any previous vascular disease (by history or electrocardiogram, ECG), and renal dysfunction (by serum creatinine, urinalysis)).

Eligible patients at randomization satisfied the following criteria: untreated systolic BP ≥ 160 mmHg or untreated diastolic BP ≥ 100 mmHg *or* treated systolic BP ≥ 140 mmHg or treated diastolic BP ≥ 90 mmHg; age 40–79 years; and ≥ 3 of 11 stipulated risk factors, e.g. male sex, age ≥ 55 years, smoking, non-insulin-dependent diabetes mellitus, ECG changes of LVH or ischaemia, peripheral vascular disease, past history of stroke ($\geq$ 3 months previously), microalbuminuria/proteinuria, total cholesterol: HDL cholesterol ratio $>$ 6, family history of premature CHD. For inclusion in the lipid lowering limb, patients also had to have serum total cholesterol $\leq$ 6.5 mmol/l and not be currently taking a statin or fibrate. Exclusion criteria included heart failure, drug treatment of angina, history of acute MI and serum triglycerides $>$ 4.5 mmol/l.

The drug treatment regimens are outlined in Table 3.2. Target BP levels are systolic BP $<$ 140 mmHg and diastolic BP $<$ 90 mmHg ($<$ 130 mmHg and $<$ 80 mmHg in diabetics). The study has 80% power (at the 5% level) to detect a relative difference of 20% in CHD end-points between the calcium channel blocker-based regimen and the beta-blocker-based regimen. The lipid-lowering limb of the study has 90% power at the 1% level to detect a relative difference of 30% in CHD end-points between groups.

Patient recruitment ended in May 2000. The demographics of the patient population are given in Table 3.3. Approximately two-thirds were taking anti-hypertensive therapy prior to randomization. Table 3.4 gives details of the risk profile of those randomized, reflecting the inclusion criteria for ASCOT.

Comment

At least 50% of high-risk hypertensive patients require two or more drugs to provide adequate BP control. Previous trials have allowed a wide range of possible drug combinations to be used making it impossible to make recommendation about specific combinations. In ASCOT, the allowed combinations are clearly specified as are subsequent add-on drugs, which are common to both limbs of the trial and the agents used have been established as producing effective 24-h BP control.

Table 3.2 Antihypertensive drug regimens in ASCOT

	Group A	Group B
Step 1	Amlodipine 5 mg	Atenolol 50 mg
Step 2	Amlodipine 10 mg	Atenolol 100 mg
Step 3	Amlodipine 10 mg	Atenolol 100 mg
	Perindopril 4 mg	BFZ 1.25 mg + K$^+$
Step 4	Amlodipine10 mg	Atenolol 100 mg
	Perindopril 8 mg (2 × 4 mg)	BFZ 2.5 mg + K$^+$
Step 5	Amlodipine 10 mg	Atenolol 100 mg
	Perindopril 8 mg (2 × 4 mg)	BFZ 2.5 mg + K$^+$
	Doxazosin GITS 4 mg	Doxazosin GITS 4 mg
Step 6	Amlodipine 10 mg	Atenolol 100 mg
	Perindopril 8 mg (2 × 4 mg)	BFZ 2.5 mg + K$^+$
	Doxazosin GITS 8 mg	Doxazosin GITS 8 mg

BFZ = bendrofluazide; GITS = Gastrointestinal Therapeutic System.
Source: Sever *et al*. (2001).

The design of ASCOT supplements that of ALLHAT. In the latter study, allowed add-on drugs are very mixed and largely outdated (reserpine, clonidine and atenolol with hydralazine as third-line therapy). However, the choice of doxazosin as third-line therapy in ASCOT poses problems in view of the premature discontinuation of that arm in ALLHAT. It remains unclear whether the relative disadvantage of alpha-blockade as first-line therapy can be extrapolated to the use of doxazosin in combination with other drugs. Nevertheless, in ALLHAT, it is likely that the majority of doxazosin-treated patients were also receiving atenolol,

Table 3.3 Baseline characteristics of randomized patients in ASCOT (mean ± SD)

	Antihypertensive limb	Lipid lowering limb
Age (years)	62.9 ± 8.5	63.1 ± 8.5
Sex (%): male	76.5	81.2
Weight (kg)		
Male	87.5 ± 14.8	87.2 ± 14.8
Female	75.2 ± 14.8	76.0 ± 15.4
SBP mmHg	165 ± 21	165 ± 20
DBP mmHg	95 ± 11	95 ± 11
Pulse beats/min	73 ± 14	72 ± 14
Caucasian (%)	95.4	94.6
Total cholesterol	6.00 ± 1.10	5.48 ± 0.69
HDL cholesterol (mmol/l)	1.29 ± 0.37	1.29 ± 0.36

SBP, systolic BP; DBP, diastolic BP.

Source: Sever *et al.* (2001).

Table 3.4 Percentage of patients with additional cardiovascular risk factors in ASCOT

	Patients (%)
No. of additional risk factors = 3	50.2
> 3	49.8

Risk factor	Patients (%)	Risk factor	Patients (%)
Age ≥ 55 years	84	Cerebrovascular event	11
Male	76	Microalbuminuria/proteinuria	62
LVH	13	Smoker	31
Abnormal ECG	14	Plasma total/HDL ≥ 6	24
NIDDM	22	Family history of coronary disease	28
Peripheral vascular disease	6		

NIDDM, non-insulin-dependent diabetes mellitus.

Source: Sever *et al.* (2001).

clonidine or reserpine. Further analysis of ALLHAT and other databases are essential before reaching conclusions.

The lipid lowering arm of ASCOT is also important. Although hypertensive individuals have been included in previous lipid lowering trials, no trials of lipid lowering carried out specifically in hypertensives have been reported. Particularly, there is little information on lipid lowering in hypertensive patients with total cholesterol ≤ 6.5 mmol/l. Again, the results of ASCOT will complement those of ALLHAT.

The Australian National Blood Pressure Study 2 (ANBP2)

Second Australian National Blood Pressure Study (ANBP2)—Progress Report.
L M H Wing, C M Reid, L J Beilin, *et al.* on behalf of the ANBP2 investigators. *J Hypertens* 2001; **19** (Suppl 2): S149.

BACKGROUND. ANBP2 is designed to compare the outcome (total cardiovascular events, fatal and non-fatal) of ACE inhibitor *vs* diuretic-based regimens for the treatment of hypertension in elderly hypertensives (aged 65–84 years) over a 5-year treatment period. Secondary aims include the identification of genetic markers related to hypertension and outcome, the association of LVH and 24-h ambulatory BP (ABPM) with outcome and the evaluation of the effects of treatment regimens on quality of life, LVH and ABPM. A health economic analysis is also being undertaken.

INTERPRETATION. ANBP2 is entering the final year of observation with an anticipated cut-off date scheduled for the last quarter of 2001.

Outcome

Patients: 6083
Planned follow-up: 5 years
Randomized treatment: ACE inhibitor, diuretic
Completion date: 2002
Entry criterion: Hypertension
Age: 64–84 years
Diastolic BP: ≥ 90 mmHg
Systolic BP: ≥ 160 mmHg
Projected events:
  CHD: 300
  Stroke: 150

The study is being conducted in over 1000 general medical practices across Australia using a PROBE design. Following completion of a screening and run-in phase to determine eligibility (average untreated sitting BP on the second and third screening visits ≥ 160 mmHg systolic or ≥ 90 mmHg diastolic and no recent cardiovascular event or other serious intercurrent illness), subjects were randomized to receive ACE inhibitor or diuretic-based therapy. Monitoring of outcomes and BP control is determined by 6-monthly reviewing of patient records.

Some 2300 (38%) newly diagnosed hypertensives and 3783 (62%) previously treated patients were randomized; 49% of the study cohort are female and the average age is 72 years with 70% being in the 65–74 year age group. Mean entry BP is 167/91 mmHg and mean BMI is 27.0 kg/m^2; 7% of subjects have diabetes; 10% have had previous CHD; 5% previous cerebrovascular disease and 7% are current cigarette smokers. Some 4897 (81%) subjects are participating in the genetic study; 1291 have had baseline echocardiographic recordings with 230 (17%) having completed the 3-year follow-up study. A total of 735 baseline ABPM studies were undertaken with 528 (71%) and 295 (40%) having undergone first and second follow-up recordings. Some 1695 subjects have participated in the quality of life project with response rates of over 90% for each of the annual follow-up questionnaires. Follow-up BP recordings indicate that 66–73% of subjects have achieved target systolic and diastolic BP levels ($<$ 140/90 mmHg), respectively. After 17 321 patient-years of follow-up, 462 major cardiovascular events (first-events only) have been confirmed (rate = 28.3/1000 patient-years).

Comment

Although a significant undertaking, it is uncertain whether ANBP2 will have sufficient power to answer the primary question. Just 1 year before projected completion, only 462 cardiovascular events have occurred. Thus, definitive conclusions are unlikely.

Studies to examine putative advantages of angiotensin receptor blockers compared with conventional or other therapy

Several studies are investigating the potential advantage of the newly introduced angiotensin receptor blockers over conventional or contemporary treatment. Some of the more important trials in this series are described.

The Losartan Intervention For End-point Reduction (LIFE) in Hypertension Study

The Losartan Intervention for End-point reduction (LIFE) in hypertension study. Rationale, design, and methods.
B Dahlöf, R Devereux, U de Faire, *et al.* for the LIFE Study Group.
Am J Hypertens 1997; **10**: 705–13.

B A C K G R O U N D . **The higher cardiovascular complication rate in treated hypertensive patients compared with normotensives is particularly evident in patients with LVH.**

Angiotensin II is an important growth factor stimulating cardiac hypertrophy and, therefore, selective angiotensin receptor blockade may reduce LVH more effectively than conventional therapy and thus improve prognosis.

INTERPRETATION. The LIFE study is a double-blind, prospective, parallel group study designed to compare the effects of an angiotensin receptor blocker, losartan, with those of the beta-blocker, atenolol, in the reduction of cardiovascular morbidity and mortality in hypertensive patients with LVH. It is the first prospective study with adequate power to link reversal of LVH to reduction in major cardiovascular events. Inclusion of patients was stopped on 30 April 1997.

Outline

Patients: 9194
Planned follow-up: 4 years
Randomized treatment: Angiotensin receptor blocker, beta-blocker
Completion date: 2001
Entry criteria: Hypertension + LVH
Age: 55–80 years
Diastolic BP: 95–115 mmHg
Systolic BP: 160–200 mmHg
Projected events:
   CHD: 693
   Strokes: 347

Although LVH is a major risk factor for all types of cardiovascular disease in hypertensive patients, the effect of regression of LVH on prognosis has not been tested in a prospective study design. The renin–angiotensin system appears to play a major part in the establishment and maintenance of LVH. Reversal of LVH with antihypertensive treatment may be related not only to the degree of BP reduction but also to changes in the components of the renin–angiotensin system. A definitive study is needed to determine whether or not antihypertensive therapy that interrupts the effects of the renin–angiotensin system more fully has a greater effect than conventional therapy on reversal of LVH, independent of BP reduction. An optimal study would also determine whether reversal of LVH is associated with a reduction in cardiovascular events.

It is postulated that losartan by blocking the action of angiotensin II will reduce cardiac morbidity and mortality to a greater extent than conventional drugs in hypertensive patients with LVH. A rigorous test of this hypothesis requires a comparison with an antihypertensive agent from a class that has been shown to reduce cardiovascular events, i.e. a diuretic or beta-blocker. The beta-blocker atenolol was selected because a beta-blocker might be better able to control the arrhythmias and coronary disease often associated with LVH and because of the established secondary prevention in high-risk patients. Thus, the major hypothesis in the LIFE study is that in patients with hypertension and LVH, losartan will be associated with reduction in cardiovascular outcomes superior to that of atenolol through a greater effect on the regression of LVH.

LIFE is a prospective, double-blind, double-dummy, randomized, parallel group study. The primary objective is to compare the long-term effects of losartan and atenolol in hypertensive patients with LVH on the combined incidence of cardiovascular morbidity and mortality—fatal and non-fatal MI, fatal and non-fatal stroke, sudden death and death due to progressive heart failure or other cardiovascular causes. Secondary and tertiary end-points include all cause mortality, regression of ECG LVH and health care resource utilization.

Hypertensive patients (sitting diastolic BP 95–115 mmHg or sitting systolic BP 160–200 mmHg after 1–2 weeks placebo), aged 55–80 years and with LVH diagnosed from a standard 12-lead ECG by the core laboratory are eligible for inclusion. Exclusion criteria include conditions that may limit long-term survival or increase the likelihood of adherence to study medication.

Approximately 830 centres in the USA, UK and Scandinavia are participating in LIFE. The first patient was enrolled in June 1995 and by 30 April 1997, when inclusion was stopped, 9194 patients had been randomized. Active treatment will continue for 4 years after the last patient was enrolled and until 1040 patients experience primary cardiovascular events.

Once-daily antihypertensive therapy is adjusted to achieve a goal BP of ≤ 140/90 mmHg at trough (24 h post-dose, range 22–24 h). The treatment regimens are based on losartan 50–100 mg or atenolol 50–100 mg supplemented by hydrochlorothiazide and other drugs (but not ACE inhibitors, angiotensin receptor blockers or beta-blockers) as necessary to achieve target BP.

With a sample size of 8300 patients, this study has 80% power to detect ≥ 15% reduction (15 *vs* 12.75%) in the combined incidence of cardiovascular morbidity and mortality when 1040 patients experience primary end-points. Interim analyses were planned after one-third and two-thirds of the expected events had occurred. The effects of regression of LVH and BP control on the incidence of cardiovascular events and the interactions between regression of LVH and BP control and treatment groups on this incidence, will be compared using Cox regression models.

Comment

The LIFE study is the first to evaluate the effect of angiotensin receptor blockade in the prevention of complications of hypertension. The study will also have the power to address prospectively the issue of whether reversal of LVH in hypertensive patients is associated with reduction of cardiovascular morbidity and mortality, as well as with a decreased cardiovascular risk independent of BP lowering *per se*. The use of simple ECG criteria for LVH will make the results readily applicable to clinical practice.

In the last year, several substudies of the main LIFE study have reported. These are summarized briefly.

LIFE substudies

Left ventricular filling patterns in patients with systemic hypertension and left ventricular hypertrophy (The Life Study).

K Wachtell, G Smith, E Gerdts, *et al. Am J Cardiol* 2000; **85**: 466–72.

Comment

Abnormal left ventricular (LV) filling may exist in early stages of hypertension. Whether this finding is related to LVH is currently controversial. This study was undertaken to assess relations between abnormal diastolic LV filling and LV geometry in a large series of hypertensive patients with ECG LVH. M-mode, two-dimensional, and pulsed Doppler echocardiographic recordings of mitral inflow velocity and isovolumetric relaxation time (IVRT) were obtained in 750 patients with stage I–III hypertension and LVH determined by ECG (sex-adjusted Cornell voltage duration criteria or Sokolow–Lyon voltage criteria) after 14 days of placebo treatment. The patients' mean age was 67 years and 44% were women. One hundred and forty patients (19%) had a normal LV geometric pattern, 79 (11%) had concentric remodelling, 342 (45%) had eccentric LVH and 189 (25%) had concentric LVH. A normal LV filling pattern was found in 116 patients (16%), abnormal relaxation in 519 (69%), 'pseudonormal' filling was found in 83 (11%) and a restrictive filling pattern in 32 (4%). Prolonged IVRT was associated with LVH ($P < 0.01$) as well as an elevated relative wall thickness ($P < 0.05$). Abnormal IVRT was highly prevalent in all LV geometric subgroups among hypertensive patients with ECG LVH, even in those with normal LV geometry determined by echocardiography. IVRT differed significantly among patient groups with different LV geometric patterns, primarily because of the association of IVRT to LV mass.

Conclusion

Although the clinical significance of prolonged IVRT and other abnormalities of LV filling have not yet fully been clarified, patients with heart failure often have apparently normal systolic LV function. Hypertension is the most common risk factor for chronic heart failure, and contributes to the pathogenesis of a large proportion of heart failure cases. Hypertensive LVH plays an important part in the development of heart failure.

The findings in this study improve our understanding of the relations between LV diastolic dysfunction and LVH caused by hypertension. They suggest that impaired LV relaxation, manifested by prolonged IVRT, could predispose to heart failure and death, thereby contributing to the morbidity and mortality associated with LVH.

The data were analysed in patients with ECG LVH, 70% of whom had echocardiographic LVH. Thus the data can be generalized to patients with echocardiographic LVH and LV mass index in the high normal range. Medication was discontinued at least 14 days before echocardiographic examination. However, some patients treated with long-acting medications may not have had their BP and cardiac function fully re-equilibrated to medication-free levels. This could have weakened relations between LV filling parameters and other variables, thus causing an understatement of some of the findings.

Effect of obesity on electrocardiographic left ventricular hypertrophy in hypertensive patients. The Losartan Intervention For End-point (LIFE) Reduction in Hypertension Study.
P M Okin, S Jern, R B Devereux, S E Kjeldsen, B Dahlöf, for the LIFE Study Group. *Hypertension* 2000; **35**: 13–18.

Comment

Obesity may limit sensitivity of ECG voltage criteria for LVH because of the attenuating effects of increased body mass on precordial voltages. However, obesity is associated with an increased prevalence of anatomic LVH, making more accurate ECG criteria in obese patients a clinical priority. ECG LVH by Cornell voltage-duration product and/or Sokolow–Lyon voltage criteria was used to select patients for the LIFE Study. Clinical and ECG data were available in 8417 patients (54% women; mean age, 67 ± 7 years); 2519 were overweight and 1573 were obese by gender-specific BMI criteria. Increased BMI had significant but directionally opposite effects on ECG LVH by these criteria. Compared with normal weight patients, obese patients had a > 2-fold higher risk of ECG LVH by the Cornell product but a 4-fold lower risk of ECG LVH by Sokolow–Lyon voltage; overweight status was associated with intermediate risks, with a 151% greater likelihood of ECG LVH by the Cornell product but only 44% of the risk of LVH by Sokolow–Lyon voltage criteria compared with normal weight individuals. Thus, Sokolow–Lyon voltage criteria underestimate the prevalence of anatomic LVH in the presence of obesity, whereas Cornell product criteria for ECG LVH appear to provide a more accurate measure of LVH in obese and overweight patients.

Conclusion

The low prevalence of ECG LVH by Sokolow–Lyon voltage and voltage-duration product criteria in overweight and obese hypertensive patients suggests that these criteria severely underestimate the presence of anatomic LVH in these patients. Use of voltage-duration products mitigates the negative impact of increased BMI on prevalence of LVH by Sokolow–Lyon criteria and increases the association between

LVH by Cornell criteria and increased BMI, suggesting that voltage-duration products may be the most accurate conventional ECG method to detect anatomic LVH, independent of body habitus. These findings suggest that true time–voltage area ECG criteria for LVH will provide the most stable and accurate test performance, independent of body habitus. Analyses in the echocardiographic substudy that enrolled > 10% of LIFE patients will provide greater insight into the impact of obesity on the accuracy of standard ECG criteria. Because the present study was, by design, limited to patients with hypertension and target organ damage, further study of this issue in normotensive and less highly selected hypertensive patients will be of importance.

Left ventricular wall stresses and wall stress–mass–heart rate products in hypertensive patients with electrocardiographic left ventricular hypertrophy: the LIFE study.

R B Devereux, M J Roman, V Palmieri, *et al.* *J Hypertens* 2000; **18**: 1129–38.

Comment

LVH on ECG strongly predicts CHD events, but the mechanisms linking increased LV mass to ischaemic vascular events is uncertain. Variables related to myocardial oxygen demand were compared among normotensive adults and patients with mild and more severe hypertension, and among groups of moderately hypertensive patients with target organ damage in relation to gender, LV geometry and LV systolic function. A total of 964 LIFE participants enrolled in an echocardiographic substudy, and groups of 282 employed hypertensive and 366 apparently normal adults were included.

In both women and men, stepwise increases from reference subjects to employed hypertensives to LIFE patients were observed for LV wall stresses, mass and stress–mass–heart rate (triple) products. LIFE men patients had slightly higher wall stresses and significantly higher triple products than women. Wall stresses were increased in patients with normal LV geometry, eccentric or concentric hypertrophy; triple products were about three and two times normal with eccentric and concentric hypertrophy, with smaller increases in other geometric groups. Patients with decreased LV fractional shortening had two times normal end-systolic stresses and three or four times normal triple products; smaller increases in stresses and triple products occurred with decreased LV mid-wall function.

Hypertensive patients with ECG LV hypertrophy have increased LV wall stresses and stress–mass–heart rate products; suggesting a contribution of high myocardial oxygen demand to increased risk in such patients. Particularly high stresses and triple products were associated with echocardiographic LV hypertrophy, and sub-normal LV chamber and mid-wall function.

Conclusion

This study provides the first information from a large population of hypertensive patients with LV hypertrophy on the level of the major determinants of myocardial oxygen demand, LV mass, wall stress and heart rate. The finding that hypertensive patients with ECG LV hypertrophy have not only increased LV mass, but also sub-stantially supranormal wall stresses and even more markedly elevated stress–mass–heart rate products provides evidence of a major demand-side predisposition to myocardial ischaemia in such patients.

Lowering of blood pressure and predictors of response in patients with left ventricular hypertrophy: The LIFE Study.

S E Kjeldsen, B Dahlöf, R B Devereux, *et al.* for the LIFE Study Group.
Am J Hypertens 2000; **13**: 899–906.

Comment

In participants in LIFE, mean baseline BP was 174.4/97.8 mmHg, age 66.9 years, BMI 28.0 kg/m^2; 54.1% were women and 12.5% had diabetes mellitus. After five scheduled visits and 12 months of follow-up, BP decreased by 23.9/12.8 mmHg to 150.5/85.1 mmHg (target < 140/90 mmHg). The mandatory titration level of ≤ 160/95 mmHg was reached by 72.1% of the patients. At the 12-month visit, 22.7% of all patients were taking blinded study drug alone, 44.3% were taking blinded drug plus hydrochlorothiazide, and 17.7% were taking blinded drugs plus hydrochlorothiazide and additional drugs. Controlling for all other variables, patients in the USA received more medication and had 2.4 times the odds of achieving BP control compared with patients in the rest of the study ($P < .001$). Previously untreated patients ($n = 2530$) had a larger initial decrease in BP com-pared with those previously treated. Diabetics ($n = 1148$) needed more medication than non-diabetics to gain BP control. Only 13.9% of the patients had discontinued blinded study drug and 1.4% missed the revisit at 12 months.

Conclusion

These data demonstrate both the successful lowering of BP during 12 months of follow-up in a large cohort of patients with hypertension and LVH on ECG, but also emphasize the need for two or more drugs to control high BP in most of these patients. Being previously treated and having diabetes were associated with lesser BP responses, whereas living in the USA indicated better BP control.

Gender differences in systolic left ventricular function hypertensive patients with electrocardiographic left ventricular hypertrophy (The LIFE Study).
E Gerdts, M Zabalgoitia, H Björnstad, T Svendsen, R B Devereux.
Am J Cardiol 2001; **87**: 980–3.

Comment

Echocardiography was performed in 944 untreated hypertensive patients (391 women and 553 men, mean age 66 years) who had ECG LVH at baseline in the LIFE study to evaluate gender-associated differences in systolic LV function. Women had significantly lower diastolic BP (175/97 *vs* 173/99 mmHg) and body surface area and a higher BMI (all $P < 0.01$). Women also had higher LV ejection fraction (EF), endocardial and mid-wall fractional shortening (63% *vs* 60%, 35% *vs* 33%, and 16% *vs* 15%, respectively, all $P < 0.01$), higher stress-corrected mid-wall fractional shortening (98% vs 96%, $P < 0.005$), and lower circumferential end-systolic wall stress (187 vs 187 kdynes/cm^2, $P < 0.01$). There was no difference in age or LV mass indexed for height, but relative wall thickness was higher in women (0.42 *vs* 0.41, $P < 0.05$). In multiple regression analyses: (a) EF and endocardial fractional shortening were 2–3% higher in women than men, independent of the effects of LV stress, BMI and height; (b) mid-wall fractional shortening was 0.5% higher in women, independent of the effects of age, BMI, circumferential end-systolic stress and absence of diabetes; and (c) stress-corrected LV mid-wall fractional shortening was 2% higher ($P = 0.004$) in women, independent of the effects of age, height, heart rate, BMI and diabetes. Thus, female gender is an independent predictor of higher systolic LV function in hypertensive patients with ECG LVH.

Conclusion

This cross-sectional survey was performed in hypertensive patients with ECG evidence of target organ damage, and hence needs replication in less severely affected populations. Furthermore, patients with moderately severe hypertension and target organ damage in a cross-sectional survey represent 'survivors,' and findings might differ in a cohort under longitudinal surveillance beginning at a point when hypertension and associated target organ damage were both milder.

Left ventricular function and hemodynamic features of inappropriate left ventricular hypertrophy in patients with systemic hypertension: the LIFE study.
V Palmieri, K Wachtell, E Gerdts, *et al. Am Heart J* 2001; **141**: 784–91.

Comment

Predicted LV mass for sex, height and haemodynamic load can be used as an intra-patient reference for the observed LV mass. The ratio of observed/predicted LV mass may allow more physiologically correct comparisons of LV geometry, systolic and diastolic functions, and haemodynamics among hypertensive patients. This was tested in 659 participants in the LIFE study with both ECG and echocardiographic LV hypertrophy (68% of the echocardiographic cohort) without previous MI. LV mass was predicted by an equation, including sex, stroke work and height were studied. Observed/predicted LV mass > 128% defined inappropriate LVH (iLVH). Relative wall thickness ≥ 0.43 defined concentric LV geometry. Systolic myocardial dysfunction was assessed by mid-wall mechanics and abnormal LV relaxation by IVRT.

Compared with patients with appropriate LVH (aLVH), those with iLVH had higher BMI, LV mass index, relative wall thickness, prevalences of systolic myocardial dysfunction and prolonged IVRT, and lower end-systolic stress and cardiac index. Patients with eccentric iLVH had the highest wall stress and lowest ejection fraction; 43% had systolic myocardial dysfunction. Of patients with concentric iLVH, 79% had systolic myocardial dysfunction but normal ejection fraction and the lowest wall stress. Systolic myocardial dysfunction was present in 12% with concentric aLVH and none with eccentric aLVH. Prevalence of prolonged IVRT was high in all four groups (65–77%). Cardiac index was similarly lower with concentric or eccentric iLVH than with aLVH. Among hypertensives with LV hypertrophy, iLVH identified cardiac phenotypes with a high prevalence of myocardial systolic dysfunction.

Conclusion

Limited echocardiography may represent a useful tool in detecting iLVH, as a target for especially intensive clinical surveillance to prevent clinically decompensated LV hypertrophy. Associations of concentric and eccentric iLVH with a high prevalence of low systolic myocardial function and abnormal LV relaxation and relatively low pump performance suggest a high risk of accelerated transition from compensatory LVH toward heart failure.

The Valsartan Antihypertensive Long-term Use Evaluation (VALUE) trial

The Valsartan Antihypertensive Long-term Use Evaluation (VALUE) trial of cardiovascular events in hypertension. Rationale and design.
J Mann, S Julius, for the VALUE Trial Group. *Blood Press* 1998; **7**: 176–83.

Gender demographics of 15 314 hypertensives with high coronary risk. The VALUE trial.

S E Kjeldsen, S Julius, H Brunner, *et al.* for the VALUE Trial Group.
J Hypertens 2001; **19** (Suppl 2): S145–6.

BACKGROUND. The role of angiotensin II on LVH, vascular hypertrophy, endothelial dysfunction and congestive heart failure is well recognized. VALUE explores whether antihypertensive therapy based on the angiotensin receptor blocker, valsartan, has advantages over therapy that does not include inhibition of angiotensin II.

INTERPRETATION. VALUE is the only ongoing trial that compares an angiotensin receptor blocker with treatment based on a contemporary drug, amlodipine. The main hypothesis is that, for an equivalent decrease in BP, valsartan will be more effective than amlodipine in decreasing cardiac mortality and morbidity. The VALUE study population consists of hypertensive patients at relatively high risk of sustaining cardiovascular events based on age, gender, risk factors and disease factors. A unique feature is the assessment of the predictive power of the risk factor scale in a large population of treated hypertensives.

Outline

Patients: 15 314
Planned follow-up: 4 years
Randomized treatment: Angiotensin receptor blocker, dihydropyridine calcium antagonist
Completion date: 2004
Entry criteria: Hypertension + cardiovascular disease risk
Age: ≥ 50 years
Diastolic BP: 95–115 mmHg
Systolic BP: 160–210 mmHg
Projected events:
  CHD: 967
  Strokes: 483

The driving scientific hypothesis is that antagonizing the renin–angiotensin system may offer clinical advantages over equivalent BP control with a long-acting calcium channel blocker, which may itself have beneficial cardiovascular protective properties. Blockade of the renin–angiotensin system by ACE inhibitors (and in some cases angiotensin receptor blockers) has beneficial action on vascular hypertrophy and LVH, atherosclerosis, endothelial dysfunction and cardiac failure. Differences in outcomes between the drug types might be expressed in rates of acute MI, congestive heart failure and cardiac deaths.

VALUE is a prospective, double-blind, randomized, parallel group comparison with a response-dependent dose titration scheme. The treatment schedule is shown in Fig. 3.2. Free add-on antihypertensive drugs exclude ACE inhibitors and drugs from the classes under study.

Eligible patients have essential hypertension, are aged ≥ 50 years and have a high cardiovascular risk profile. Hypertension is defined as systolic BP 160–210 mmHg and/or diastolic BP 95–115 mmHg in the untreated state. Randomized patients are treated to a goal BP < 140/90 mmHg.

VALUE assesses cardiovascular risk by risk factors and predisposing conditions, and by disease factors, which can be documented by invasive and/or non-invasive techniques (Table 3.5). Using these data it will be possible to assess the predictive power of a contemporary cardiovascular risk scale in a large population of hypertensive patients considered to be at high risk. Risk assessment is stratified according to age (Table 3.6).

The main exclusion criteria are renal artery stenosis, pregnancy, acute MI, coronary angioplasty or bypass in the previous 3 months, severe hepatic disease or chronic renal failure, congestive heart failure. Patients taking beta-blockers for angina and hypertension are also excluded.

The primary outcome variable is time to first cardiac morbidity or mortality event. Secondary variables include all-cause mortality, cardiac mortality, cardiac morbidity (including silent MI), serious arrhythmias, stroke and end-stage renal failure.

A total of 14 400 patients equally allocated to each treatment is required to provide end-points in 1450 patients, giving a power of 90% to detect a 15% difference between the groups with a two-sided P-value of 0.05. When randomization was completed in December 1999, 15 314 patients had been randomized in 31 countries world-wide. VALUE is a maximum information trial, which means it will end when 1450 patients have reached the primary end-point.

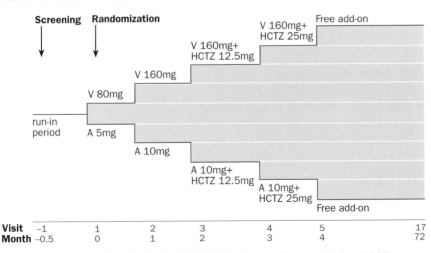

Fig. 3.2 Treatment allocation in the VALUE trial. Source: Mann and Julius (1998).

Table 3.5 Risk factors and disease factors in the VALUE trial

Risk factors
- Diabetes mellitus (defined as overnight fasting plasma glucose concentration > 7.8 mmol (140 mg/l) on at least two separate occasions or as chronic intake of hypoglycaemic agents with or without occasional intake of insulin)
- Current smoking (defined as smoking 'at least 10 cigarettes/day on a regular basis for at least 5 years prior to inclusion in the study; if the patient has quit smoking, he/she will be considered a smoker if he/she stopped less than 12 months before inclusion')
- High total cholesterol (> 240 mg/dl)
- Left ventricular hypertrophy (LVH) as per ECG (Sokolow–Lyon criteria or Cornell criteria)
- Proteinuria (I+ or more on dipstick in a morning urine specimen)
- Serum creatinine > 1.7 mg/dl

Disease factors
- History of MI verified by Q-wave ECG and/or hospital records, and/or cardiovascular revascularization
- CHD verified by angiography and/or hospital records
- History of peripheral arterial occlusive disease, verified by angiography or Doppler or hospital records or statement of angiologist
- History of stroke, TIA, verified by angiography or Doppler or PET or Cat-scan or LVH with strain pattern (ST segment depression)

ECG = electrocardiogram; MI = myocarial infarction; CHD = coronary heart disease; TIA = transient ischaemic attack; PET = positron emission tomography.

Source: Mann and Julius (1998).

Table 3.6 Risk assessment in the VALUE trial. Stratification according to age.

Age 50–59 years	
Male	≥ 3 risk factors or 1 disease
Female	≥ 2 risk factors and 1 disease
Age 60–69 years	≥ 2 risk factors or 1 disease
Age > 70 years	≥ 1 risk factor or 1 disease

Source: Mann and Julius (1998).

Follow-up is expected to continue for an average of 4–5 years per patient. Two equally spaced interim analyses of the primary end-point are planned.

Patients recruited to VALUE had a mean BP of 154.7/87.5 mmHg at the time of randomization. More than 92% of those randomized had been treated for hypertension for at least 6 months when screened. The population comprises 57.6% men, 89.1% Caucasians, mean age 67.2 years, mean BMI 28.6 kg/m². The gender demographics of the participants are shown in Table 3.7. Men qualified with more diseases and women with more risk factors.

Comment

VALUE compares outcomes in high-risk hypertensive patients treated with two different contemporary antihypertensive strategies. Although there is little out-

Table 3.7 Gender demographics at randomization in the VALUE trial.

	Men ($n = 8816$)	Women ($n = 6497$)	Total ($n = 15\,314$)
Qualifying risk factors (%)			
Serum cholesterol > 6.2 mmol/l	23.9	45.2	33.0
Diabetes mellitus (mostly type 2)	29.8	34.2	31.7
Current smoking	26.7	20.3	24.0
Proteinuria	22.1	23.2	22.5
Left ventricular hypertrophy	9.2	16.3	12.2
Serum creatinine > 150 µmol/l	4.7	2.1	3.6
Qualifying disease factors (%)			
CHD	53.5	35.4	45.8
Stroke or transient ischaemic attack	21.1	17.9	19.8
Peripheral arterial disease	15.5	11.6	13.9
LVH with strain pattern	6.2	6.0	6.1

Source: Mann and Julius (1998).

come data with either angiotensin receptor blockers or calcium channel blockers in hypertension, the latter class and particularly amlodipine is rapidly becoming the most widely prescribed antihypertensive agent. Therefore, amlodipine is a valid pragmatic comparator for the new agent, valsartan.

The study will provide important and overdue data on how well amlodipine performs against an alternative therapy in the long term. As well as comparison of cardiac outcomes, it will be of clinical relevance to examine how these strategies compare with regard to tolerability.

The Study on COgnition and Prognosis in Elderly patients with hypertension (SCOPE)

Cognition and quality of life at baseline in SCOPE (Study on COgnition and Prognosis in the Elderly).
L Hansson. On behalf of the SCOPE Study Group. *J Hypertens* 2001; **19** (Suppl 2): S147.

Baseline characteristics according to age groups and gender in the Study on COgnition and Prognosis in the Elderly (SCOPE).
L Hansson. On behalf of the SCOPE Study Group. *J Hypertens* 2001; **19** (Suppl 2): S150–1.

BACKGROUND. SCOPE will assess the effect of candesartan on major cardiovascular events and cognitive function in elderly patients with mild hypertension.

INTERPRETATION. SCOPE is one of the largest outcome studies in the very elderly. It is expected to report its findings in the first half of 2002.

Outline

Patients: 4964
Planned follow-up: 3 years
Randomized treatment: Angiotensin receptor blocker, placebo
Completion date: 2002
Entry criteria: Hypertension
Age: 70–89 years
Diastolic BP: 90–99 mmHg
Systolic BP: 160–179 mmHg
Projected events:
  CHD: 60
  Strokes: 30

SCOPE is a multicentre, prospective, randomized, double-blind study that will evaluate the effect of the angiotensin receptor blocker candesartan (8–16 mg daily) vs placebo on major cardiovascular events, cognitive impairment and incidence of dementia in elderly patients (70–89 years) with mild hypertension. A total of 4964 patients was recruited and will be followed for a minimum of 3 years. Hydrochlorothiazide is allowed as an add-on therapy for the control of BP.

The mean age of patients was 76 years, the average BP was 166/90 mmHg with 30% of the patients having isolated systolic hypertension (systolic BP $\geq$ 140 mmHg, diastolic BP $<$ 90 mmHg). The mean Mini Mental State Examination (MMSE) score was 28. There were approximately twice as many women as men ($n = 3200$ and $n = 1764$, respectively). The occurrence of previous cardiovascular disease was higher among men than women: MI 7.8 and 2.7%, stroke 4.8 and 3.3% and atrial fibrillation 4.9 and 2.9%, respectively. A similar proportion of men (12.4%) and women (11.4%) had diabetes. Although the majority of patients in SCOPE were aged 70–79 years ($n = 3909$), a large proportion were 80 years or older ($n = 1055$). The prevalence of previous MI was similar among the 70–79 year olds and those aged 80 or more (4.4 and 4.9%, respectively). However, the prevalence of stroke (5.9% in $>$ 80 years group, 3.3% in 70–79 years group), atrial fibrillation (5.9% vs 3.0%) and diabetes (13.7% vs 11.2%) was higher in the older group than in the younger group.

A total of 2680 patients (976 men and 1704 women), with a mean age of 76.4 years, with mild hypertension were included in the cognitive function study. Two validated psychological tests, the MMSE and the Psychological General Well-Being (PGWB) index, were completed at baseline. In the MMSE, a total score of 30 is the maximum. An MMSE score of $\geq$ 24 was required as inclusion criteria in this study (range in the study group 24–30). In the PGWB index, a total score of 132 is the maximum, 22 the minimum and a normal score approximately 105.

The effect for MMSE score at a baseline was highly significant ($P < 0.0001$), i.e. high performance in cognitive functioning (for men M = 28.7 and for women M = 28.6) was associated with high values in well-being for both men (M = 110.2) and women (M = 103.1). In addition, increasing age was associated with decreasing PGWB scores ($P < 0.005$). Patents who were chronically treated with psychopharmacological drugs scored significantly ($P < 0.0001$) lower (M = 95.7) on the PGWB than patients who were not treated with these agents M = 10.6.7).

Comment

The baseline characteristics in SCOPE indicate that the target population has been achieved. The overall pattern and findings at baseline suggests that there may be a relationship between well-being and cognitive function in an elderly group of patients with mild hypertension.

Study on Evaluation of Candesartan cilexetil after REnal Transplantation (SECRET)

SECRET—a multinational trial of candesartan cilexetil on mortality, cardiovascular morbidity and kidney graft failure in renal transplant patients.

Th Phillip, Ch Legendre, S Nisse-Durgeat, G Kiel. On behalf of the investigators of SECRET. *Hypertens* 2001; **19** (Suppl 2): S150.

BACKGROUND. SECRET will study the effect of candesartan *vs* placebo on all-cause mortality, cardiovascular morbidity and loss of graft in hypertension and normotensive patients with a kidney allograft. The effect on LVH in a subgroup of patients will also be recorded by echocardiography.

INTERPRETATION. SECRET is designed to evaluate the cardioprotective and nephroprotective value of candesartan in a subset of patients with a high cardiovascular risk. The long-term data on the clinical course provided by SECRET will help to improve the care of hypertensive patients with a kidney graft.

Outline

Patients: 750
Planned follow-up: 3 years
Randomized treatments: Angiotensin receptor blocker, placebo
Completion date: 2004
Entry criteria: Renal transplantation ± diabetes mellitus
Age: 30–70 years
Diastolic BP: Any
Systolic BP: Any
Projected events: Not stated

SECRET is a prospective, randomized, double-blind, placebo-controlled clinical trial underway at 36 sites in Germany, France and Austria. The primary outcome is a composite index of all causes of mortality, cardiovascular morbidity and graft failure. Secondary outcomes include cardiovascular mortality, renal function, protein excretion, incidence of nephrotic syndrome (urine protein > 3.5 g/24-h), lipid blood levels and number of erythropoietin doses required. Seven hundred and fifty outpatients with a renal allograft at least 1 year and up to 15 years after transplantation or retransplantation will be recruited with a minimum of follow-up of 3 years. Patients will be stratified on the basis of diabetes as a comorbid condition. Normotensive and hypertensive patients, aged between 30 and 70 years, with stable renal function (creatinine clearance ≥ 25 ml/min) and no evidence of renal artery stenosis are eligible for this study. Patients requiring chronic treatment with an ACE inhibitor or an angiotensin II receptor antagonists for a non-renal indication or with an overt proteinuria (≥ 2.0 g/24-h) are excluded. The two treatment groups are to achieve equivalent BP control, with the study drug as primary therapy given add on to antihypertensive drugs, excluding ACE inhibitors and angiotensin receptor blockers. Study medication is titrated stepwise from 4 mg up to 16 mg whereas diuretics, beta-blockers, long-term-acting calcium channel blockers, centrally acting sympatholytic drugs and beta-blockers as an additional therapy can be added or discontinued to achieve the target BP defined as seated systolic BP < 135 mmHg and diastolic BP < 85 mmHg at each visit.

Comment

This study has the potential to clarify the role of angiotensin receptor blockers in individuals who have undergone renal transplants. The mechanism of action of these agents, selective angiotensin AT_1 receptor blockade and angiotensin AT_2 receptor stimulation, may be particularly appropriate in such patients. However, the small size of SECRET may limit interpretation.

Evaluation of newer drugs in patients with high-risk Perindopril Protection against Recurrent Stroke Study (PROGRESS)

PROGRESS: Perindopril Protection Against Recurrent Stroke Study: status in July 1996.
PROGRESS Management Committee. *J Hypertens* 1996; **14** (Suppl 6): S47–51.

BACKGROUND. Among individuals with a history of cerebrovascular disease, the association between BP and secondary stroke is steep and continuous. Small trials of BP lowering in patients with a history of cerebrovascular disease suggest a reduction of stroke risk. Although the proportional reduction on stroke risk appears to be similar in patients with and without cerebrovascular disease, further large prospective studies are required in patients with a history of stroke or transient ischaemic attacks.

INTERPRETATION. PROGRESS is designed to resolve the persisting clinical uncertainty about the benefits of lowering BP in patients who have suffered a cerebrovascular event, a population with a very high risk of stroke. The primary aim is to determine precisely the balance of benefits and risks of treatment with an ACE inhibitor-based BP-lowering regimen. As epidemiological data suggest there should be worthwhile benefits across a wide range of BP from as low as 75 mmHg (diastolic), PROGRESS is being conducted in both normotensive and hypertensive subjects with a history of cerebrovascular disease.

Outline

Patients: 6000
Projected follow-up: 5 years
Randomized treatment: ACE inhibitor, diuretic, placebo
Completion date: 2001
Entry criteria: Stroke or transient ischaemic attack
Age: Any
Diastolic BP: Any
Systolic BP: Any
Projected events:
  CHD: 600
  Strokes: 300

The primary objective of PROGRESS is to determine reliably the efficacy of lowering BP for the prevention of stroke in patients with a history of cerebrovascular disease. PROGRESS is a randomized, double-blind, placebo-controlled trial investigating the effects of treatment with ACE inhibitor, perindopril, alone and in combination with the diuretic, indapamide on the incidence of stroke and other major cardiovascular events and dementia.

The study population comprises 6000 normotensive or hypertensive patients with a history of stroke or transient ischaemic attack within the previous 5 years. The study is being conducted in over 160 centres in seven regions: Australia and New Zealand, The People's Republic of China, France and Belgium, Italy, Japan, Sweden and the UK. Recruitment is managed so that approximately one-half of the patients have a history of hypertension and about one-half of the patients randomized to active therapy receive combination treatment with perindopril (4 mg daily) and indapamide (2.5 mg daily or 2 mg daily in Japan).

The primary study outcome is fatal and non-fatal stroke. Secondary study outcomes include fatal and total cardiovascular events (stroke, MI, cardiovascular death), cognitive function and dementia, and disability and dependency. Treatment and follow-up is scheduled to continue for a minimum of 4 years after randomization.

The study sample size of 6000 was estimated on the basis of 1.5–2% annual stroke rate among control patients over 4 years of follow-up and on average difference in diastolic BP between active treatment and placebo of $\geq$ 4 mmHg throughout the follow-up. The projected event rate will provide at least 200 strokes among patients assigned to the placebo group and ≥ 90% power to detect a 30% reduction in total stroke incidence (at 2 $P = 0.05$).

Comment

PROGRESS addresses the important clinical issue of whether symptomatic reduction of BP in survivors of cerebrovascular events confers benefits. The protocol requires all subjects to be challenged with perindopril and only those who tolerate the drug can proceed to randomization. Although intended to identify before randomization those patients who might be likely to withdraw, this introduces a bias in favour of ACE inhibition. This weakness, together with the absence of a positive control group, means that PROGRESS can only provide information on the benefits (or otherwise) of BP reduction rather than those concerning a particular therapeutic regimen.

The HYpertension in the Very Elderly Trial (HYVET)

The Hypertension in the Very Elderly Trial: the importance of the pilot trial and modifications to the protocol.
C J Bulpitt on behalf of the HYVET Investigators. *Eur Heart J Suppl* 1999; **1** (Suppl P): P9–P12.

The rationale for the HYpertension in the Very Elderly Trial (HYVET).
N S Beckett, A E Fletcher, C J Bulpitt. *Eur Heart J Suppl* 1999; **1** (Suppl P): P13–P16.

Number of patients achieving blood pressure targets in 12 months in the HYpertension in the Very Elderly Trial (HYVET) pilot.
N S Beckett, J D Cooke, A E Fletcher, C J Bulpitt. On behalf of the HYVET Pilot Investigators. *J Hypertens* 2001; **19** (Suppl 2): S103–4.

BACKGROUND. BP increases with age and elevated levels of BP are common in the elderly. The elderly is a high-risk group for cardiovascular disease, which is the leading cause of death in European countries for individuals aged ≥ 80 years. Major outcome trials have either excluded specifically those over the age of 80 years or recruited too few subjects to establish the benefits or risks of treatment in this group. Deaths from non-vascular disease and the inability of the very old to gain many extra years of life may lessen or negate any reduction in mortality. However, a reduction in morbidity and improvement in quality of life would be worthwhile, although this may not be achieved if adverse events limit the benefit or if the benefits are not large.

INTERPRETATION. Outcome trials in elderly patients with hypertension have consistently found a reduction in cardiac mortality greater than that expected from the results of trials in middle-aged subjects. This may be due to the elderly being particularly at risk of dying from congestive heart failure as a consequence of hypertension. If the latter is true, the very elderly should similarly experience a fall in cardiac mortality with antihypertensive treatment. The benefit–risk comparison from active treatment needs to be determined in the very elderly, and HYVET has been designed to address this issue.

Outline

Patients: 2100
Planned follow-up: 5 years
Randomized treatment: ACE inhibitor, diuretic, placebo
Completion date: 2003
Entry criteria: Hypertension
Age: > 80 years
Diastolic BP: 90–109 mmHg
Systolic BP: 160–179 mmHg
Projected events:
   CHD: 683
   Strokes: 341

It may well be that treatment of hypertensive patients > 80 years is a balance between benefit in terms of a reduction in stroke and heart failure, each a major cause of disability in this age group, and the possible adverse effect of an increase in mortality. The over-80s are survivors and are unlikely to benefit significantly from a gain in life-years. However, a reduction in disability, maintenance of independence and quality of life would clearly be of benefit. There is a need for a well-designed, randomized, controlled trial in this age group to assess the benefits of treatment and the level of risk.

HYVET is a randomized, double-blind, placebo-controlled trial. The main objective is to investigate the primary and secondary prevention of fatal and non-fatal strokes. It is designed to determine whether or not a 35% difference in stroke events (fatal and non-fatal) occurs between placebo and active treatment in hypertensive patients aged > 80 years; this is consistent with results from previous trials in hypertension in the elderly. The trial has 90% power to detect such a difference at the 1% level of significance. Secondary outcome measures include total mortality, cardiovascular mortality and stroke mortality.

A total of 2100 patients > 80 years are to be recruited from centres in the UK, Bulgaria, Finland, Romania, Spain, Lithuania, Ireland, Poland, Greece and Serbia. Follow-up will be for 5 years. Patients will be eligible for the trial if, while on single blind placebo treatment, sustained systolic BP is 160–199 mmHg and/or diastolic BP is 90–109 mmHg. The active treatment group will receive sustained release indapamide 1.5 mg daily with perindopril 2–4 mg daily being added to achieve the target BP < 150/80 mmHg. Recruitment started in January 1999 and the trial will end late in 2003.

A pilot study demonstrated the feasibility of HYVET. The HYVET pilot was a randomized open trial of treating hypertensive patients aged 80 or more. Entry criteria were a sitting BP of 160–219 mmHg systolic and 90–109 mmHg diastolic. Patients were randomized to either no treatment (NT), low-dose diuretic (D) or ACE-inhibitor (A). Diltiazem could be added as second-line treatment. Target BP was < 150 mmHg systolic and < 80 mmHg diastolic in the sitting position.

A total of 1283 patients was recruited (mean age 84 years, women 63.5%). There was no difference in baseline mean sitting BP between the three groups: NT, 181/100 mmHg; D, 182/100 mmHg; and A, 182/100 mmHg. At 6 months the readings were: NT ($n = 414$) 175/96 mmHg; D ($n = 413$) 156/86 mmHg; and A ($n = 408$) 155/85 mmHg ($P < 0.001$). At 12 months the readings were: NT ($n = 167$) 175/97 mmHg; D ($n = 184$) 148/83 mmHg; and A ($n = 183$) 148/83 mmHg ($P < 0.001$). At 6 months 89% were on monotherapy in both groups D and A and at 12 months 89% of group D and 91% of group A. At 6 months 1.9% in group NT had reached target BP compared with 24% in group D and 26% in group A. At 12 months the figures were 1.2%, 28% and 33%, respectively.

In this open pilot trial a satisfactory difference of 20/11 mmHg between active treatment and no treatment was achieved at 6 months and 27/12 mmHg at 12 months. At 1 year 30% of actively treated patients had achieved the target BP. These are encouraging results for the main trial, which is expected to run for 5 years. As it is a placebo-controlled double-blind trial, the differences in this trial may be less owing to the placebo effect. It is expected, however, that over 60% in the main trial will achieve target BP by 5 years.

Comment

Information from HYVET should aid clinicians in assessing the benefits and risks of treating hypertensive patients aged > 80 years. Subgroup analysis of earlier trials have suggested that for patients in this age range, treatment reduces stroke events (fatal and non-fatal) but may increase all-cause mortality. Thus, further reliable data are needed.

Action in Diabetes and Vascular Disease—PreterAx and DiamicroN MR Controlled Evaluation (ADVANCE)

ADVANCE: Action in Diabetes and Vascular disease— PreterAx and DiamicroN MR Controlled Evaluation.
J Chalmers, S MacMahon on behalf of the ADVANCE Management Committee. *J Hypertens* 2001; **19** (Suppl 2): S149–50.

BACKGROUND. **Patients with diabetes have increased risk of macrovascular and microvascular diseases, both of which have been shown to be reduced by the control**

of raised BP in hypertensive individuals. The microvascular complications have also been shown to be reduced by intensive glycaemic control.

INTERPRETATION. ADVANCE aims to determine the overall balance of benefits and risks associated with a BP-lowering regimen (based on a fixed low-dose ACE inhibitor–diuretic combination) and an intensive glucose-lowering regimen (based on modified-release gliclazide) targeting a haemoglobin A_{1c} level $\leq 6.5\%$ among high-risk hypertensive or non-hypertensive individuals with type 2 diabetes.

Outline

Patients: 10 000
Planned follow-up: 4.5 years
Randomized treatment: ACE inhibitor, diuretic, placebo
Factorial assignment: Sulphonylurea, standard guideline-based diabetic control
Completion date: 2006
Entry criteria: Diabetes, high cardiovascular risk
Age: ≥ 55 years
Diastolic BP: Any
Systolic BP: Any
Projected events: Not stated

ADVANCE is a factorial, randomized controlled trial among 10 000 individuals aged ≥ 55 years with type 2 diabetes and at high risk of vascular disease. Following a 6-week run-in phase, patients will be randomized to receive the fixed low-dose perindopril-indapamide combination or matching placebo. Patients will also be randomized to receive modified-release gliclazide based on intensive glucose lowering or standard guidelines-based glucose control. Mean scheduled period of treatment and follow-up will be 4.5 years. A number of substudies are planned, including an economic and quality of life substudy, and a genetic substudy. The study will be conducted in about 200 collaborating clinical centres in some 20 countries in Asia, Australasia, Europe and North America.

The two primary outcomes are the composite macrovascular end-points of non-fatal stroke, non-fatal MI, and death from any cardiovascular cause; and the composite microvascular end-points of new or substantially worsening nephropathy or microvascular eye disease. Final results are expected in 2006.

Comment

The need for multifactorial interventions to reduce the risk of cardiovascular and other complications in patients with type 2 diabetes mellitus is more well-established. ADVANCE should clarify the relative benefits of rigorous BP and tight glycaemic control. However, the design of the study will preclude identification of the particular advantages of individual drugs.

Overview of ongoing trials

Protocol for prospective collaborative overviews of major randomized trials of blood-pressure-lowering treatments.

World Health Organization—International Society of Hypertension Blood Pressure Lowering Treatment Trialists' Collaboration. *J Hypertens* 1998; **16**: 127–37.

BACKGROUND. **Prospectively planned overviews (meta-analyses) of the ongoing randomized trials of BP-lowering drugs should facilitate the generation of reliable data on the effects of newer classes of drugs on major causes of cardiovascular mortality and morbidity for a variety of patient groups. A registry has been established to collate information from over 30 trials. By 2003, data from at least 195 000 patients and 899 000 patient-years of follow-up should be available. An estimated 8000 strokes, 12 000 CHD events and 23 000 cardiovascular events should provide sufficient statistical power to detect even modest cause-specific differences in the incidence of the main study outcomes.**

INTERPRETATION. This project should provide more reliable information about the effects of newer BP-lowering drugs than would any one study alone. The use of data from individual patients in the overviews will facilitate the investigation of the separate effects of various drug regimens in treating members of the major patient subgroups.

Individually, the ongoing trials are not likely to resolve all the current uncertainties about the effects of regimens based on the various agents. Systematic overviews should provide more reliable information about any differences in cardiovascular outcomes with different regimens than that from any one trial alone.

Trials are potentially eligible for inclusion if they satisfy one of the following criteria: random allocation of patients between antihypertensive regimens based on various BP-lowering agents; random allocation between a BP-lowering treatment and placebo (or other inactive control condition); or randomization of patients between various BP goals. In addition, eligible trials must have a planned minimum of 1000 patient-years of follow-up for patients in each randomly allocated treatment group.

A registry has been established to identify all major ongoing and planned randomized trials of BP-lowering agents. Data requested from each participating trial will include baseline characteristics, selected measurements performed during follow-up and details of the occurrence of all pre-defined study outcomes during the scheduled follow-up period (Table 3.8).

The study outcomes chosen for inclusion in these overviews represent the main cardiovascular disease outcomes likely to be affected by BP-lowering treatment regimens and the main non-cardiovascular disease outcomes for which questions about the safety of some newer agents have arisen, e.g. cancer with calcium channel

Table 3.8 Treatment Trialists' Collaboration. Baseline, follow-up and outcome data from each patient.

Baseline (at or before randomization)	Follow-up (at annual or similar intervals)	Outcomes (all events in each category recorded during scheduled follow-up period)
Patient identifier	Systolic blood pressure	Ischaemic stroke
Date of randomization	Diastolic blood pressure	Cerebral haemorrhage
Treatment allocation	Weight	Subarachnoid haemorrhage
Date of birth/age	Serum cholesterol level	Other stroke (including
Sex	Serum creatinine level	unknown)
Ethnicity	Smoking status	Myocardial infarction
Systolic blood pressure	Compliance	Hospitalization for heart failure
Weight		Hospitalization for renal disease
Height		Hospitalization or transfusion for
Smoking status		non-cerebral haemorrhage
Serum total cholesterol level		Arterial revascularization procedure
Serum creatinine level		Bone fracture
Regular use of		Major cancer (site-specific)
aspirin/anti-platelet drug		Admission to hospital for any other
Use of other blood pressure-		cause
lowering drug		Death (cause-specific)
History of		Date for each event
Diabetes		Date of last follow-up for fatal
Left ventricular hypertrophy		events
Heart failure		Date of last follow-up for non-fatal
Cerebrovascular disease		events
Coronary heart disease		
Peripheral vascular disease		
Planned end of scheduled		
treatment and follow-up		

Source: World Health Organization—International Society of Hypertension Blood Pressure Lowering Treatment Trialists' Collaboration (1998).

blockers. Two sets of primary comparisons have been specified in advance. The first concerns the overview of trials comparing regimens based on newer (ACE inhibitor or calcium channel blocker) and older (diuretic or beta-blocker) based BP-lowering treatments that produce similar reductions in BP. In addition, comparisons of ACE inhibitor-based treatment *vs* calcium antagonist-based treatment will be performed. The second set of primary comparisons concerns the overview of trials comparing BP-lowering regimens (ACE inhibitor or calcium antagonist based) *vs* control.

Ongoing trials eligible for inclusion in the overviews are listed in Table 3.9. These include 17 trials comparing various drug regimens and 17 trials comparing at least one regimen with an untreated or less treated control condition. Eighteen trials are exclusively in hypertension and 18 in selected patients with coronary disease, cardiovascular disease, renal disease or diabetes.

Table 3.9 Characteristics of trials identified as eligible for inclusion in overviews

Title	Acronym	Patients (n)	Planned follow-up (years)	Randomized treatments (factorial assignments)	Patient characteristics — Completion date	Patient characteristics — Entry criteria	Age (years)	Diastolic blood pressure	Systolic blood pressure	Projected events — CHD	Projected events — Strokes
African American Study of Kidney Disease and Hypertension	AASK	1200	5	ACE, β-blocker, DCA (more, less)	2001	HBP plus renal disease	18–70	≥95	Any	144	72
Appropriate Blood Pressure Control in Diabetes Trial	ABCD	950	5	ACE, DCA	1998	Diabetes	40–74	Any	No ISH	119	59
Antihypertensive Therapy and Lipid-Lowering Heart Attack Prevention Trial	ALLHAT	40 000	6	ACE, α-blocker, DCA diuretic (CHOL, open)	2002	HBP plus CVD risk	>55	90–109	140–179	2580	2790
Australian National Blood Pressure Study 2	ANBP2	6000	5	ACE, diuretic	2002	HBP	65–84	≥90	≥160	300	150
Anglo-Scandinavian Cardiac Outcomes Trial	ASCOT	18 000		DCA with/without ACE, β-blocker with/without diuretic (CHOL, placebo)	2003	HBP plus CVD risk	40–79	≥90	≥140	1150	400
Bergamo Nephrology Diabetes Complication Trial	BENEDICT	2400	3	ACE, NCA, placebo	2001	Diabetes	≥40	≥90	≥140	200	100
Captopril Prevention Project	CAPPP	10 800	5	ACE, β-blocker/diuretic	1998	HBP	25–66	≥100	Any	324	162
Controlled Onset Verapamil Investigation for Cardiovascular Endpoints	CONVINCE	15 000	5	NCA, β-blocker/diuretic	2001	HBP plus CVD risk	≥55	90–109	140–189	1250	750
Collaborative Study Group Trial on Effect of Irbesartan	CSGTEI	1650	3	AIIA, DCA, placebo	2000	Diabetes plus proteinuria	30–70	≥85	≥135	124	62
Diabetes Hypertension Cardiovascular Morbidity – Mortality and Ramipril	DIAB-HYCAR	4000	3	ACE, placebo	1999	Diabetes plus proteinuria	>50	Any	Any	300	150
European Lacidipine Study of Atherosclerosis	ELSA	2251	4	DCA, β9-blocker	2000	HBP	45–75	95–115	150–209	89	44
Hypertension in Diabetes Study	HDS	1148	8.2	ACE, β-blocker, open (insulin, sulphonamide, diet)	1998	HBP plus diabetes	25–75	≥85	≥150	244	122
Heart Outcomes Prevention Evaluation Study	HOPE	9541	4.7	ACE, placebo (vitamin E, placebo)	2000	CVD risk	≥55	Any	Any	1200	550
Hypertension Optimal Treatment study	HOT	19 196	3.5	More, less (aspirin, placebo)	1997	HBP	50–80	100–115	Any	552	276
Hypertension in the Very Elderly Trial	HYVET	2100	5	ACE, diuretic, placebo	2001	HBP	>80	90–109	160–219	683	341

Study	Acronym	N	Years	Treatment	Year	Entry criteria	Age	DBP	SBP		
International Nifedipine Gastrointestinal Therapeutic System Study Intervention as a Goal in Hypertension Treatment	INSIGHT	6592	3	DCA, diuretic	1999	HBP plus CVD risk	55–80	≥95	≥150	246	123
Losartan Intervention for Endpoint Reduction in Hypertension	LIFE	9194	4	AIIA, β-blocker	2001	HBP plus LVH	55–80	95–115	160–200	693	347
National Intervention Cooperative Study in Elderly Hypertensive	NICS-EH	1000	5	DCA, diuretic	1997	HBP	≥60	<115	160–219	30	15
Nordic Diltiazem Study	NORDIL	11 000	5	NCA, β-blocker/diuretic	2002	HBP	50–69	≥100	Any	360	180
Prevention of Atherosclerosis with Ramipril	PART2	617	4	ACE, placebo	1998	Atherosclerosis	18–75	Any	Any	40	14
Plaque Hypertension Lipid-Lowering Italian Study	PHYLLIS	450	3	ACE, placebo (CHOL, placebo)	2000	CIT	45–70	95–115	151–210	7	4
Prospective Randomized Evaluation of Vascular Effects of Norvasc	PREVENT	825	5	DCA, placebo	1997	ACHD	30–80	Any	Any	20	6
Perindopril Protection Against Recurrent Stroke Study	PROGRESS	6000	5	ACE, placebo	2000	Stroke or TIA	Any	Any	Any	600	300
Quinapril Ischaemia Event Trial	QUIET	1750	3	ACE, placebo	1996	ACHD	18–75	Any	Any	500	350
Randomized Evaluation of Non-insulin-dependent Diabetes Mellitus with the Angiotensin II Antagonist Losartan	RENAAL	1500	4	AIIA, placebo	2002	Diabetes	31–70	<110	<200	100	50
Study of Cognition and Prognosis in Elderly Patients with Hypertension	SCOPE	4000	2.5	AIIA, placebo	2003	HBP	70–89	90–99	160–179	60	30
Systolic Hypertension in the Elderly Lacidipine Long-Term Study	SHELL	4800	3.5	DCA, diuretic	1999	HBP	≥60	<95	161–219	101	50
Swedish Trial in Old Patients with Hypertension	STOP-2	6628	4	ACE, β-blocker/diuretic, DCA	1998	HBP	70–84	≥105	≥180	318	167
Systolic Hypertension in Europe Multicentre Trial	SYST-EUR	4695	1.6	DCA, placebo	1997	ISH	≥60	<95	160–219	500	250
Verapamil in Hypertension Atherosclerosis Study	VHAS	1414	2	NCA, diuretic	1996	HBP	40–65	≥95	≥160	40	20

ACE = angiotensin-converting enzyme inhibitor; AIIA = angiotensin II antagonist; ACHD = angiographic coronary heart disease; CHOL = cholesterol lowering; CIT = carotid intimal thickness; CVD = cardiovascular disease; DCA = dihydropyridine calcium antagonist; HBP = high blood pressure; ISH = isolated systolic hypertension; less = less intensive blood pressure lowering; LVH = left ventricular hypertrophy; more = more intensive blood pressure lowering; NCA = non-dihydropyridine calcium antagonist; open = open control; TIA = transient ischaemic attack.

Source: World Health Organization—International Society of Hypertension Blood Pressure Lowering Treatment Trialists' Collaboration (1998).

The total planned recruitment is 194 701 patients, the mean projected follow-up is 4.6 years and the total projected number of patient-years of follow-up is 898 643. The total number of patients planned in the trials comparing various treatment regimens is 132 177 of whom 67 876 will be randomly allocated between ACE inhibitor-based treatments and diuretic or beta-blocker-based treatments, 81 421 between dihydropyridine calcium antagonist-based treatments and diuretic or beta-blocker-based treatments and 27 414 between verapamil- or diltiazem-based treatments and diuretic or beta-blocker-based treatments. The total number of patients planned in trials comparing a BP-lowering treatment with an untreated or less treated control condition is 62 022 of whom 28 006 will be randomly allocated between ACE inhibitor-based therapy and control, and 9570 will be randomly allocated between calcium antagonist-based therapy and control.

Estimates of the statistical power for the principal comparisons of treatment effects on stroke incidence, major CHD events and total cardiovascular events are given in Table 3.10. For comparisons of newer *vs* older treatment regimens (and ACE inhibitors *vs* calcium antagonist regimens) all calculations assume minimum detectable differences of 15% (relative risk 0.85) and for comparisons between treatment and untreated or less actively treated control conditions, the calculations assume minimum detectable differences of 20% (relative risk 0.80). By 2003, the estimated number of events accrued will be about 8000 strokes, 12 000 CHD events and 23 000 cardiovascular events. The available data should provide sufficient power to detect modest differences in the incidence of each of the principal outcomes for the main treatment comparisons.

Comment

This project should provide reliable data about the effects of newer classes of anti-hypertensive agents on major classes of cardiovascular morbidity and mortality for a variety of groups of patients who have high risk of cardiovascular disease events. The prospective overview approach should reduce random errors and avoid bias. The results of a planned preliminary analysis are summarized in Chapter 1.

The Trialists' Collaboration will accumulate a formidable body of data in terms of patient numbers and events. It is sobering to appreciate the size of comparisons required to provide adequate power to reliably detect important differences between active treatments. The limitation of individual trials, even when appropriately designed and adequately powered, is manifest.

Conclusion

As we move into the new millennium, the emphasis in management of hypertension has advanced decisively towards evidence-based medicine. It is no longer sufficient to demonstrate that an antihypertensive agent reduces BP. Today, evidence must be provided that the drug reduces real outcome measures, such as CHD events. Furthermore, new drugs have to demonstrate at least equivalence to,

Table 3.10 Estimates of statistical power for principal prespecified comparisons

Comparison	n	Estimated number of events			Estimated power (%) ($\alpha = 0.05$)		
		CHD	Strokes	CVD	CHD	Strokes	CVD
Data available in 1999							
Newer versus older regimens							
ACE versus β-blocker/diuretic	15 977	697	354	1156	54	30	77
Calcium antagonists versus β-blocker/diuretic	19 174	748	378	1239	57	32	80
DCA versus β-blocker/diuretic	17 760	708	358	1173	55	30	78
NCA versus β-blocker/diuretic	1414	40	20	66	5	1	7
ACE versus calcium antagonist	4419	212	111	356	19	11	31
More versus less or none							
Active versus placebo/control	33 181	1875	1077	3247	100	93	100
ACE versus placebo	7157	1008	598	1766	94	75	100
Calcium antagonist versus placebo	5520	120	106	249	19	16	37
Data available in 2003							
Newer versus older regimens							
ACE versus β-blocker/diuretic	47 407	3055	2398	5998	99	97	100
Calcium antagonist versus β-blocker/diuretic	89 230	5173	3406	9436	100	100	100
DCA versus β-blocker/diuretic	61 816	3523	2456	6576	100	98	100
NCA versus β-blocker/diuretic	27 414	1650	950	2860	90	68	99
ACE versus calcium antagonist	23 644	1524	1402	3218	87	84	100
More versus less or none							
Active versus placebo/control	62 022	4893	3286	8997	100	100	100
ACE versus placebo	26 148	3304	2466	3242	100	100	100
Calcium antagonist versus placebo	8220	336	214	605	48	32	75

ACE = angiotensin-converting enzyme; DCA = dihydropyridine calcium antagonist; NCA = non-dihydropyridine calcium antagonist; CHD = non-fatal myocardial infarctions plus deaths from coronary heart disease; Strokes = non-fatal strokes plus deaths from cerebrovascular disease; CVD = 1.1 × (CHD plus Strokes). *Calculations assume minimum detectable differences of 15% (relative risk 0.85) for comparisons between newer versus older (and ACE inhibitor versus calcium antagonist) treatment regimens, and of 20% (relative risk 0.80) for comparisons between treatment and an untreated or less actively treated control condition.

Source: World Health Organization—International Society of Hypertension Blood Pressure Lowering Treatment Trialists' Collaboration (1998).

and preferably superiority over conventional therapy. In response, there is an epidemic of ongoing outcome trials.

This is a welcome development. However, even large, well-designed individual trials are unlikely to answer all the outstanding relevant questions reliably and decisively. Thus, meta-analyses of the available outcome data will be required. It is encouraging that overviews have been planned prospectively. At the conclusion of the current round of ongoing trials the management of hypertension should have a much more secure base.

References

1. Collins R, MacMahon S. Blood pressure, antihypertensive drug treatment and the risks of stroke and of coronary heart disease. *Br Med Bull* 1994; **50**: 272–98.

2. Staessen JA, Fagard R, Thijs L, Celis H, Arabidze GG, Birkenhäger WH, Bulpitt CJ, de Leeuw PW, Dollery CT, Fletcher AE, Forette F, Leonetti G, Nachev C, O'Brien ET, Rosenfield J, Rodicio JL, Tuomilehto J, Zanchetti A, and for the Systolic Hypertension in Europe (Syst-Eur) Trial Investigators. Randomized double-blind comparison of placebo and active treatment for older patients with isolated systolic hypertension. *Lancet* 1997; **350**: 757–64.

3. Gong L, Zhang W, Zhu Y, Zhu J, 11 collaborating centres in the Shanghai area, Kong D, Page V, Ghadirian P, LeLorier J, Hamet P. Shanghai trial of nifedipine in the elderly (STONE). *J Hypertens* 1996; **14**: 1237–45.

4. Hansson L, Lindholm LH, Ekbom T, Dahlöf B, Lanke J, Schersten B, Wester PO, Hedner T, de Faire U. Randomized trial of old and new antihypertensive drugs in elderly patients: cardiovascular mortality and morbidity the Swedish Trial in Old Patients with Hypertension-2 Study. *Lancet* 1999; **354**: 1751–6.

5. Hansson L, Lindholm LH, Niskanen L, Lanke J, Hedner T, Niklason A, Luomanmäki K, Dählöf B, de Faire U, Mörlin C, Karlberg BE, Wester PO, Björck J-E, for the Captopril Prevention Project (CAPPP) Study Group. Effect of angiotensin-converting enzyme inhibition compared with conventional therapy on cardiovascular morbidity and mortality in hypertension: the Captopril Prevention Project (CAPPP) randomized trial. *Lancet* 1999; **353**: 611–16.

6. Neaton JD, Grimm RH, Prineas RJ, Stamler J, Gandits GA, Elmer PJ, Cutler JA, Flack JM, Schoenberger JA, McDonald R, Lewis CE, Liebson PR. Treatment of Mild Hypertension Study. Final results. *JAMA* 1993; **270**: 713–14.

Part II

Interface: hypertension and other cardiovascular risk factors

4

Hypertension, diabetes and cardiovascular risk

Introduction

Hypertension and diabetes mellitus are independent risk factors for the development of cardiovascular disease. The two conditions often coexist and hypertension is twice as prevalent in diabetic patients than in the general population; however, the evolution of hypertension differs slightly in type 1 compared with type 2 diabetes mellitus. In type 1 diabetes, hypertension and diabetic nephropathy tend to develop in parallel: in type 2 diabetes, while hypertension may again be coincident with an evolving diabetic nephropathy, it is frequently a component part of the metabolic syndrome ('insulin resistance'), which also includes obesity and dyslipidaemia. In either case, there also is the possibility of a chance association between diabetes mellitus and essential hypertension, especially in those with a family history of hypertension.

In past years, 'tight' glycaemic control was invariably emphasized in both type 1 and type 2 diabetes mellitus with little attention (relatively) being directed towards blood pressure (BP) reduction or lipid modification. It is interesting to note, however, that it is only within the past 10 years that confirmation of the benefits of tight glycaemic control have been confirmed by clinical outcome studies. The landmark study by the Diabetes Control and Complications Trial Research Group (DCCT) confirmed these benefits in type 1 diabetes mellitus, particularly in relation to microvascular complications, and a smaller scale study produced corresponding evidence in type 2 diabetes mellitus, albeit with an intensified insulin regimen rather than oral hypoglycaemic drugs [1,2].

The results of recent clinical outcome trials, albeit in patients with hypertension and/or coronary heart disease (CHD; rather than 'uncomplicated' diabetes) have provoked a significant shift in therapeutic emphasis for current practice. These results, and the current focus on the treatment of high-risk patients, has directed the treatment strategy in both types 1 and 2 diabetes towards BP control and overall risk factor management, rather than glycaemic control *per se*.

Blood pressure control

At present, 'tight' control of BP might be considered the dominant factor in the management of the hypertensive diabetic patient. Several recent clinical outcome trials have involved cohorts of patients with hypertension and diabetes mellitus.

UK Prospective Diabetes Study

The UK Prospective Diabetes Study (UKPDS) was a long-running (about 20 years from its inception) clinical outcome trial designed to address issues relating to the optimal treatment of type 2 diabetes. The principal objectives of the original study design focused upon glycaemic targets and the selection of the most appropriate therapeutic strategy, but a number of other issues of practical importance and clinical relevance were also addressed.

Between 1977 and 1991, 5102 newly diagnosed type 2 diabetic patients (58% male) were recruited into the main study, which was designed to address the following issues:

1. Does intensive treatment with oral antidiabetic agents or insulin reduce the risk of microvascular and macrovascular disease relative to less intensive, conventional measures, i.e. diet.

2. Is any particular treatment advantageous? Or disadvantageous?

In 1987 a subgroup was identified for the Hypertension in Diabetes Study and this was incorporated into the main study via a factorial design to compare 'tight' BP control (target less than 150/85 mmHg) compared with 'less tight' BP control (target less than 180/105 mmHg). A total of 1148 patients were randomized in this study with a further subdivision in the 'tight' control group to a treatment regimen based either upon an angiotensin-converting enzyme (ACE) inhibitor (captopril) or upon a beta-blocker (atenolol).

Main study—UKPDS 33: intensive glycaemic control

Intensive blood-glucose control with sulphonylureas or insulin compared with conventional treatment and risk of complications in patients with type 2 diabetes: UKPDS 33.
United Kingdom Prospective Diabetes Study Group. *Lancet* 1998; **352**: 837–53.

BACKGROUND. Improved blood glucose control decreased the progression of diabetic microvascular disease, but the effect on macrovascular complications is unknown. There is concern that sulphonylureas may increase cardiovascular mortality in patients with type 2 diabetes and that high insulin concentrations may enhance atheroma formation. **We compared the effects of intensive blood glucose control with either sulphonylurea or insulin and conventional treatment on the risk of macrovascular complications in patients with type 2 diabetes in a randomized controlled trial.**

INTERPRETATION. Intensive blood glucose control by either sulphonylureas or insulin substantially decreases the risk of microvascular complications, but not macrovascular disease, in patients with type 2 diabetes. None of the individual drugs had an adverse effect on cardiovascular outcomes. All intensive treatment increased the risk of hypoglycaemia.

Comment

Over 10 years the mean HbA_{1C} was significantly less at 7% in the intensive treatment group *vs* 7.9% for the diet group ($P < 0.0001$), but there was no difference between the different intensive treatment subgroups. This improvement in glycaemic control was associated with a 12% risk reduction for any diabetes-related end-point and this was mainly attributable to a 25% reduction in microvascular end-points ($P < 0.005$). Although there was a 16% reduction in fatal and non-fatal myocardial infarction (MI) in the intensive group this failed to achieve conventional statistical significance ($P = 0.052$), but sudden death was significantly reduced ($P < 0.05$). No differences were attributable to the three principal agents—chlorpropamide, glybenclamide and insulin—although, interestingly, the reduction in the risk of progression of retinopathy was less pronounced for chlorpropamide. However, BP was significantly higher throughout the study in the chlorpropamide-treated patients.

Overweight subgroup—UKPDS 34: diet versus metformin

Effect of intensive blood glucose control with metformin on complications in overweight patients with type 2 diabetes: UKPDS 34.
United Kingdom Prospective Diabetes Study Group. *Lancet* 1998; **352**: 854–65.

BACKGROUND. **In patients with type 2 diabetes, intensive blood glucose control with insulin or sulphonylurea therapy decreases the progression of microvascular disease and may also reduce the risk of heart attack. This study investigated whether intensive glucose control with metformin has any specific advantage or disadvantage.**

INTERPRETATION. As intensive glucose control with metformin appears to decrease the risk of diabetes-related end-points in overweight diabetic patients, and is associated with less weight gain and fewer hypoglycaemic attacks than are insulin and sulphonylureas, it may be the first-line pharmacological therapy of choice in these patients.

Comment

HbA$_{1C}$ was significantly lower at 7.4% in the metformin group compared with 8% in the diet only group. Significant risk reductions were observed for all-cause mortality, diabetes-related death and all diabetes-related end-points. For all macro-vascular events, there was a 30% risk reduction for metformin compared with conventional dietary treatment ($P = 0.02$) with a 30% risk reduction for MI ($P = 0.01$).

Blood pressure study—UKPDS 38: 'tight' versus 'less tight' blood pressure control

Tight blood pressure control and risk of macrovascular and microvascular complications in type 2 diabetes: UKPDS 38.

United Kingdom Prospective Diabetes Study Group. *BMJ* 1998; **317**: 703–13.

B ACKGROUND. **The objective of this study was to determine whether tight control of BP prevents macrovascular and microvascular complications in patients with type 2 diabetes.**

I NTERPRETATION. Tight BP control in patients with hypertension and type 2 diabetes achieves a clinically important reduction in the risk of deaths related to diabetes, complications related to diabetes, progression of diabetes retinopathy and deterioration in visual acuity.

Comment

The mean achieved BP was significantly less at 144/82 mmHg in the 'tight' control group compared with 154/87 mmHg in the 'less tight' BP control group ($P < 0.0001$). This difference of 10/5 mmHg was associated with significant reductions in macrovascular and microvascular events (Table 4.1): all diabetes end-points

Table 4.1 Tight blood pressure control in type 2 diabetes: events per 1000 patient years

	BP control		Relative risk	
	Tight	Less	Reduction	
Any diabetes-related end point	50.9	67.4	−24%	$P < 0.005$
All-cause mortality	22.4	27.2	−18%	
Myocardial infarction	18.6	23.5	−21%	
Stroke	6.5	11.6	−44%	$P < 0.02$
Microvascular disease	12.0	19.2	−37%	$P < 0.01$

Source: UKPDS 38 (1998).

were significantly reduced by 24% as was stroke by 44% and microvascular disease by 37%.

The reduction in microvascular complications was predominantly attributable to a reduced risk of retinopathy and its progression.

Blood pressure control—UKPDS 39: atenolol versus captopril

Efficacy of atenolol and captopril in reducing risk of macrovascular and microvascular complications in type 2 diabetes: UKPDS 39.

United Kingdom Prospective Diabetes Study Group. *BMJ* 1998; **317**: 713–20.

BACKGROUND. The objective of this study was to determine whether tight control of BP with either a beta-blocker or an ACE inhibitor has a specific advantage or disadvantage in preventing the macrovascular and microvascular complications of type 2 diabetes.

INTERPRETATION. BP lowering with captopril or atenolol was similarly effective in reducing the incidence of diabetic complications. This study provided no evidence that either drug has any specific beneficial or deleterious effect, suggesting that BP reduction in itself may be more important than the treatment.

Comment

Unfortunately, this aspect of the UKPDS was not statistically empowered to address a very important issue relating to potential additional benefits that might be attributable to an individual drug treatment. In this substudy, treatment regimens based upon captopril 25–50 mg twice daily (400 patients) or upon atenolol 50–100 mg daily (358 patients) were compared: there were no significant differences but the overall trends consistently favoured atenolol (Table 4.2 and Fig. 4.1). Thus, captopril and atenolol were equally effective in reducing the incidence of diabetic complications in the 'tight' BP control group. It is important to recognize, however, that single drug therapy was capable of providing 'tight' control in less than half the patients and that multiple drug treatments (3 or more agents) were required in 29% of patients. Furthermore, after 9 years of treatment, only just over half of the 'tight' control group (56%) had attained the target BP of less than 150/85 mmHg.

Incidentally, in the light of reports suggesting that ACE inhibitors may predispose to hypoglycaemia while beta-blockers may delay recovery from hypoglycaemia there were no differences in the rates for hypoglycaemic episodes in this study.

Table 4.2 Captopril *vs* atenolol diabetes-related end-points

Clinical end-point	Patients with aggregate end-points		*P*	Relative risk for captopril
	Captopril (*n* = 400)	Atenolol (*n* = 358)		
Any end-point	141	118	0.43	1.10
Deaths	48	34	0.28	1.27
Acute MI	61	46	0.35	1.20
Stroke	21	17	0.74	1.12
Peripheral vascular disease	5	3	0.59	1.48
Microvascular disease	40	28	0.30	1.29

Source: UKPDS 39 (1998).

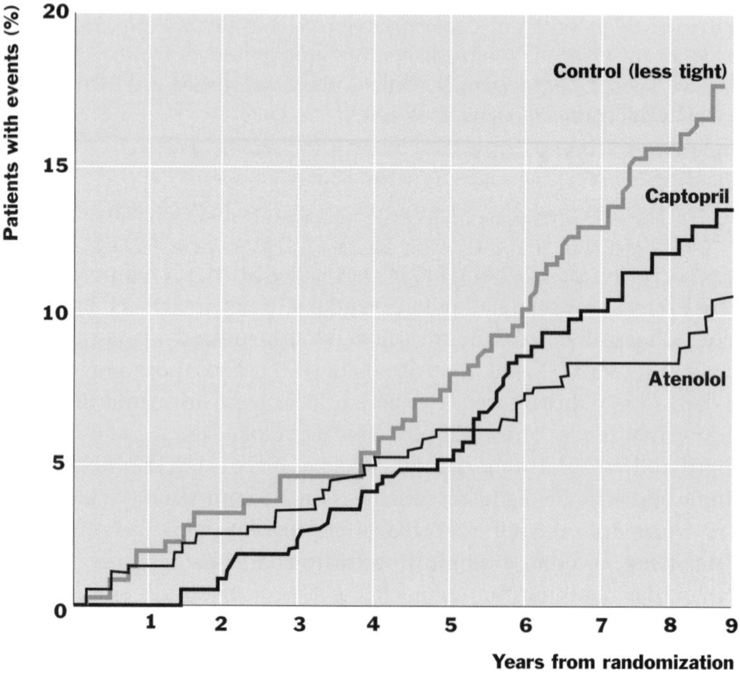

Fig. 4.1 Cumulative event rates (%) in patients randomized to 'less tight' control and to 'tight' control with either captopril or atenolol (UKPDS). Source: UKPDS 39 (1998).

Association of systolic blood pressure and vascular complications

Association of systolic blood pressure with the macrovascular and microvascular complications of type 2 diabetes (UKPDS 36): prospective observational study.

A I Adler, I M Stratton, H A Neil, *et al*. on behalf of the UK prospective Diabetes Study Group. *BMJ* 2000; **321**: 415–19.

B A C K G R O U N D. To determine the relationship between systolic BP over time and the risk of macrovascular or microvascular complications in patients with type 2 diabetes.

I N T E R P R E T A T I O N. In patients with type 2 diabetes the risk of diabetic complications was strongly associated with raised BP. Any reduction in BP is likely to reduce the risk of complications, with the lowest risk being in those with systolic BP less than 120 mmHg.

Comment

This was a further analysis from the UKPDS database derived from 4801 patients of white, Asian-Indian and Afro-Caribbean origin of whom 3842 were included in the analyses of relative risk. The primary end-point was predefined as any complications or deaths related to diabetes and all-cause mortality. Secondary end-points included MI, stroke, severe peripheral vascular disease and microvascular disease (predominantly retinal photocoagulation). The incidence of clinical complications was significantly associated with systolic BP whereby for each 10 mmHg reduction in systolic BP there was a 12% reduction in any complication related to diabetes (Fig. 4.2). For individual end-points there was 15% reduction in deaths related to diabetes, an 11% reduction in MI and a 13% reduction in microvascular complications.

Conclusion

Although this is essentially a confirmatory study it emphasizes a number of important issues. First, there is a direct relationship between systolic BP and the risk of the complications of diabetes over time. There was no BP threshold for a substantive change in risk and there was a twofold increase in risk over the range of achieved systolic BPs from less than 120 mmHg to more than 160 mmHg. Thus, the rate for MI increased from 18 per 1000 patient years in the group with the lowest systolic BP to 33 per 1000 patient years in the group with BP greater than 160 mmHg. Correspondingly, the lowest risk of complications was associated with the lowest systolic BP to a level of less than 120 mmHg.

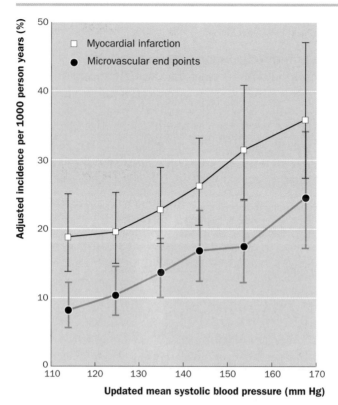

Fig. 4.2 Relationship between achieved systolic BP and the incidence of MI and microvascular end-points. Source: Adler *et al.* (2000).

Association between glycaemic control and vascular complications

Association of glycaemia with macrovascular and microvascular complications of type 2 diabetes (UKPDS 35): prospective observational study.

I M Stratton, AI Adler, H A Neil, *et al.* on behalf of the UK prospective Diabetes Study Group. *BMJ* 2000; **321**: 405–12.

BACKGROUND. **To determine the relationship between exposure to glycaemia over time and the risk of macrovascular or microvascular complications in patients with type 2 diabetes.**

INTERPRETATION. In patients with type 2 diabetes the risk of diabetic complications was strongly associated with previous hyperglycaemia. Any reduction in HbA$_{1c}$ is likely to reduce the risk of complications, with the lowest risk being in those with HbA$_{1c}$ values in the normal range ($< 6.0\%$).

Comment

This further analysis from the UKPDS was closely similar to the systolic BP analysis with slight differences in patient numbers. The analysis was adjusted in the conventional statistical fashion for confounding variables and the salient results were that there was a 21% reduction for any end-point related to diabetes in association with each 1% reduction in achieved mean HbA$_{1c}$ (Fig. 4.3). Thus, there was a 21% reduction in death related to diabetes, a 14% reduction in MI and a 37% reduction in microvascular complications.

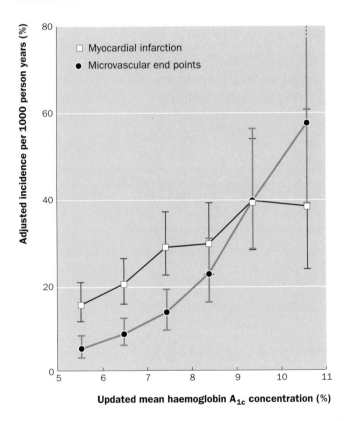

Fig. 4.3 Relationship between achieved glycaemic control and the incidence of MI and microvascular end-points. Source: Stratton *et al.* (2000).

Conclusion

Once again, these results are confirmatory rather than unexpected whereby there is direct relationship between glycaemia and the risk of the complications of diabetes over time. There was no threshold for any substantial change in risk and the lower the level of glycaemia the lower the risk of complications.

Summary

The UKPDS has been the subject of some criticism but, nevertheless, the findings are entirely consistent with the results from other studies leading to important practical messages for the treatment of type 2 diabetes mellitus. Thus, glycaemic control appears to be particularly important for microvascular disease and BP control for macrovascular disease, including coronary artery disease and its complications. As for essential hypertension, the focus should be on achieving tight control of BP and systolic BP, in particular, with a suggested systolic BP target of less than 120 mmHg.

Captopril Prevention Project (CAPPP)

Effect of angiotensin-converting-enzyme inhibition compared with conventional therapy on cardiovascular morbidity and mortality in hypertension: the Captopril Prevention Project (CAPPP) randomized trial.
L Hansson, L H Lindholm, L Niskanen, *et al. Lancet* 1999; **353**: 611–16.

BACKGROUND. ACE inhibitors have been used for more than a decade to treat high BP, despite the lack of data from randomized intervention trials to show that such treatment affects cardiovascular morbidity and mortality. CAPPP is a randomized intervention trial to compare the effects of ACE inhibition and conventional therapy on cardiovascular morbidity and mortality in patients with hypertension.

INTERPRETATION. Captopril and conventional treatment did not differ in efficacy in preventing cardiovascular morbidity and mortality. The difference in stroke risk is probably due to the lower levels of BP obtained initially in previously treated patients randomized to conventional therapy.

Comment

This was a prospective, randomized, open, blinded end-point trial in 10 985 hypertensive patients allocated to a treatment regimen based upon an ACE inhibitor (captopril) or upon traditional antihypertensive drugs (thiazide diuretics or beta-blockers). Overall, for the primary end-point, which was a composite of fatal and non-fatal MI, stroke and other cardiovascular deaths there was no difference between the treatment groups.

However, the most controversial finding was derived from the subgroup analysis of the patients with hypertension and diabetes mellitus. First, and not surprisingly, the treatment regimen based upon the thiazides or beta-blockers was more likely to result in new cases of diabetes albeit in small numbers with 43 cases arising during 30 000 patient years of treatment. Thus, the well recognized adverse effects of these traditional agents on carbohydrate metabolism was confirmed.

In the subgroup of patients with diabetes mellitus prior to entry into the study there was no difference between treatment based upon the traditional treatments and captopril. Thus, there was no evidence of any benefit beyond BP reduction in the captopril-treated patient group. It must be recognized, however, that only 572 patients were included in this study and it is therefore completely under-powered in statistical terms to draw any definitive conclusions. Furthermore, captopril was administered only once daily in about 50% of patients and this regimen is unlikely to provide full 24-h BP control. Thus, the captopril-treated patients may not have had the full benefit of intensive BP reduction.

Systolic Hypertension in Europe trial (SYST-EUR): diabetic cohort

Effects of calcium channel blockade in older patients with diabetes and systolic hypertension.
J Tuomilehto, D Rastenyte, W H Berkenhager, *et al. N Engl J Med* 1999;
340: 677–84.

BACKGROUND. Recent reports suggest that calcium channel blockers may be harmful in patients with diabetes and hypertension. These authors previously reported that antihypertensive treatment with the calcium channel blocker nitrendipine reduced the risk of cardiovascular events. This *post hoc* analysis compared the outcome of treatment with nitrendipine in diabetic and non-diabetic patients.

INTERPRETATION. Nitrendipine-based antihypertensive therapy is particularly beneficial in older patients with diabetes and isolated hypertension. Thus our findings do not support the hypothesis that the use of long-acting calcium channel blockers may be harmful in diabetic patients.

Comment

Increasingly, the message for intensive BP control in diabetic hypertensives is being reinforced through the subgroup analyses of clinical outcome trials. An important additional component to this basic message is the emphasis on BP control through drug treatment combinations rather than monotherapy and, while an ACE inhibitor would undoubtedly be incorporated into the treatment regimen, the balance of evidence favours aggressive BP reduction rather than reliance upon the pharmacological characteristics of any individual drug or class. For example, in the SYST-EUR study of 4695 patients aged 60 years or older an antihypertensive treatment regimen based upon a calcium antagonist was found to be particularly beneficial. These were older patients with systolic BP between 160 and 219 mmHg and diastolic BP less than 95 mmHg. The diabetic cohort in this study comprised 492 patients and after 2 years of follow-up systolic and diastolic BP had been reduced by 8.6/3.9 mmHg in the treatment group relative to the patient group. The treatment group received the dihydropyridine derivative nitrendipine but ultimately more than half of the patients were on drug combination treatments to produce this BP reduction. After adjusting for confounding factors, the treated group had a 76% reduction in overall mortality from cardiovascular disease, a 73% reduction in fatal and non-fatal strokes and a 63% reduction in all cardiac events combined (Table 4.3). The magnitude of the benefits were significantly greater in the diabetic versus the non-diabetic patients for all cardiovascular events and for cardiovascular mortality. This emphasises the benefits of BP reductions in high risk patients.

Hypertension Optimal Treatment (HOT) study: diabetic cohort

Effects of intensive blood pressure lowering and low-dose aspirin in patients with hypertension: principal results of the Hypertension Optimal Treatment (HOT) randomized trial.

L Hansson, A Zanchetti, S G Carruthers, *et al. Lancet* 1998; **351**: 1755–62.

BACKGROUND. Despite treatment, there is often a higher incidence of cardiovascular complications in patients with hypertension than normotensive individuals. Inadequate reduction of their BP is a likely cause, but the optimum target BP is not known. The impact of acetylsalicylic acid (aspirin) has never been investigated in patients with hypertension. This study aimed to assess the optimum target diastolic BP and the potential benefit of low-dose acetylsalicylic acid in the treatment of hypertension.

Table 4.3 Reduction in mortality and cardiovascular events in diabetics *vs* non-diabetics

	Diabetic patients (*n* = 492)	Non-diabetic patients (*n* = 4203)
All strokes	73%	38%
All cardiac end-points	63%	21%
All cardiovascular end-points	69%*	26%
Total mortality	55%	6%
Cardiovascular mortality	76%*	13%

*$P < 0.05$ for diabetic *vs* non-diabetic patients.

Source: Tuomilehto *et al.* (1999).

INTERPRETATION. Intensive lowering of BP in patients with hypertension was associated with a low rate of cardiovascular events. The HOT study shows the benefits of lowering the diastolic BP down to 82.6 mmHg. Acetylsalicylic acid significantly reduced major cardiovascular events, with the greatest benefit seen in MI. There was no effect on the incidence of stroke or fatal bleeds, but non-fatal major bleeds were twice as common.

Comment

A cohort of 1501 patients with diabetes mellitus were identified within the 18 790 patients who participated in the HOT study with treatment based upon another dihydropyridine calcium channel blocker, felodipine. Overall, there was a significant reduction in major cardiovascular events in relation to the 'tightness' of the BP control. In the group randomized to less than 80 mmHg the risk of major cardiovascular events was halved in comparison with that of the target group randomized to less than 90 mmHg (Fig. 4.4). The cardiovascular event rates were generally reduced in the group targeted for less than 80 mmHg, relative to the group targeted for less than 90 mmHg, although conventional statistical significance was not always achieved in each category.

Once again, multiple drug treatments were required with only 26% of patients targeted to < 80 mmHg continuing with the single drug treatment. Interestingly, although reported adverse events increased with the number of administered drugs, there was no difference in relation to the BP target. In other words, 'tight' control caused no excess of side-effects.

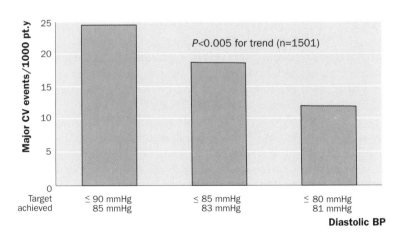

Fig. 4.4 Major cardiovascular event rates according to the target BP category in the HOT study. Source: Hansson *et al.* (1998).

Systolic Hypertension in the Elderly Programme (SHEP) study: diabetic cohort

Effect of diuretic-based antihypertensive treatment on cardiovascular disease risk in older diabetic patients with isolated systolic hypertension.

D Curb, S L Pressel, J A Cutler, *et al. JAMA* 1996; **276**: 1886–92.

BACKGROUND. The objective of this study was to assess the effects of low-dose, diuretic-based antihypertensive treatment on major cardiovascular disease event rates in older, non-insulin-treated diabetic patients with isolated systolic hypertension, compared with non-diabetic patients.

INTERPRETATION. Low-dose diuretic (chlorthalidone) treatment is effective in preventing major cardiovascular disease events, cerebral and cardiac, in both non-insulin-treated diabetic and non-diabetic older patients with isolated systolic hypertension.

Comment

The results of the studies published within the past 12 months or so are entirely confirmatory to those first identified in hypertensive patients with type 2 diabetes mellitus. A total of 4736 men and women aged 60 years and older with isolated systolic hypertension participated in this clinical outcome trial based upon low-dose thiazide diuretic (chlorthalidone). Within this study there were 583 non-insulin-dependent diabetic patients who were randomly assigned to receive either placebo or an active antihypertensive treatment regimen based on low-dose (12.5 or 25 mg) chlorthalidone. For both diabetic and non-diabetic patients there was a similar 34% reduction in major cardiovascular events for active treatment compared with placebo. However, the absolute risk reduction was twice as great for diabetic *vs* non-diabetic patients (101 per 1000 participants at the 5-year follow-up *vs* 51 per 1000 participants) reflecting the higher risk of diabetic patients.

   In retrospect, this study highlighted two important points. First, that antihypertensive treatment and significant BP reductions lead to improved cardiovascular outcomes in high-risk patients who attained the greatest absolute benefits. Secondly, although thiazide diuretics have been implicated in causing adverse metabolic effects, including the precipitation of diabetes mellitus, there was no suggestion that the cardiovascular benefits were compromised.

Conclusion

As hypertension is common in patients with diabetes, particularly type 2 diabetes mellitus, and is a major contributor to the development and progression of micro-vascular and macrovascular complications, the results of the UKPDS have clearly demonstrated the importance of intensive antihypertensive treatment and 'tight' BP control. These results accord with the findings from recently published trials involving diabetic hypertensive patients with clear outcome benefits in such high-risk patients. However, these benefits have been obtained with regimens based upon different types of antihypertensive drug and there is no clear evidence that any individual drug or drug class is superior. The primary target is to attain BP control with values of 140/90 mmHg or less (135/85 mmHg or less has also been recommended). Frequently this will require multiple drug treatments.

Heart Outcomes Prevention Evaluations (HOPE) and Microalbuminuria and Renal Outcomes-HOPE (MICRO-HOPE) study

Effects of ramipril on cardiovascular and microvascular outcomes in people with diabetes mellitus: results of the HOPE study and MICRO-HOPE substudy.

Heart Outcomes Prevention Evaluations (HOPE) Study Investigators.
Lancet 2000; **355**: 253–9.

BACKGROUND. Diabetes mellitus is a strong risk factor for cardiovascular and renal disease. We investigated whether the ACE inhibitor ramipril can lower these risks in patients with diabetes.

INTERPRETATION. Ramipril was beneficial for cardiovascular events and overt nephropathy in people with diabetes. The cardiovascular benefit was greater than that attributable to the decrease in BP. This treatment represents a vasculoprotective and renoprotective effect for people with diabetes.

Comment

The HOPE study included 3577 patients with diabetes, aged 55 years or more, with a previous cardiovascular event or at least one other cardiovascular risk factor. Patients were randomly assigned to ramipril (10 mg daily) or placebo and the combined primary outcome was MI, stroke or cardiovascular death. The study was stopped after 4.5 years (6 months prematurely) by the Independent Safety and Monitoring Board because of a consistent benefit of ramipril compared with placebo. Ramipril lowered the risk of the combined primary outcome by 25% with significant relative reductions in the incidence of MI by 22%, stroke by 33%, cardiovascular death by 37% and total mortality by 24%. It was calculated that, after adjustment for the changes in systolic BP (2.4 mmHg) and diastolic BP (1.0 mmHg), ramipril still lowered the risk of the combined primary outcome by 25%.

Conclusion

This substudy in patients with diabetes mellitus reinforces the message of the main study, which was undertaken in patients at high cardiovascular risk in so far as 90%

had evidence of pre-existing CHD. There is no doubt that this additional drug treatment is of benefit, but the debate continues as to whether or not this was specific to ramipril, or applicable to ACE inhibitors in general because of some 'protective' effect of ACE inhibition, or simply a reflection of the benefits of even small BP reductions in very high-risk patients.

Swedish Trial in Old Patients with Hypertension-2 (STOP-2): elderly diabetic cohort

Comparison of antihypertensive treatments in preventing cardiovascular events in elderly diabetic patients: results from the Swedish Trial in Old Patients with Hypertension-2.

L H Lindholm, L Hansson, T Ekbom, *et al.* for the STOP Hypertension-2 Study Group. *J Hypertens* 2000; **18**: 1671–5.

BACKGROUND. The benefits of treating hypertension in elderly diabetic patients, in terms of achieving reductions in cardiovascular morbidity and mortality, have been documented in several recent prospective trials. There has, however, been some controversy regarding the effect of different antihypertensive drugs on the frequency of MI in this group of patients.

INTERPRETATION. Treatment of hypertensive diabetic patients with conventional antihypertensive drugs (diuretics, beta-blockers, or both) seemed to be as effective as treatment with newer drugs such as calcium antagonists for ACE inhibitors.

Comment

This subgroup analysis from the STOP-2 study was derived from 719 elderly patients, mean age 75.8 years, who were randomly assigned to one of three treatment strategies. Conventional antihypertensive drugs (diuretics or beta-blockers), calcium channel blockers or ACE inhibitors. Blood pressure reductions were similar in the three treatment groups and the prevention of cardiovascular mortality was also similar. Cardiovascular mortality was 37.3 with conventional treatment, 34.1 with ACE inhibitor treatment and 28.9 per 1000 patient years with calcium channel blockers. There were some differences, however, in the overall pattern of events, whereby significantly fewer MIs occurred during ACE inhibitor treatment, relative to calcium channel blocker treatment, and there was a non-significant trend for more strokes to occur with ACE inhibitor treatment relative to calcium channel blocker treatment.

Conclusion

The results of this substudy are essentially confirmatory albeit extending the benefits of antihypertensive drug treatment into patients in the age range 70–84 years. The broad conclusions that BP reduction and the attainment of tight BP control are entirely consistent from other similar studies, with this study extending the observation into another high-risk group, i.e. the elderly. The additional observation that there were no significant differences between 'newer' treatments (ACE inhibitors and calcium channel blockers) and 'conventional' treatments (thiazide diuretics and beta-blockers) is probably the most important additional practical message. The debate continues as to whether any class of antihypertensive drug is particularly effective and, although the ACE inhibitor group appeared to have some advantages relating to CHD events, it should be noted that the total number of events was small, that the statistical power was weak and that multiple statistical tests were employed.

Cholesterol reduction

Dyslipidaemia tends to occur more frequently in patients with diabetes mellitus, although total and low-density lipoprotein (LDL) cholesterol levels are often similar to those of people without diabetes. However, these apparent similarities may mask underlying differences in lipid particle size and lipid composition, which in turn are influenced by the type of diabetes and the adequacy of the glycaemic control. In type 2 diabetes mellitus, even with adequate metabolic control triglyceride levels tend to be elevated and high-density lipoprotein (HDL) levels reduced.

The extent to which cardiovascular complications can be modified by conventional risk factor interventions (other than BP reduction) has also been confirmed through cholesterol reduction in the CARE study.

Cholesterol and Recurrent Events (CARE): diabetic subgroup

Cardiovascular events and their reduction with pravastatin in diabetic and glucose-intolerant myocardial infarction survivors with average cholesterol levels: subgroup analyses in the Cholesterol and Recurrent Events (CARE) trial.

R B Goldberg, M J Mellies, F M Sacks, *et al. Circulation* 1998; **98**: 2513–19.

BACKGROUND. Although diabetes is a major risk factor for CHD, little information is available on the effects of lipid-lowering in diabetic patients. We determined whether lipid-lowering treatment with pravastatin prevents recurrent cardiovascular events in diabetic patients with CHD and average cholesterol levels.

INTERPRETATION. Diabetic patients and non-diabetic patients with impaired fasting glucose are at high risk of recurrent coronary events that can be substantially reduced by pravastatin treatment.

Comment

A subgroup of 586 patients were identified among the 4159 patients participating in the CARE trial, which was a secondary prevention trial investigating the impact of cholesterol reduction (with pravastatin) over a 5 year follow-up period. The diabetic patients were older, more obese and more hypertensive but their baseline lipid concentrations were similar to the non-diabetic group. Similarly, the reductions in LDL cholesterol were similar at 27 and 28% in the diabetic and non-diabetic groups, respectively.

In the diabetic cohort there was a 25% relative risk reduction for all major coronary events (death from CHD, non-fatal MI or revascularization procedure) in the pravastatin-treated group compared with the placebo group. The relative risk of coronary artery by-pass or percutaneous transluminal coronary angioplasty was reduced by 32%. Overall, cholesterol reduction with pravastatin treatment reduced the absolute risk of coronary events by 8.1% in the diabetic patients and by 5.2% in the non-diabetic patients: the relative risk reductions were respectively 25% ($P = 0.05$) and 23% ($P < 0.001$), respectively. Of additional interest, were the 342 patients who had impaired fasting glucose on entry to the study (of the 3553 patients who were not categorized as diabetic: these patients had a higher rate of recurrent coronary events than those with normal fasting glucose, e.g. 13% compared with 10% suffered a non-fatal MI.

Conclusion

This *post hoc* subgroup analysis supports the general view that lipid-lowering treatment is beneficial for patients who fall into high-risk categories and particularly those with evidence of pre-existing cardiovascular disease with prior MI or angina. Whether or not it is necessary to prescribe lipid-lowering drug treatment for diabetics who have no evidence of clinical cardiovascular disease remains unanswered.

Effects of fenofibrate on progression of coronary artery disease in type 2 diabetes: the Diabetes Atherosclerosis Intervention Study, a randomized study.

Diabetes Atherosclerosis Intervention Study Investigators. *Lancet* 2001; **357**: 905–10.

BACKGROUND. Atherosclerosis is the most common complication of diabetes. Correction of hyperglycaemia helps to prevent microvascular complications but has little effect on macrovascular disease. *Post-hoc* analyses of diabetic subpopulations in lipid intervention trials suggest that correction of lipoprotein abnormalities will lead to a decrease in coronary artery disease. The Diabetes Atherosclerosis Intervention Study (DAIS) was specifically designed to assess the effects of correcting lipoprotein abnormalities in coronary atherosclerosis in type 2 diabetes.

INTERPRETATION. DAIS suggests that treatment with fenofibrate reduces the angiographic progression of coronary artery disease in type 2 diabetes. This effect is related, at least partly, to the correction of lipoprotein abnormalities, even those previously judged not to need treatment.

Comment

This is an interesting study on 731 patients with type 2 diabetes who were randomly assigned to fenofibrate or placebo to assess the impact on angiographic measures of coronary atherosclerosis. Fenofibrate was associated with the expected changes in the lipid profile with a modest reduction of LDL cholesterol of about 5%, an increase in HDL cholesterol of about 5% and reductions in triglycerides of about 30% relative to the placebo treatment). There were corresponding improvements in the angiographic findings with a significantly smaller increase in percentage diameter stenosis, a significantly smaller decrease in minimum lumen diameter and a non-significantly smaller decrease in mean segment diameter in the group assigned fenofibrate compared with placebo. Although the trial was not powered to examine clinical end-points it was noted that there were 38 events in the fenofibrate group compared with 50 events in the placebo group.

Pravastatin and the development of diabetes mellitus: evidence for a protective treatment effect in the West of Scotland Coronary Prevention Study.

D J Freeman, J Norrie, N Sattar, *et al. Circulation* 2001; **103**: 357–62.

BACKGROUND. We examined the development of new diabetes mellitus in men aged 45–64 years during the West of Scotland Coronary Prevention Study.

INTERPRETATION. We concluded that the assignment to pravastatin therapy resulted in a 30% reduction ($P = 0.042$) in the hazard of becoming diabetic. By lowering plasma triglyceride levels, pravastatin therapy may favourably influence the development of diabetes, but other explanations, such as the anti-inflammatory properties of this drug in combination with its endothelial effects, cannot be excluded with these analyses.

Comment

This was a further analysis from the West of Scotland Coronary Prevention Study (WOSCOPS) |3| involving 5974 subjects (of 6595) of whom 139 subsequently developed diabetes mellitus. In the multivariate analysis, body mass index, trigly-cerides (log concentration) and blood glucose were all predictive for the subsequent development of diabetes mellitus, whereas pravastatin therapy was 'protective'. There is interesting speculation by the authors regarding possible mechanisms, including the triglyceride-lowering effect of pravastatin therapy; the effect of prava-statin on cytokines, which are known to affect insulin responsiveness adversely, and the effect on endothelial function, which may also lead to an improvement responsiveness.

This is an interesting finding and the mechanism proposed by the authors are plausible and consistent with findings of other studies. However, it was a retrospective analysis and the interpretation must be viewed with caution until it is confirmed by the results of prospective studies.

Conclusion

Increasingly the management of the diabetic patient is becoming the management of a high-risk patient and these studies have confirmed the concept that high-risk individuals benefit from multifactorial intervention strategies.

Intensified multifactorial intervention

The evidence that BP reduction and cholesterol reduction can independently improve outcome was extended through the findings of a smaller study that explored the multiple risk factor approach, whereby hypertension was targeted in conjunction with intensive treatment for hyperglycaemia, dyslipidaemia and microalbuminuria.

Steno

Intensified multifactorial intervention in patients with type 2 diabetes mellitus and microalbuminuria: The Steno type 2 randomized study.
P Gaede, P Vvedel, H-H Parving, O Pederson. *Lancet* 1999; **353**: 617–22.

BACKGROUND. In type 2 diabetes mellitus the aetiology of long-term complications is multifactorial. The authors carried a randomized trial of stepwise intensive treatment or standard treatment of risk factors in patients with microalbuminuria.

INTERPRETATION. Intensified multifactorial intervention in patients with type 2 diabetes and microalbuminuria slows progression to nephropathy, and progression of retinopathy and autonomic neuropathy. However, further studies are needed to establish the effect of intensified multifactorial treatment on macrovascular complications and mortality.

Comment

Eighty patients were randomized to standard treatment and 80 patients were randomized to intensive treatment to assess the impact on the primary end-point of development/progression of nephropathy. The mean age of these patients was 55 years and they were followed up for an average of 3.8 years. Patients receiving intensive treatment had significantly lower rates for progression to nephropathy with a reduction by 73% for this primary end-point and similar reductions in the secondary end-points with progression of retinopathy reduced by 55% and progression of autonomic neuropathy reduced by 68%. To achieve these benefits 48 of 76 patients received antihypertensive treatment in the standard group compared with 71 of 73 patients in the intensive group who finished the study. Correspondingly, lipid-lowering drugs administered to 33 of 73 patients in the intensive group compared with only two in the standard group. Furthermore, aspirin was administered to 31 in the intensive group but only 17 in the standard group. Overall, the results for the major risk factors were as follows. There was a significantly greater reduction in BP in the intensive group by 8/7 mmHg compared with 4/5 mmHg but there were also significant reductions in cholesterol by 0.6 mmol/l compared with 0.2 mmol/l, in glycated haemoglobin with a reduction by 0.8% in the intensive group compared with an increase of 0.2% in the standard group and a reduction in fasting glucose by 2.7 mmol compared with 0.3 mmol/l.

Although not a primary end-point of the study it is interesting to note that these multifactorial interventions were also associated with a trend towards improved outcome with mortality and major macrovascular events numbering 26 in the intensive group compared with 42 in the standard group.

Conclusion

Preservation of renal function remains an important component of the treatment strategy in diabetic hypertensives. As with atherosclerotic cardiovascular disease itself, improvement in all the major cardiovascular risk factors produces the greatest overall benefit.

Microalbuminuria and diabetic nephropathy

It is well recognized that BP reduction is necessary for the preservation of renal function in most types of renal impairment particularly diabetic nephropathy. Diabetes, usually complicated by hypertension, continues to be numerically the most important cause of end-stage renal failure and much recent research has focused attention on how best to maintain renal function and improve patient outcome. There remains considerable debate, however, about the 'best' treatment regimen and whether or not different drug types have specifically beneficial or adverse properties. Despite the evidence from the UKPDS that BP reduction is beneficial in these high-risk patients, there also remain questions about the optimal BP targets and the most effective drug treatment strategies for not only preserving renal function but also improving patient outcome in terms of reducing cardiovascular morbidity and mortality.

The overall treatment emphasis in both type 1 and type 2 diabetes mellitus remains good BP control but the debate continues as to whether or not ACE inhibitors have benefits beyond the haemodynamic. It has been suggested that this is particularly important in type 1 diabetes and of potential importance even in patients who are normotensive. This concept of preserving kidney function and delaying the progression from microalbuminuria to frank diabetic nephropathy has recently been further studied with captopril.

Randomized controlled trial of long-term efficacy of captopril on preservation of kidney function

Randomized controlled trial of long-term efficacy of captopril on preservation of kidney function in normotensive patients with insulin-dependent diabetes and microalbuminuria.
E R Mathieson, E Hommel, H P Hansen, U M Smidt, H-H Parving.
BMJ 1999; **319**: 24–5.

BACKGROUND. In patients with insulin-dependent diabetes, ACE inhibition delays the progression from microalbuminuria to diabetic nephropathy, but previous studies have been too short to show a preservation of kidney function.

INTERPRETATION. This study assessed the effectiveness of ACE inhibition to preservation of kidney function in an 8-year prospective, randomized controlled trial.

Comment

This is a small-scale but well conducted study of 44 normotensive patients with type 1 diabetes who were followed up for a period of 8 years. The treatment group ($n = 21$) received captopril (100 mg per 24 h) and bendrofluazide (2.5 mg per 24 h), whereas the untreated group ($n = 23$) continued without antihypertensive medication. Glomerular filtration rate declined by 11.8 ml/min in the untreated group and by 1.4 ml/min in the captopril group ($P = 0.09$) and the proportion of patient who progressed to diabetic nephropathy was 40% in the control group and 10% in the captopril group ($P = 0.019$). These authors concluded that the ACE inhibitor had a clinically significant effect on the preservation of normal glomerular filtration rate by virtue of the prevention of progression from micro-albuminuria to diabetic nephropathy. Unfortunately, the question as to whether or not there are benefits beyond the haemodynamic cannot be clearly answered by this study. In particular, although the patients were defined as normotensive, no information is provided about the baseline and achieved BP values in either group.

Conclusion

The established facts are that intensive antihypertensive treatment and 'tight' BP control improve both renal and cardiovascular outcome in patients with diabetic nephropathy. It is assumed that similar 'tight' BP control will also improve outcome in other forms of renal disease. On the basis of the available evidence it appears that an appropriate treatment target is a BP of less than 135/85 mmHg.

The choice of antihypertensive drug

An ACE inhibitor is generally regarded as the first choice antihypertensive agent for a patient with diabetes and hypertension. In contrast, there has been considerable controversy about the role of calcium channel blockers with some reports of adverse outcomes, particularly in two recent small-scale clinical trials.

Outcome results of the Fosinopril versus Amlodipine Cardiovascular Events randomized Trial (FACET) in patients with hypertension and NIDDM.

P Tatti, M Pahor, R P Byington, *et al*. *Diabetes Care* 1998; **21**: 597–603.

BACKGROUND. ACE inhibitors and calcium antagonists may favourably affect serum lipids and glucose metabolism. The primary aim of the Fosinopril versus Amlodipine Cardiovascular Events randomized Trial (FACET) was to compare the effects of fosinopril and amlodipine on serum lipids and diabetes control in non-insulin-dependent diabetes mellitus patients with hypertension.

INTERPRETATION. Fosinopril and amlodipine had similar effects on biochemical measures, but the patients randomized to fosinopril had a significantly lower risk of major vascular events, compared with patients randomized to amlodipine.

Comment

FACET was not designed or statistically empowered to assess treatment-related differences in cardiovascular outcomes. The salient result was that the ACE inhibitor treatment (fosinopril) was associated with a significantly lower cardiovascular event rate than the calcium channel blocker group (amlodipine) (Table 4.4). However, this combined end-point was a secondary end-point and, once the data were correctly adjusted for multiple statistical comparisons, this difference lost its statistical significance.

Table 4.4 FACET trial: post-randomization analysis

	Amlodipine *n* = 141	Fosinopril *n* = 131	Combination *n* = 108
MI	13	7	3
Stroke	10	3	1
Hospitalized angina	4	0	0
All major events	27*	10	4

*$P < 0.01$ *vs* fosinopril *vs* combination.

Source: Tatti *et al*. (1998).

Interestingly, and importantly, the combination of the calcium channel blocker and the ACE inhibitor, relative to the effectiveness of either agent alone, appeared to be the most effective for reducing cardiovascular events. Overall, therefore, it seems unlikely that this long-acting calcium channel blocker was inherently dangerous for diabetic hypertensives.

The effect of nisoldipine as compared with enalapril on cardiovascular outcomes in patients with non-insulin-dependent diabetes and hypertension.

R O Estacio, B W Jeffers, W R Hiatt, *et al. N Engl J Med.* 1998; **338**: 645–52.

BACKGROUND. It has recently been reported that the use of calcium channel blockers for hypertension may be associated with an increased risk of cardiovascular complications. Because this issue remains controversial, the authors studied the incidence of such complication in patients with non-insulin-dependent diabetes mellitus and hypertension who were randomly assigned to treatment with either the calcium channel blocker nisoldipine or the ACE inhibitor enalapril as part of a larger study.

INTERPRETATION. In this population of patients with diabetes and hypertension, there was a significantly higher incidence of fatal and non-fatal MI among those assigned to therapy with the calcium channel blocker nisoldipine than among those assigned to receive enalapril. As these findings are based on a secondary end-point, they will require confirmation.

Comment

The Appropriate Blood Pressure Control in Diabetes Trial contained a hypertensive cohort and a normotensive cohort. The hypertensive study was terminated prematurely on the basis of apparently adverse outcomes in the patients receiving a calcium channel blocker (nisoldipine) rather than an ACE inhibitor (enalapril). However, a close scrutiny of the statistical analysis reveals that two significant differences had been identified between the two treatments in respect of the primary and secondary end-points. However, this represented two differences out of 36 end-points tested and this is precisely what would be expected to occur by chance.

Conclusion

These two trials must be interpreted with caution. The results are certainly compatible with the prevailing view that ACE inhibitors are probably to be preferred as first-line antihypertensive agents for the hypertensive diabetic. However, there is no convincing evidence that calcium channel blockers are actually harmful and, as 'tight' BP control will require multiple drug treatments, there is some evidence that the combination of an ACE inhibitor and a calcium channel blocker is effective and beneficial. Furthermore, the effectiveness of treatment regimens based upon dihydropyridine calcium channel blockers has already been confirmed in the subgroup analysis of large-scale prospective clinical outcome trials such as SYST-EUR and HOT.

Insulin responsiveness and treatment effects

Insulin resistance is recognized as a feature of type 2 diabetes mellitus, and also of untreated essential hypertension and it is generally accepted that conventional doses of thiazide diuretics and beta-blockers may further worsen this problem and amplify the underlying metabolic disturbances of lipid and glucose metabolism. In contrast there is a popular belief that ACE inhibitors have beneficial effects on insulin responsiveness. Although numerous studies in the literature have reported beneficial effects of ACE inhibition on aspects of glucose metabolism, only one published trial has incorporated all of the following features:

1. A double blind placebo controlled cross-over design.

2. Assessment of insulin responsiveness (sensitivity) using a highly reproducible technique.

3. Adequate statistical power for avoiding clinically important type 2 errors.

4. Reliable exclusion of potentially confounding carry-over effects.

Captopril does not improve insulin action in essential hypertension: a double-blind placebo-controlled study.
M I Wiggam, S J Hunter, A B Atkinson, *et al. J Hypertens* 1998; **16**: 1651–7.

BACKGROUND. The objective of this study was to compare the effect of captopril with that of placebo on peripheral and hepatic insulin action in essential hypertension, in the light of evidence that insulin resistance is associated with cardiovascular risk.

INTERPRETATION. Captopril therapy in uncomplicated essential hypertension has no effect on peripheral or hepatic insulin sensitivity.

Comment

This was a double blind placebo-controlled study designed to evaluate the effect of captopril on peripheral and hepatic insulin action in patients with essential hypertension. Eighteen hypertensive, non-diabetic patients, aged under 65 years, received captopril 50 mg twice daily or placebo for two 8-week treatment periods separated by a 6-week washout phase. For the 14 patients who completed the study there were no differences in fasting levels of glucose and insulin and postabsorptive hepatic glucose production was similar. During the hyperinsulinaemic euglycaemic clamp it was shown that hepatic glucose production was suppressed to comparable levels after captopril and after placebo and the glucose uptake rates were also similar at 30.0 ± 2.6 with captopril and 30.3 ± 2.6 mmol/kg per min with placebo. These authors concluded that captopril treatment had no effect on peripheral or hepatic insulin sensitivity.

Conclusion

Despite the early reports that ACE inhibitor drugs improve insulin responsiveness the accumulated evidence suggests that this is not the case. The majority of these studies have had methodological shortcomings and there are more negative or neutral reports than positive reports. Furthermore, glycaemic control and hypo-glycaemic episodes were no different in the captopril group compared with the atenolol group in UKPDS.

Conclusion

In the light of recent reports, there has been a clear change in emphasis in the treat-ment of hypertensive diabetic patients in so far as 'tight' BP control is considered to be essential and the benefits of BP reduction have now been confirmed in a number of clinical outcome trials. Of additional interest is the emerging concept that, while ACE inhibition will remain as the cornerstone of antihypertensive drug treatment in this patient group, the maximum benefits may be achieved through 'tight' BP control and pronounced BP reductions independently of the pharmacological characteristics of any particular antihypertensive drug. However, it is not only BP control that is important. Intensive management of all risk factors safely and effec-tively reduces the risk of the chronic complications of diabetes.

References

1. DCCT Research Group. The effect of intensive treatment of diabetes on the development and progression of long-term complications insulin-dependent diabetes mellitus. *N Engl J Med* 1993; **329:** 977–86.
2. Ohkubo Y, Kishikawa H, Araki E, Miyata T, Isami S, Motoyoshi S, Kojima Y. Intensive insulin therapy prevents the progression of diabetic microvascular complications in Japanese patients with non-insulin-dependent diabetes mellitus: a randomized prospec-tive 6-year study. *Diabetes Res Clin Pract* 1995; **28:** 103–17.

3. Shepherd J, Cobbe SM, Ford I, Isles CG, Lorimer AR, Macfarlane PW, McKillop JH, Packard CJ. Prevention of coronary heart disease with pravastatin in men with hypercholesterolaemia. *N Engl J Med* 1995; **333**: 1301–7.

5

Lipid-lowering treatment: status report

Introduction

The benefits of lipid-lowering drug treatment, particularly with 'statins', are well established in the primary and secondary prevention of coronary artery disease. Since the publication of the 'landmark' Scandinavian Simvastatin Survival Study (4S) |1| in 1994 there have been further major clinical outcome studies in both:

- Primary prevention: West of Scotland Coronary Prevention Study (WOSCOPS; 1995), |2| Air Force/Texas Coronary Atherosclerosis Prevention Study (AFCAPS/TexCAPS; 1998);

- Secondary prevention: Cholesterol and Recurrent Events (CARE; 1996) and Long-term Intervention with Pravastatin in Ischaemic Disease Study (LIPID; 1998).

Of additional and particular interest have been several recent studies investigating underlying pathophysiological mechanisms and also the benefits of cholesterol reduction in specific patient groups. Unfortunately, particularly in the UK, the widespread applicability of this important therapeutic strategy continues to be complicated by issues of cost and cost-effectiveness. While there is no dispute about the fundamental merit of targeting resources to those patients at greatest risk, there continues to be considerable debate about the appropriate 'cut-off' level of risk for which drug treatment can and should justifiably be prescribed.

Clinical outcome trials

Primary prevention

Primary prevention of acute coronary events with lovastatin in men and women with average cholesterol levels.
J R Downs, M Clearfield, S Weis, *et al. JAMA* 1998; **279**: 1615–22.

BACKGROUND. Although cholesterol-reducing treatment has been shown to reduce fatal and non-fatal coronary disease in patients with coronary heart disease (CHD), it is unknown whether benefit from the reduction of low-density lipoprotein (LDL) cholesterol in patients without CHD extends to individuals with average serum cholesterol levels, women and older persons. Its aim was to compare lovastatin with placebo for prevention of the first acute major coronary event in men and women without clinically evident atherosclerotic cardiovascular disease with average total cholesterol (TC) and LDL cholesterol levels and below-average high-density lipoprotein (HDL) cholesterol levels.

INTERPRETATION. Lovastatin reduces the risk for the first acute major coronary event in men and women with average TC and LDL cholesterol levels and below-average HDL cholesterol levels. These findings support the inclusion of HDL cholesterol in risk factor assessment, confirm the benefit of LDL cholesterol reduction to a target goal, and suggest the need for reassessment of the National Cholesterol Education Program guidelines regarding pharmacological intervention.

Comment

This primary prevention study—AFCAPS/TexCAPS—was a randomized double-blind placebo-controlled trial involving 6605 subjects (of whom 997 were women) who had 'average' lipid levels. The average age of the participants was 58 years with 22% aged 65 years or more. All subjects were advised to continue with a low saturated fat, low cholesterol diet and then they were randomly assigned to lovastatin (20–40 mg daily) or placebo. After an average follow-up of 5.2 years there were significant reductions in all the major end-points, both primary and secondary (Table 5.1).

Table 5.1 Primary and secondary endpoints in AFCAPS/Tex CAPS

End-points	Event rate (per 1000 patient years)		Relative risk reduction	P
	Placebo	Lovastatin		
Primary (fatal/non-fatal MI, unstable angina, sudden cardiac death)	10.9	6.8	37%	< 0.001
Secondary				
Cardiovascular events	15.3	11.5	25%	< 0.003
CHD Events	12.8	9.6	25%	< 0.006
Revascularization	9.3	6.2	33%	< 0.001
MI	5.6	3.3	40%	< 0.002
Unstable angina	5.1	3.5	32%	< 0.02
Fatal Cardiovascular events	1.4	1.0	–	–
Fatal CHD events	0.9	0.6	–	–

Source: Downs *et al.* (1998).

Overall, the reductions in CHD events and coronary intervention procedures by 40% and 33%, respectively, in AFCAPS/TexCAPS were remarkably similar to the corresponding reductions of 31% and 37% in the WOSCOPS study. Also remarkably similar were the percentage changes in lipid fractions (see Fig. 5.1) even although the average pre-treatment cholesterol values were different: 7.0 and 5.7 mmol/l in WOSCOPS and AFCAPS/TexCAPS, respectively.

The results of this study are confirmatory and reassuring. First, this is the first primary prevention study to include women (albeit, in the minority) and it is important to note that women benefited from treatment to at least as great an extent as men. Secondly, benefit was apparent across all baseline levels (tertiles) of cholesterol (across the range 2.33–6.0 mmol/l) with no evidence to suggest a threshold level. Of additional interest was the finding that absolute benefit was greatest in those at greatest risk: for example, the event rate was approximately twice as great in those with concomitant hypertension and the relative risk reduction for a first primary end-point event tended to be greater at 39% in the hypertensives compared with 27% in the normotensive subjects.

Finally, however, even in patients with low absolute CHD risk (less than 10% per 10 years) there was a statistically significant reduction in the number of end-points. In terms of 'evidence', therefore, patients with a CHD risk of as low as 7% per 10 years would benefit from statin treatment.

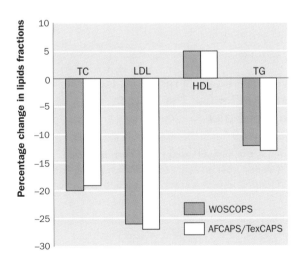

Fig. 5.1 Comparison of percentage changes in lipid fractions in WOSCOPS and AFCAPS/TexCAPS. TC = total serum cholesterol; LDL = low-density lipoprotein; HDL = high-density lipoprotein; TG = triglyceride. Source: Downs *et al.* (1998).

Secondary prevention

Early statin treatment following acute myocardial infarction and 1-year survival.

U Stenestrand, L Wallentin, for the Swedish Register of Cardiac Intensive Care. *JAMA* 2001; **285**: 430–6.

BACKGROUND. Randomization trials have established statin treatment as secondary prevention in coronary artery disease, but it is unclear whether early treatment with statins following acute myocardial infarction (MI) influences survival.

INTERPRETATION. Early initiation of statin treatment in patients with acute MI is associated with reduced 1-year mortality. These results emphasize the importance of implementing the results of randomized statin trials in unselected acute MI patients.

Comment

This was a prospective cohort study in almost 20 000 patients who had been admitted to the coronary care units of hospitals in Sweden during 1995 through 1998. The principal outcome measure was the mortality at 1 year in those patients younger than 80 years who were discharged alive from hospital following a first recorded acute MI. At or before discharge, 5528 patients had received statins whereas 14 071 patients had not. In the no-statin group the unadjusted mortality was 9.3% compared with 4% in the statin treatment group. After adjustment for confounding factors, there was a 25% relative risk reduction in association with early statin treatment and this benefit was independent of age, sex, baseline characteristics, previous disease manifestations and other medications.

Effects of atorvastatin on early recurrent ischemic events in acute coronary syndromes. The MIRACL study: a randomised controlled trial.

G G Schwartz, A G Olsson, M D Ezekowitz, *et al. JAMA* 2001; **285**: 1711–18.

BACKGROUND. Patients experience the highest rate of death and recurrent ischaemic events during the early period after an acute coronary syndrome, but it is not known whether early initiation of treatment with a statin can reduce the occurrence of these early events.

INTERPRETATION. For patients with acute coronary syndrome, lipid-lowering therapy with atorvastatin, 80 mg/day, reduces recurrent ischaemic events in the first 16 weeks, mostly recurrent symptomatic ischaemia requiring rehospitalization.

Comment

MIRACL (Myocardial Ischaemia Reduction with Aggressive Cholesterol Lowering) was a randomized double-blind study in 3086 patients who were hospitalized for unstable angina or non-Q wave MI. Within 24–96 h after admission patients were randomly assigned to a conventional lipid-lowering diet and placebo or to the diet plus atorvastatin 80 mg daily for 16 weeks. Relative to the placebo group, atorvastatin treatment was associated with a 34% reduction in TC, a 52% reduction in LDL cholesterol and a 9% increase in HDL cholesterol. There was a significant relative risk reduction by 16% in the primary efficacy measure that comprised non-fatal MI, resuscitated cardiac arrest and worsening angina. The cumulative incidence of a primary end-point event was 17.4% over 16 weeks in the placebo group and 14.8% in the atorvastatin group. Of additional interest was the fact that there were also significant benefits for stroke prevention albeit in a small number of patients, with a 50% relative risk reduction.

While the results of this study are interesting and important in themselves, there is the additional consideration that MIRACL provided information that 'fills a gap' in the spectrum of coronary artery disease treatment. Thus, the picture is completed between so-called primary prevention with no history of coronary artery disease (as studied in the WOSCOPS and AFCAPS/TexCAPS studies) through to CARE, LIPID and 4S, which investigated patients with established coronary artery disease. Furthermore, the results of MIRACL not only confirm that lipid lowering is an effective treatment for patients with acute coronary syndromes, who arguably are at an early stage of the atherosclerotic process, but also that statins are safe and effective when initiated within the first few days of the acute coronary event.

Pravastatin therapy and the risk of stroke.

H D White, J Simes, N E Anderson, *et al. J Med* 2000; **343**: 317–26.

BACKGROUND. Several epidemiological studies have concluded that there is no relation between TC levels and the risk of stroke. In some studies that classified strokes according to cause, there was an association between increasing cholesterol levels and the risk of ischaemic stroke and a possible association between low cholesterol levels and the risk of haemorrhagic stroke. Recent reviews of trials of 3-hydroxy-3-methylglutaryl-coenzyme A reductase inhibitors have suggested that these agents may reduce risk of stroke.

INTERPRETATION. Pravastatin has a moderate effect in reducing the risk of stroke from any cause and the risk of non-haemorrhagic stroke in patients with previous MI or unstable angina.

Comment

This was a substudy within LIPID (1998) that assessed the impact of pravastatin treatment on stroke, which was a secondary end-point. A total of 9014 patients with known CHD were entered into this double-blind trial and over a follow-up period of 6 years there were 419 strokes among 373 patients. A total of 309 strokes were classified as ischaemic, 31 as haemorrhagic and 79 of unknown cause: 74%,

7% and 19% of stroke events, respectively. There was an overall, significant relative reduction by 19% with an incidence of 3.7% in those patients receiving pravastatin compared with 4.5% in those receiving placebo. For non-haemorrhagic stroke there was an overall significant relative reduction of 23% with incidences of 3.4 and 4.4.% in the pravastatin and placebo groups, respectively. Pravastatin had no effect on haemorrhagic stroke, albeit in small numbers of patients, with an incidence of 0.4% in the pravastatin group compared with 0.2% in the placebo group.

This result is entirely consistent with the findings in other secondary prevention studies. For example, in the 4S study |3| there was a 28% relative reduction in the combined end-point of stroke and transient ischaemic attack. In the CARE study, there was a 32% relative reduction in the incidence of stroke |4|. These benefits were achieved whether the rate of aspirin use was low (as in 4S) or high (as in LIPID and CARE). Furthermore, these results are consistent with previous meta-analyses of trials in statins in which there was a significantly lower rate of stroke (24–32% lower) in secondary prevention trials and a non-significantly lower rate (15–30%) in primary prevention trials |5,6|.

Conclusion

These recent studies have confirmed that improved lipid profiles, particularly in response to treatment with statins lead to cardiovascular benefits. It might now be considered that we have the final 'seal of approval' for lipid-lowering treatment in patients known to have CHD. The only significant medical issues that remain the subject of debate are 'What is the optimal target concentration for total and/or LDL cholesterol?' and 'How important are the concentrations of HDL cholesterol and trigyclerides?'.

From clinical trials to clinical practice

Despite the progressive accumulation of evidence that lipid-lowering drug treatment is particularly beneficial in high-risk patients, and especially in secondary prevention in patients known to have CHD, there continues to be a discrepancy between 'recommendation' and 'implementation' with respect to the prescription of lipid-lowering drugs in routine clinical practice. This applies not only in the UK but it is also apparent in the USA and in western Europe and in Asia.

Clinical reality of coronary prevention guidelines: a comparison of EUROASPIRE I and II in nine countries.
EUROASPIRE I and II Group. *Lancet* 2001; **357**: 995–1001.

B A C K G R O U N D . Patients with CHD are the top priority for preventative cardiology. The first EUROASPIRE survey among patients with established CHD in nine countries in 1995–96 showed substantial potential for risk reduction. A second survey

(EUROASPIRE II) was done in 1999–2000 in the same countries to see whether preventive cardiology had improved since the first. We compared the proportion of patients in both studies who achieved the life-style, risk factor and therapeutic goals recommended by the Joint European Societies report on coronary prevention.

INTERPRETATION. The adverse life-style trends among European CHD patients are a cause for concern, as is the lack of any improvement in blood pressure management, and the fact that most CHD patients are still not achieving the cholesterol goal of less than 5 mmol/l. There is a collective failure of medical practice in Europe to achieve the substantial potential among patients with CHD to reduce the risk of recurrent disease and death.

Comment

A total of 3569 were interviewed in the 1995–96 survey and 3379 patients in the 1999–2000 survey. In summary, the prevalence of smoking remained almost unchanged at 19.4% *vs* 20.8%, but the prevalence of obesity (body mass index > 30 kg/m^2) had increased substantially from 25.3% to 32.8%. The proportion of patients with high blood pressure (> 140/90 mmHg) remained essentially unchanged at about 55%, whereas the prevalence of high TC concentrations (>5 mmol/l) had decreased substantially from 86.2% to 58.8%. With particular respect to lipid-lowering drugs and the attainment of the goal of a TC of less than 5 mmol/l there had been an increase from 20.9% to 49.2% but cholesterol targets were attained in less than 45% of high-risk patients with known CHD.

Secondary prevention in 24 431 patients with coronary heart disease: survey in primary care.
A J B Brady, M A Oliver, J B Pittard. *BMJ* 2001; **322**: 1463.

BACKGROUND. Prevention of further cardiovascular events in patients with established CHD is a priority for public health. The Health-wise Survey was conducted in primary care throughout Britain to identify the prevalence of recorded coronary disease and to examine whether progress had been made in secondary preventive measures.

INTERPRETATION. Lipids were much less well managed than blood pressure. Most patients were hypercholesterolaemic or had been tested. Only a few were taking statins, despite evidence that these drugs are effective. It is also disappointing that so few patients with a previous MI were receiving beta-blockers, drugs that are proved to reduce ventricular tachycardia, and that about half of the patients with heart failure in this study were prescribed angiotensin-converting enzyme inhibitors.

Comment

This survey was undertaken in 548 UK practices in patients known to have a diagnosis of coronary disease. In this high-risk population 35% of men and 52% of women had no recorded cholesterol measurement and 47% of men and 40% of women had a TC greater than 5 mmol/l. Only 18% and 13% of women were receiving treatment with a statin.

Lipid concentrations and the use of lipid lowering drugs: evidence from a national cross sectional survey.
P Primatesta, N R Poulter. *BMJ* 2000; **321**: 1322–5.

BACKGROUND. To evaluate the prevalence of the use of lipid-lowering agents and its relation to blood lipid concentrations in English adults.

INTERPRETATION. Despite the high prevalence of dyslipidaemia in English adults, the proportion of adults taking lipid-lowering drugs in 1998 was only 2.2%. Rates of treatment were low among high-risk patients eligible for primary prevention with lipid-lowering drugs, and less than one-third of patients with established cardiovascular disease received such treatment.

Comment

This was a cross-sectional survey undertaken throughout England in 1998 and involving 13 586 adults. In the survey, 385 adults were eligible for lipid-lowering treatment because of a history of CHD but only 30% were taking lipid-lowering treatment and of those on drug treatment only 44% had a total concentration of less than 5 mmol/l. Correspondingly, of those 117 patients who were eligible for a lipid-lowering drug treatment because of a 10-year risk of CHD of greater than 30% only four (3%) were receiving lipid-lowering treatment.

Conclusion

Although there is some evidence of improvement, these results are essentially disappointing. In EUROASPIRE and in the survey in England less than 50% of high-risk patients achieved target. Perhaps of greater concern, is that the emphasis on high-risk patients (secondary prevention) may be detracting from the primary prevention strategy in so far as only 3% of eligible patients were receiving treatment.

Practical aspects of lipid-lowering strategies

The volume and consistency of the evidence derived from studies of different 'statin' drugs underlies their position as the most commonly prescribed lipid-lowering medication. In contrast, the early clinical outcome trials with bile acid sequestrant resins (cholestyramine) and fibrates (clofibrate and gemfibrozil) created a confused picture. Nevertheless, despite the recent positive evidence with statins, a number of important practical issues remain to be definitively resolved and clarified. For example, although the magnitude of the reductions in TC and

LDL cholesterol achieved with statins is generally superior to those obtained through dietary efforts, dietary modifications or life-style intervention continue to be recommended as the initial and cornerstone approach to improving lipid profiles. At present, the following are among the major practical issues:

1. The role of dietary modification.

2. The relevance of hypertriglyceridaemia and other lipid-lowering treatments.

3. The threshold and target levels for TC and LDL cholesterol treatment.

4. The choice of the optimal, or most cost-effective, statin treatment.

Dietary modifications

Systematic review of dietary intervention trials to lower blood total cholesterol in free-living subjects.

J L Tang, J M Armitage, T Lancaster, *et al. BMJ* 1998; **316**: 1213–20.

BACKGROUND. To estimate the efficacy of dietary advice to lower blood and TC concentration in free-living subjects and to investigate the efficacy of different dietary recommendations.

INTERPRETATION. Individualized dietary advice for reducing cholesterol concentration is modestly effective in free-living subjects. More intensive diets achieve a greater reduction in serum cholesterol concentrations. Failure to comply fully with dietary recommendations is the likely explanation for this limited efficacy.

This analysis indicates that the effectiveness of dietary intervention, in the patient with 'average' motivation is of modest effectiveness, with TC reductions in the range of 5–10%, at best. This result does not negate the value of dietary modification but places it in a practical perspective.

Despite good compliance, very low fat diet alone does not achieve recommended cholesterol goals in outpatients with coronary heart disease.

R Aquilani, R Tramarin, R F E Pedretti, *et al. Eur Heart J* 1999; **20**: 1020–9.

BACKGROUND. A low saturated fat, low cholesterol diet is important in the treatment of hypercholesterolaemia in patients with CHD. The aim of this study was to investigate the efficacy of a very low fat diet to achieve a targeted serum LDL cholesterol level ≤ 2.59 mmol/l in outpatients with CHD.

INTERPRETATION. Diet alone does not allow patients with CHD to achieve the recommended blood cholesterol levels, even if its fat content is highly reduced.

This is an interesting study in 126 male patients who were all ex-smokers and with known CHD. They were carefully assessed in terms of energy expenditure and then assigned to four different treatment groups: group A were instructed in a low fat diet (related to their energy expenditure); group B were on a standard low fat diet as described by the National Cholesterol Education Programme (step 2 diet); and groups C and D had the corresponding diets augmented by simvastatin 10 mg daily. All patients were set a target LDL cholesterol of < 2.59 mmol/l and the effectiveness of the different treatment regimens was assessed after 6 months.

The average decrease in serum LDL cholesterol did not differ between group A and group B but neither of these dietary regimens proved capable of reaching the target. The only significant difference between the two diets was that there was a significant increase by 29% in HDL cholesterol in group A, which obviously led to a significant reduction in the LDL/HDL cholesterol ratio. Obviously the drug treatments were more effective in reducing TC and LDL cholesterol than dietary intervention alone.

Comment

The target of LDL cholesterol < 2.59 mmol/l set a very demanding test for the efficacy of dietary modification to reduce cholesterol. The average changes in TC and LDL cholesterol were modest in the two dietary regimens, –13 and –18%, respectively, in the more rigorous diet and –5 and –6%, respectively, on the standard step 2 diet. None of these patients with dietary restriction alone achieved the primary target of LDL cholesterol < 2.59 mmol/l. The step 2 diet corresponds approximately to the 'usual' lipid-lowering diets that are widely applied and the reduction of 5% for TC and 6% for LDL cholesterol is typical of what has been reported elsewhere. For the target LDL cholesterol of < 3.37 mmol/l, in this study, only 26% achieved target with the rigorous diet and 0% (again) reached target with the standard step 2 diet.

Conclusion

In an apparently well conducted study in a relatively well motivated patient group, the effectiveness of standard dietary intervention was modest at best. The overall conclusion from each of these publications is that dietary modification may be sufficient in an individual patient to produce a worthwhile reduction in cholesterol but, and especially if rigorous targets are set, drug treatment will inevitably be required for the great majority of patients.

Dietary fat intake and prevention of cardiovascular disease: systematic review.
L Hooper, C D Summerbell, J P T Higgins, *et al. BMJ* 2001; **322**: 757–63.

BACKGROUND. To assess the effect of reduction or modification of dietary fat intake on total and cardiovascular mortality and cardiovascular morbidity.

INTERPRETATION. There is a small but potentially important reduction in cardiovascular risk with reduction or modification of dietary fat intake, seen particularly in trials of longer duration.

This was a systematic review of 27 randomized controlled trials with the stated aim of reducing or modifying fat/cholesterol intake in healthy adult participants. Overall, alterations of dietary fat intake were associated with a significant reduction in total mortality and cardiovascular mortality, by 2% and 9%, respectively, and a 14% reduction in cardiovascular events. However, in trials with at least 2 years follow up there was a significant 24% reduction in cardiovascular events.

Comment

Dietary change is likely to be useful but not definitive for reducing cholesterol in the majority of 'at-risk' patients. Nevertheless, the result in any single (motivated) individual may be sufficiently effective to avoid the need for drug treatment. The role of dietary modification, therefore, may be more important as a mechanism for 'involving' the patient in the overall risk reduction strategy.

Other lipid-lowering drugs

The fibrate drugs principally decrease serum triglycerides (often by about 30–40%) by several mechanisms one of which involves enhanced triglyceride clearance from the circulation by a process involving interaction of the fibrate with hepatic and adipocyte peroxisomal proliferator activator receptors. The effect on cholesterol is less than the effect on triglycerides and less than that obtained with statins. The results of further trials to define patients who may benefit more from a fibrate than a statin are awaited and, in the meantime, the principal indication for a fibrate is the treatment of severe hypertriglyceridaemia and for a fibrate–statin combination in some patients who are at particularly high coronary risk through elevations of both cholesterol and triglycerides. Combination treatment, however, must be closely monitored because of potential problems with adverse effects and the increased risk of myositis.

Gemfibrozil for the secondary prevention of coronary heart disease in men with low levels of high-density lipoprotein cholesterol.
H B Rubins, S J Robins, D Collins, *et al. N Engl J Med* 1999; **341**: 410–18.

BACKGROUND. Although it is generally accepted that lowering elevated serum levels of LDL cholesterol in patients with CHD is beneficial, there are a few data to guide decisions about therapy for patients whose primary lipid abnormality is a low level of HDL cholesterol.

INTERPRETATION. Gemfibrozil therapy resulted in a significant reduction in the risk of major cardiovascular events in patients with CHD whose primary lipid abnormality was a low HDL cholesterol level. The findings suggest that the rate of coronary events is reduced by raising HDL cholesterol levels and lowering levels of triglycerides without lowering LDL cholesterol levels.

Comment

Fibrates retain a role in the management of these patients with 'mixed' or severe dyslipidaemia, particularly where low HDL cholesterol concentrations are featured.

Conclusion

While the weight of evidence has clearly shown that reductions in LDL cholesterol lead to reductions in cardiovascular morbidity and mortality it must be borne in mind that approximately 40% of CHD patients do not have elevated levels of LDL cholesterol and many of them have low levels of HDL cholesterol. In fact, about 25% of patients with coronary disease have a low HDL cholesterol in the absence of an elevated LDL cholesterol [7] . This study with gemfibrozil introduces a further dimension to our approaches to the management of dyslipidaemia. Thus, even in the presence of a total of LDL cholesterol measurement that might be considered to be low or normal there was clear benefit from a drug treatment that increased the HDL concentration. In this study there was no change in LDL cholesterol, whereas HDL cholesterol was increased by 6% and triglycerides were reduced by 31%. This translated to a 22% relative reduction in non-fatal MI and cardiac death and a 29% reduction in stroke. Of particular interest was the high prevalence of features of the metabolic syndrome (insulin resistance, glucose intolerance or diabetes mellitus, hypertension and obesity). Again this finding is consistent with previous studies, such as the Helsinki Heart Study, which identified that the treatment effect of gemfibrozil as a primary preventative strategy was largely confined to patients who were overweight or who had low HDL cholesterol and high triglycerides [8].

Treatment targets

There is strong evidence to support the use of lipid-lowering drugs, and statins in particular, in those patients at high absolute risk of CHD. Once the treatment decision has been made, the target should be a cholesterol of less than 5 mmol/l in both primary and secondary prevention.

The evidence of benefit is strongest in secondary prevention in those patients known to have CHD and a TC value of greater than 5 mmol/l or LDL cholesterol of greater than 3 mmol/l.

Patients with other major atherosclerotic disease (in the absence of overt coronary disease), for example, those with peripheral vascular disease or cerebro-vascular disease should be managed in the same way as those with overt CHD (i.e. secondary prevention), although there is no direct clinical trial evidence of benefit. Thus, the benefits in high-risk CHD patients, which are supported by evidence, are extrapolated to other high-risk patients with established atherosclerotic cardio-vascular disease.

Table 5.2 Cardiovascular risk factor

Cardiovascular risk factor	Threshold for initiation of dietary therapy		Threshold for initiation of drug therapy risk factor	
	Total cholesterol mg/dl (mmol/l)	LDL cholesterol mg/dl (mmol/l)	Total cholesterol mg/dl (mmol/l)	LDL cholesterol mg/dl (mmol/l)
0 or 1 risk factors	240 (6.24)	160 (4.16)	275 (7.15)	190 (4.94)
2 or more risk factors	200 (5.2)	130 (3.38)	240 (6.24)	160 (4.16)
Established cardiovascular disease	160 (4.16)	100 (2.6)	200 (5.2)	130 (3.38)

Source: Knopp (1999).

Drug treatment of lipid disorders.
R H Knopp. *N Engl J Med* 1999; **341**: 498–510.

B A C K G R O U N D . **Arteriosclerosis of the coronary and peripheral vasculature is the leading cause of death among men and women in the USA and world-wide.**

I N T E R P R E T A T I O N . Cardiovascular disease accounts for nearly 50% of all deaths in the USA. Clinical trials and pathophysiological evidence support the use of aggressive therapy in patients with arteriosclerotic vascular disease and in those with several risk factors for the disease. Combination therapy with lipid-lowering drugs is advisable, especially in patients with combined hyperlipidaemia.

Comment

This review article summarizes the evidence to date and recommends treatment according to the thresholds shown in Table 5.2. It is likely that these thresholds will be revised to lower values in the near future and, although there are not yet prospective studies from which targets can be clearly defined, the general view is 'the lower the better'.

Attaining United States and European guideline LDL-cholesterol levels with simvastatin in patients with coronary heart disease (the GOALLS study).
F Garmendia, A S Brown, I Reiber, P C Adams. *Curr Med Res Opin* 2000; **16**: 208–19.

BACKGROUND. The effectiveness and safety of simvastatin in reducing LDL cholesterol to target levels in patients with CHD were evaluated in the GOALLS (Getting to Appropriate LDL cholesterol Levels with Simvastatin) study.

INTERPRETATION. These goals were similarly achieved for a variety of high-risk subgroups (hypertensive, diabetes and elderly patients).

Comment

This was a prospective study in 198 patients with documented CHD. Patients received dietary advice for 6 weeks prior to assignment to a 14-week period of treatment with simvastatin. Patients were commenced on 20 mg daily with dose titration up to 80 mg daily if the LDL cholesterol remained above 100 mg/dl (2.6 mmol/l) at weeks six and ten. After 14 weeks of simvastatin (20–80 mg), approximately 90% of the patients achieved the LDL cholesterol goals according to the US and European guidelines (87% and 94%, respectively). An estimated 14% of the patients required titration to the 80 mg dose. Overall, the mean reductions in TC and LDL cholesterol were 28% and 41%, respectively. The increase in HDL cholesterol was approximately 4%.

An assessment of the efficacy of atorvastatin in achieving LDL cholesterol target levels in patients with coronary heart disease: a general practice study.

H Neil, G Fowler, H Patel, Z Eminton, S Maton. *Int J Clin Pract* 1999; **53**: 422–6.

BACKGROUND. Adherence to evidence-based guidelines for the secondary prevention of CHD has been shown to be poor in a number of surveys.

INTERPRETATION. Achieving LDL cholesterol targets (with atorvastatin) without the need for dose titration simplifies clinical management and should encourage better adherence to evidence-based recommendations for secondary prevention of CHD.

Comment

This was an open label, non-comparative study in 399 patients with existing CHDs and an LDL cholesterol concentration greater than 3.4 mmol/l. The simple target of a reduction to less than 3.4 mmol/l was achieved by 94% of patients on the initial dosages of 10 mg daily. Half of the 23 patients titrated to higher doses of atorvastatin achieved the target LDL cholesterol after 17 weeks.

Which statin? The choice of the optimal, or most cost-effective statin treatment

This is a topical issue because of the potential cost implications if all at-risk patients are prescribed lipid-lowering drug treatment. Unfortunately, there are no definitive, comparative studies, although the balance of evidence suggests that, across the recommended dose ranges, atorvastatin is the most effective.

Comparative dose efficacy study of atorvastatin, lovastatin, and fluvastatin in patients with hypercholesterolaemia (the CURVES study).

P Jones, S Kafonek, I Laurora, D Hunnginghake. *Am J Cardiol* 1998; **81**: 582–7.

BACKGROUND. The objective of this multicentre, randomized, open-label, parallel group, 8-week study was to evaluate the comparative dose efficacy of the 3-hydroxy-3-methyl-glutaryl coenzyme A reductase inhibitor atorvastatin 10, 20, 40 and 80 mg compared with simvastatin 10, 20 and 40 mg, pravastatin 10, 20 and 40 mg, lovastatin 20, 40 and 80 mg, and fluvastatin 20 and 40 mg.

INTERPRETATION. Atorvastatin 10, 20 and 40 mg produced a greater ($P \leq 0.01$) reduction in LDL cholesterol (–38%, –46% and –51%, respectively) than the milligram equivalent dose of simvastatin, pravastatin, lovastatin and fluvastatin. Atorvastatin 10 mg produced LDL cholesterol reductions comparable with or greater than simvastatin 10, 20 and 40 mg ($P < 0.02$), pravastatin 10, 20 and 40 mg, lovastatin 20 and 40 mg, and fluvastatin 20 and 40 mg. Atorvastatin 10, 20 and 40 mg produced greater reductions in TC ($P < 0.01$) than the milligram equivalent doses of simvastatin, pravastatin, lovastatin and fluvastatin. All reductase inhibitors studied had similar tolerability. There was no incidence of persistent elevations in serum transaminases or myositis.

Comment

This study evaluated the responses to five different agents in a total of 534 hyper-cholesterolaemic patients. The principal results are shown in Fig. 5.2 where it can be seen that fluvastatin consistently produced the smallest reductions in LDL cholesterol, whereas atorvastatin consistently produced the greatest reductions in LDL cholesterol. While it might be assumed that atorvastatin is the most powerful lipid-lowering agent it is necessary to modify this conclusion with the rider of 'at the doses studied'. Thus, it may simply be a reflection of the fact that the recom-mended dose range for atorvastatin appears to have encompassed the lipid-lowering potential of this agent, whereas the dose ranges of most of the other agents may be at relatively and inappropriately low points on their dose–response curves.

Atorvastatin compared with simvastatin-based therapies in the management of severe familial hyperlipidaemias.

A S Wierzbicki, P J Lumb, Y Semra, *et al. Q J Med* 1999; **92**: 387–94.

BACKGROUND. We compared atorvastatin with simvastatin-based therapies in a prospective observational study of 201 patients with severe hyperlipidaemia.

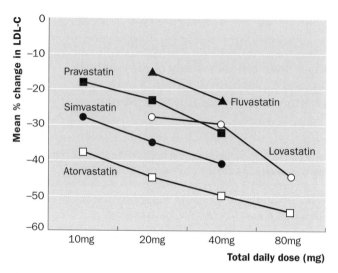

Fig. 5.2 Comparative dose efficacy of atorvastatin, fluvastatin, lovastatin, pravastatin and simvastatin in patients with hypercholesterolaemiaLDL-C = low-density lipoprotein cholesterol. Source: CURVES study, Jones *et al.* (1998).

INTERPRETATION. These data suggest that atorvastatin is more effective than current simvastatin-based therapies in achieving treatment targets in patients with familial hypercholesterolaemia but at the expense of a possible increase in side-effects. This issue needs further study in randomized controlled trials.

Comment

It is well recognized that patients with severe hyperlipidaemias, and typically those with familial hypercholesterolaemia or combined hyperlipidaemia, have a poor prognosis because of the difficulties of achieving aggressive and effective cholesterol reductions. In this study, treatment based on atorvastatin (10–20 mg daily) proved superior to simvastatin (20–40 mg) treatment in so far as it reduced LDL cholesterol by more than twice as much as simvastatin, with or without the addition of choles-tyramine. However, although atorvastatin is generally considered to be similar to other statins in respect of its profile of adverse effects, the results in this study indicated a slightly greater incidence. Depending upon the dose, 10–36% of patients reported adverse effects with atorvastatin. These authors concluded that, although atorvastatin was more effective, and particularly more effective at lower doses than simvastatin, there is an increased likelihood of adverse effects particu-larly with the highest dose of 80 mg.

Safety of low-density lipoprotein cholesterol reduction with atorvastatin versus simvastatin in a coronary heart disease population (the TARGET TANGIBLE trial).

W März, H Wollschläger, G Kleinm, A Neiß, M Wehling. *Am J Cardiol* 1999; **84**: 7–13.

BACKGROUND. Reduction in plasma lipids has been recognized as one of the primary cardiovascular risk reduction strategies in the secondary prevention of CHD. The primary end-points of TARGET TANGIBLE were the safety (adverse events and laboratory measurements) and efficacy (responder rates) of therapy with atorvastatin *vs* simvastatin with the aim of achieving LDL cholesterol lowering to ≤ 100 mg/dl (2.6 mmol/l).

INTERPRETATION. Atorvastatin resulted in a significantly greater number of patients reaching their LDL cholesterol goal than those treated with simvastatin, with 67% of atorvastatin patients and 53% of simvastatin patients reaching target LDL cholesterol level of ≤ 100 mg/dl (2.6 mmol/l) ($P < 0.001$). Some 2856 patients (of 3748 screened) with LDL cholesterol above 3.4 mmol/l were randomly assigned to treatment with atorvastatin or simvastatin for 14 weeks. These were patients with known CHD and treatment was generally well tolerated with only 2% of the atorvastatin patients and 3% of the simvastatin patients reporting serious adverse events. Overall adverse event rates were equivalent for atorvastatin and simvastatin at 36.3% and 35.7%, respectively. The principal efficacy measure showed that a significantly greater number of patients reached the LDL cholesterol goal with atorvastatin: 67% of atorvastatin patients compared with 53% of simvastatin reached the target LDL cholesterol level of < 2.6mmol/l. Correspondingly, significantly fewer patients in the atorvastatin group required titration to 40 mg: 38% of atorvastatin patients *vs* 54% of simvastatin patients.

Comment

This is an interesting study, which again demonstrates the overall efficacy and good tolerability of the statin group of drugs. On a milligram for milligram basis there is accumulating evidence that atorvastatin is the most effective of the currently available drugs. However, it remains unclear whether or not atorvastatin is intrinsically more potent, or whether it simply is a reflection that different statins have different effective dose ranges.

Efficacy of atorvastatin compared with simvastatin in patients with hypercholesterolaemia.

M Farnier, J-J Portal, P Maigret. *J Cardiovasc Pharmacol Ther* 2000; **5**: 27–32.

BACKGROUND. Atorvastatin, a new enantiomerically pure synthetic statin, has shown a marked LDL cholesterol reduction at doses ranging from 10 to 80 mg/day.

This trial was designed to compare the efficacy of atorvastatin 10 mg with simvastatin 10 mg and 20 mg, the latter dose being commonly used in some countries.

INTERPRETATION. In primary hypercholesterolaemia, atorvastatin 10 mg was more effective and non-equivalent to simvastatin 20 mg and significantly more effective than simvastatin 10 mg for reducing LDL cholesterol levels.

Comment

This was a parallel group comparison in 272 patients of atorvastatin 10 mg daily, simvastatin 10 mg daily and simvastatin 20 mg daily. The salient results were that atorvastatin 10 mg led to a 37% reduction in LDL cholesterol, whereas the corresponding values were 33.8% and 28.9% for simvastatin 20 mg and simvastatin 10 mg, respectively.

Conclusion

These studies illustrate the difficulties inherent in making simplistic assumptions about the comparability of different drugs especially when the doses may not be comparable on a milligram per milligram basis and especially when cost considerations assume an over-riding importance. Whether or not atorvastatin is the most effective of the available agents remains to be clearly established because, on the basis of current evidence, it may simply be that the recommended dosages for atorvastatin are more appropriately within the effective therapeutics range than the currently recommended dosages of comparator drugs.

The role of aggressive lipid-lowering treatment

Aggressive lipid-lowering therapy compared with angioplasty in stable coronary artery disease.
B Pitt, D Waters, W V Brown, et al. N Engl J Med 1999; **341**: 70–6.

BACKGROUND. Percutaneous coronary revascularization is widely used in improving symptoms and exercise performance in patients with ischaemic heart disease and stable angina pectoris. In this study, percutaneous coronary revascularization was compared with lipid-lowering treatment for reducing the incidence of ischaemic events.

INTERPRETATION. In low-risk patients with stable coronary artery disease, aggressive lipid-lowering therapy is at least as effective as angioplasty and usual care in reducing the incidence of ischaemic events.

Comment

This study in more than 300 patients with known coronary artery disease investigated the efficacy of medical treatment with atorvastatin (80 mg daily) or percutaneous coronary transluminal angioplasty with a follow-up period of 18 months during which 'usual care' was permitted in the intervention group, including lipid-lowering treatment. Aggressive lipid-lowering treatment led to a 46% reduction in LDL cholesterol and was accompanied by ischaemic events in 13% of patients. In contrast, 21% of patients who underwent percutaneous coronary transluminal angioplasty had an ischaemic event despite an 18% reduction in LDL cholesterol. As compared with the patients treated with angioplasty followed by usual care, the patients who received atorvastatin and obtained pronounced reductions in LDL cholesterol had a significantly longer time to the first ischaemic event.

These results support other corresponding studies that have shown that aggressive medical treatment was at least as effective as conventional cardiological intervention.

Conclusion

The evidence of benefit from lipid-lowering strategies is virtually indisputable. Treatment of patients at high cardiovascular risk is now mandatory and the only real debate relates to the 'optimal' target levels and the 'optimal' drug treatment. While the studies are not definitive there is evidence to suggest that, at the usually recommended doses, atorvastatin is the most effective of the agents currently available. Whether or not the new 'super-statins' prove to be more effective (and more cost-effective) remains to be seen. Elsewhere, the issues relate to cost-effectiveness because of the (potentially) huge number of patients at relatively low risk who might nevertheless benefit, in the long term, from primary prevention of cardiovascular disease through drug treatment to reduce cholesterol.

References

1. Scandinavian Simvastatin Survival Study Group. Randomized trial of cholesterol lowering in 4444 patients with coronary heart disease; the Scandinavian Survival Study. *Lancet* 1994; **344**: 1383–9.

2. Shepherd J, Cobbe SM, Ford I, Isles CG, Lorimer AR, MacFarlane PW, McKillop JH, Packard CJ, for the West of Scotland Coronary Prevention Study Group. Prevention of coronary heart disease with pravastatin in men with hypercholesterolaemia. *N Engl J Med* 1995; **333**: 1301–7.

3. Pedersen TR, Olsson AG, Faergeman O, Kjekshus J, Wedel H, Berg K, Wilhelmsen L, Haghfelt T, Thorgeirsson G, Pyorala K, Miettinen T, Christophersen B, Tobert JA, Musliner TA, Cook TJ. Lipoprotein changes and reduction in the incidence of major coronary heart disease events in the Scandinavian Simvastatin Survival Study (4S). *Circulation* 1998; **97**: 1453-60.

4. Sacks FM, Pfeffer MA, Moye LA, Rouleau JL, Rutherford JD, Cole TG, Brown L, Warnica JW, Arnold JM, Wun CC, Davis BR, Braunwald E. The effect of pravastatin on coronary events after myocardial infarction in patients with average cholesterol levels. *N Engl J Med* 1996; **335**: 1001–9.

5. Hebert PR, Gaziano JM, Hennekens CH. An overview of trials of cholesterol lowering and risk of stroke. *Arch Intern Med* 1995; **155**: 50-5.

6. Crouse JR, Byington RP, Bond MG, Espeland MA, Craven TE, Sprinkle JW, McGovern ME, Furberg CD. Pravastatin, lipids, and atherosclerosis in the carotid arteries (PLAC-II). *Am J Cardiol* 1995; **75**: 455-9.

7. Rubins HR, Robins SJ, Collins D, Iranmanesh A, Wilt TJ, Mann D, Mayo-Smith M, Faas FH, Elam MB, Rutan GH, *et al.* Distribution of lipids in 8500 men with coronary artery disease. *Am J Cardiol* 1995; **75**: 1196-201.

8. Tenkanen L, Manttari M, Manninen V. Some coronary risk factors related to the insulin resistance syndrome and treatment with gemfibrozil. Experience from the Helsinki Heart Study. *Circulation* 1995; **92**: 1779-85.

6

Hormone replacement therapy and cardiovascular risk

Introduction

The incidence of atherosclerotic cardiovascular disease is low in pre-menopausal women; it increases in postmenopausal women; and, reportedly, is reduced to pre-menopausal levels in those women who receive hormone replacement therapy with oestrogen [hormone replacement therapy (HRT) or o/estrogen replacement therapy (ERT)] after the menopause. Additionally, HRT has been reported to be particularly beneficial for secondary prevention with hormone users having between 35 and 80% fewer recurrent events than non-users. However, the lower rates of coronary heart disease (CHD) in women taking HRT have been generally identified in observational studies and, relative to the available evidence, two important issues arise: first, can the beneficial effects of HRT be clearly demonstrated in prospective randomized large-scale clinical outcome trials; and, secondly, if HRT is beneficial, can the underlying mechanisms be clearly identified.

Effects of HRT on cardiovascular disease and cancer

Observational studies have shown a reduction in cardiovascular disease risk and mortality in postmenopausal women on ERT but there remains some debate about the extent to which this reduction results from selection bias. With respect to hormone-dependent cancers, the increased risk of endometrial cancer has been greatly decreased or almost eliminated by the addition of progestogen to ERT |**1**|, but opinions are still divided on the association between ERT and an increased risk of breast cancer |**2**|.

Cardiovascular and cancer morbidity and mortality and sudden cardiac death in postmenopausal women on oestrogen replacement therapy (ERT).
L Sourander, T Rajala, I Räihä, *et al. Lancet* 1998; **352**: 1965–9.

BACKGROUND. Advantages and disadvantages of postmenopausal ERT are still not clear. Its aim was to analyse the relation between postmenopausal ERT, cardiovascular disease and cancer.

INTERPRETATION. Current ERT reduced primarily sudden cardiac death and predicted reduced cardiovascular mortality, but did not reduce morbidity. ERT did not increase the risk of breast cancer, but was associated with an increased risk of endometrial cancer. This Finnish community-based prospective study investigated cardiovascular disease mortality and the associated risk of breast and endometrial cancer in postmenopausal women taking ERT. During 1987–88, 8164 women (mean age 61 years) were invited to participate in a free mammography screening programme for breast cancer: 7944 women participated in the study and completed detailed questionnaires about a wide range of health-related issues, including the use of HRT. At baseline, 988 women were identified as current users of HRT, 757 as former users and 5572 as never users, and all women were followed up until 1995.

Compared with never users, there was a significant reduction for cardiovascular mortality with a risk ratio of 0.21 (adjusted for other risk factors). There were significant differences in absolute risk for death from CAD at 0 in current HRT users, 0.81 in former HRT users and 1 per 1000 woman-years for never users. The corresponding figures for sudden cardiac death were 0, 1.0 and 1.6 per 1000 woman-years. There was a similar trend for deaths related to acute MI at 0.45, 1.2 and 1.1 per 1000 woman-years, respectively, but this did not attain a statistical significance. There were, however, significant reductions in death from stroke with figures of 0.15, 1 and 1.2 per 1000 woman-years, respectively. However, in contrast to the mortality results there were no significant differences for morbidity from CAD or stroke.

The incidence of endometrial cancer, but not breast cancer, was increased among current users (although most use unopposed oestrogen) with values of 5.06, 1.27 and 1 in the current users, former users and never users, respectively.

Comment

Hormone replacement therapy reduced cardiovascular mortality but not morbidity during this period of approximately 8 years of follow up. The conclusion was drawn that HRT might be more likely to interfere with the progression of existing coronary disease than primarily to prevent it. Although this is an important study and, although the conclusions may be valid and correct, the study design cannot eliminate selection bias in relation, for example, to the reasons for taking or not taking HRT, or for responding or not, to the invitation for breast screening.

Conclusion

This study illustrates the nature of the current debate. There appear to be cardiovascular benefits but concerns remain about the potential increase in risk from hormone-dependent cancers. Unfortunately, more recent studies have not yet provided definitive answers.

HRT, cardiovascular risk factors and vascular effects

Mechanistic studies have suggested that oestrogen has a vasodilator effect on arteries, including coronary arteries, and this has been attributed to both calcium channel blockade and augmented nitric oxide mechanisms. Anti-ischaemic and anti-anginal effects have also been described. These benefits in combination with a positive effect on lipid metabolism have been proffered as the explanation for the positive cardiovascular effects of HRT. With regards to blood pressure (BP) itself, there are some inconsistencies in the published literature but the results of most studies suggest that HRT is associated with a reduction in BP.

Risk factors

A randomized trial on effects of hormone therapy on ambulatory blood pressure and lipoprotein levels in women with coronary artery disease.
U Pripp, G Hall, G Csemiczky, *et al. J Hypertens* 1999; **17**: 1379–86.

BACKGROUND. To investigate 1-year effects of HRT on ambulatory BP (ABP) and lipoprotein levels in postmenopausal women with coronary artery disease (CAD).

INTERPRETATION. One year of HRT in patients with CAD does not influence ABP. Oral HRT induces beneficial effects on lipoprotein levels. Sixty postmenopausal women, mean age 59 years, were randomized to three treatment groups to receive either conjugated equine oestrogen ($n = 20$), transdermal oestradiol ($n = 20$) or placebo ($n = 20$) during repeated 28-day cycles for 1 year. Each monotherapy was administered for 18 days and then combined with medroxyprogesterone for the remaining 10 days of each cycle. The ABP results in the three groups are summarized in Table 6.1. Overall, there was a small but non-significant trend for BP to reduce during the 12 cycles of active treatment and placebo: average daytime BP was 125/78 mmHg in the 32 women receiving HRT compared with 125/75 mmHg in the 13 women assigned to placebo. After 12 months of treatment the corresponding daytime averages were 125/76 in the HRT group and 124/72 in the placebo group. Corresponding figures for night-time BP showed overall decreases from baseline, which were statistically significant. With respect to the lipid parameters there were no changes in triglyceride levels but the increases in high-density lipoprotein (HDL) cholesterol and decreases in low-density lipoprotein (LDL) cholesterol did achieve statistical significance.

The effects of different types and doses of oestrogen replacement therapy on clinic and ambulatory blood pressure and the renin–angiotensin system in normotensive postmenopausal women.
P J Harvey, L M Wing, J Savage, D Molloy. *J Hypertens* 1999, **17**: 405–14.

BACKGROUND. The effect on BP of oral 'replacement' doses of oestrogen may depend on the type and dose of oestrogen administered. This study was designed to compare with placebo the effect of once daily treatment with a 'natural' oestrogen, piperazine oestrone sulphate, in two different doses and a semisynthetic oestrogen, ethinyloestradiol, on clinic BP and ABP, and the renin–angiotensin system in postmenopausal women.

Table 6.1 Average ambulatory BP values

BP		Oral systolic	HRT diastolic	Transdermal systolic	HRT diastolic	Placebo (n = 13) systolic	diastolic
Baseline	Daytime	123.3 ± 14.0	75.9 ± 5.8	127.5 ± 14.2	80.4 ± 8.1	124.5 ± 12.3	74.8 ± 8.3
	Night-time	109.4 ± 16.3	62.9 ± 7.0	115.4 ± 17.0	69.1 ± 10.1	112.2 ± 20.1	62.2 ± 9.2
12 cycle	Daytime	124.3 ± 16.3	74.8 ± 7.0	126.8 ± 15.0	78.6 ± 9.5	124.1 ± 19.7	72.2 ± 10.1
	Night-time	99.0 ± 14.4	64.0 ± 10.1	101.4 ± 15.9	65.6 ± 5.9	91.5 ± 13.1	57.8 ± 19.5

INTERPRETATION. In normotensive postmenopausal women, replacement doses of natural and semisynthetic oestrogen reduce night-time ABP with either no change or a small reduction in clinic BP. Reduction in BP is not explained by reduced activity of the renin–angiotensin system but could have a component of reduced central sympathetic drive consistent with the decreased heart rate. This was a randomized double blind cross-over study involving 24 normotensive postmenopausal women, aged 47–60 years, who received four different treatments, each for 4 weeks' duration. The treatments were a 'natural' oestrogen in two different doses: a semi-synthetic oestrogen and placebo. There were no significant effects on daytime ABP but night-time BP, both systolic and diastolic, was significantly reduced by two of the oestrogen preparations. There were no significant differences between treatments for the clinic systolic BPs but two of the oestrogen preparations were associated with significant reductions in diastolic BP relative to the placebo phase.

Comment

These two studies, albeit with some limitations in methodology and poor statistical power, provide reassurance that HRT does not increase BP. In fact, the published literature now shows an overall consistency in reporting small reductions in BP and beneficial trends in lipid measures.

Vascular effects

Estrogen improves abnormal norepinephrine-induced vasoconstriction in postmenopausal women.

B H Sung, M Ching, J L.Izzo Jr, P Dandona, M F Wilson. *J Hypertens* 1999, **17**: 523–8.

BACKGROUND. **An exaggerated BP response to mental stress in postmenopausal women has been reported but the underlying mechanism is not clear. In the present study, the role of oestrogen in the BP response to mental stress was examined.**

INTERPRETATION. Healthy, normotensive postmenopausal women showed an exaggerated BP response to noradrenaline and loss of oestrogen-mediated vasodilation may contribute to the increased BP response to stress in postmenopausal women without ERT.

Withdrawal of hormone therapy for 4 weeks decreases arterial compliance in postmenopausal women.

T K Waddell, C Rajkumanr, J D Cameron, *et al. J Hypertens* 1999; **17**: 413–18.

BACKGROUND. **A previous cross-sectional study demonstrated that arterial compliance is elevated in postmenopausal women taking oestrogen-containing** hormonal therapy, which may partially account for the reduction in cardiovascular events.

INTERPRETATION. These data suggest that hormonal modulation of distal arterial vascular tone may account for short-term changes in arterial compliance associated with oestrogen-containing hormonal therapy.

Comment

The improvements in arterial compliance, in relation to oestrogen treatment, are entirely consistent with the improvements reported in the clinical BP studies.

Hormone replacement improves haemodynamic profile and left ventricular geometry in hypertensive and normotensive postmenopausal women.
K Light, A Hinderliter, S West, *et al. J Hypertens* 2001; **19**: 269–78.

BACKGROUND. Postmenopausal oestrogen replacement, with or without progestin, has been related to lower cardiovascular risks.

INTERPRETATION. These findings suggest that oestrogen-mediated reductions in haemodynamic load on the heart may contribute to the reduced risk of cardiovascular events in relatively healthy postmenopausal women who use hormone replacement. This was a 6-month double blind study in 69 women who were randomized to receive either conjugated oestrogens alone, oestrogens plus medroxyprogesterone or placebo. Both groups on active hormone replacement showed similar decreases in vascular resistance and modest BP reductions, which differed from the unchanged responses from those on placebo. Women receiving hormone replacement showed increased stroke volume and cardiac index at 6 months and there were significant but small decreases in echocardiographic measures of left ventricular mass index and relative wall thickness. Hormone replacement was also associated with decreases in plasma noradrenaline.

Comment

This is an interesting study that appears to add further weight to the potential mechanisms underlying the purported cardiovascular benefits of HRT. Unfortunately, this is a relatively small study and, for example, only 53 of the 69 women were able to complete the echocardiographic measures. Additionally, the statistical analysis assessed changes from baseline and, with the variability in many of the measurements, it would be surprising if there were any statistically significant differences in the achieved BP, haemodynamic and other variables at the end of the 6-month treatment. In short, these are interesting results that are consistent with those of other studies but not sufficiently robust in statistical terms to be considered definitive evidence.

Estrogen stimulates delayed mitogen-activated protein kinase activity in human endothelial cells via an autocrine loop that involves basic fibroblast growth factor.

S Kim-Schulze, W L Lowe, W Schnaper. *Circulation* 1998; **98**: 413–21.

B ACKGROUND. Oestrogen plays a significant role in protecting pre-menopausal women from cardiovascular disease. It was found that oestradiol augments endothelial cell activities related to vascular healing and that human coronary artery and umbilical vein endothelial cells express oestrogen receptors. Classically, the oestrogen receptor functions as a transcription factor, but the cytoplasmic targets of this genomic effect have not been defined for endothelial cells. In the present study, the potential role of the mitogen-activated protein (MAP) kinase ERK1 and ERK2 as mediators of oestrogen action was examined.

INTERPRETATION. These data describe an autocrine mechanism for E2 induction of ERK1/2 in human umbilical vein endothelial cells. Because our previous studies suggested that certain cardioprotective effects of oestrogen are genomic in nature, the results are consistent with the hypothesis that autocrine stimulation of endothelial ERK1/2 activity by basic fibroblast growth factor may play a part in the beneficial effects of oestrogen on cardiovascular biology.

Comment

This is an interesting experimental study that seeks to explore the mechanisms underlying the vascular effects of oestrogen. In short, the addition of oestrogen to human umbilical vein endothelial cells was associated with an improvement in endothelial cell function. These findings are consistent with the small changes in BP and in arterial compliance that have been seen in clinical studies.

Conclusion

Overall, from molecular biology to clinical studies, there is a consistent message that oestrogen has beneficial modulating effects on endothelial function, vascular resistance and BP.

HRT and cardiovascular outcomes

Prospective trials

 Randomized trial of estrogen plus progestin for secondary prevention of coronary heart disease in postmenopausal women.

S Hulley, D Grady, T Bush, *et al.* for the Heart and Estrogen/progestin Replacement Study (HERS) Research Group. *JAMA* 1998; **280**: 605–13.

BACKGROUND. Observational studies have found lower rates of CHD in postmenopausal women who take oestrogen than in women who do not, but this potential benefit has not been confirmed in clinical trials. The objective was to determine if oestrogen plus progestin therapy alters the risk for CHD events in postmenopausal women with established coronary disease.

INTERPRETATION. During an average follow-up of 4.1 years, treatment with oral conjugated equine oestrogen plus medroxyprogesterone acetate did not reduce the overall rate of CHD events in postmenopausal women with established coronary disease. Based on the finding of no overall cardiovascular benefit and a pattern of early increase of risk of CHD events, the authors do not recommend this treatment for the purpose of secondary prevention of CHD. However, given the favourable pattern of CHD events after several years of therapy it could be appropriate for women already receiving this treatment to continue.

This was a randomized, blinded, placebo-controlled secondary prevention trial in 2763 women younger than 80 years (mean age 66.7 years) who were known to have CHD and who were postmenopausal with an intact uterus. Follow-up averaged 4.1 years, with 82% of those assigned to HRT taking it at the end of 1 year and 75% at the end of 3 years. Overall, there was no significant difference between groups in the primary outcomes [non-fatal myocardial infarction (MI) or CHD death] or in any of the secondary cardiovascular outcomes. MI or CHD death occurred in 172 women receiving HRT and in 176 receiving placebo. The lack of any overall beneficial effect occurred despite a net reduction of 11% in LDL cholesterol and a net 10% increase in HDL cholesterol in the HRT group ($P < 0.001$). Within the overall null effect, however, there was a statistically significant time trend with more CHD events in the HRT group during year 1 and fewer events in years 4 and 5. Furthermore, the HRT group had more episodes of venous thromboembolic events (34 *vs* 12) and gall bladder disease (84 *vs* 62 events).

Comment

The Heart and Estrogen/progestin Replacement Study (HERS) was a landmark study because it was the first double-blind randomized trial of HRT in women with pre-existing CHD. Unfortunately, there was a highly significant increase in CHD events during the first year of oestrogen treatment with a relative increase for any CHD event by 2.3 in months 0–4, 1.46 in months 5–8, and 1.18 in months 9–12.

The overall lack of benefit occurred despite significant and beneficial changes in both HDL and LDL cholesterol. Total mortality was similar in both groups at 131 deaths in the HRT group and 123 deaths in the placebo group.

Effects of estrogen replacement on the regression of coronary artery atherosclerosis.
D Herrington, D Reboussin, B Brosnihan, *et al. N Engl J Med* 2000; **343**: 522–9.

BACKGROUND. **Heart disease is a major cause of illness and death in women. To understand better the role of oestrogen in the treatment and prevention of heart disease, more information is needed about its effect on coronary atherosclerosis and the extent to which concomitant progestin therapy may modify these effects.**

INTERPRETATION. Neither oestrogen alone nor oestrogen plus medroxyprogesterone acetate affected the progression of coronary atherosclerosis in women with established disease. These results suggest that such women should not use oestrogen replacement with an expectation of cardiovascular benefit. A total of 309 women with angiographically confirmed CAD were randomized to receive unopposed oestrogen, oestrogen plus progestogen, or placebo. During the 3 years of follow up the women receiving HRT showed significant reductions in LDL cholesterol by 9.4% and 16.5% in the oestrogen and oestrogen plus medroxyprogesterone groups, respectively, and corresponding significant increases in HDL cholesterol by 18.8% and 14.2%, respectively. However, neither hormonal treatment altered the progression of coronary atherosclerosis as measured by coronary angiography.

Conclusion

To some extent these two important studies simply complicate the debate about the role of HRT in primary and secondary prevention. For example, the Nurses' Health Study reinforces previous findings that examined life-style related risk factors to show that there was an 83% lower risk of coronary events in those women who were non-smokers, not overweight, who exercised regularly and had a healthy diet (although, in fact, this was only 3% of the study population!) These observational studies do not, however, constitute definitive proof for the prospective benefits of HRT.

In the secondary prevention study, the short-term use of HRT was not associated with any beneficial changes in coronary artery measurements despite favourable changes in the lipid profile. It can be argued that such measurements constitute a poor surrogate and that the treatment period was of insufficient duration in patients with established CAD. However, although ostensibly a negative study it is important to note that there was no deterioration and no difference in event rates in this study, which might be considered to provide some reassurance in respect of the increased rate of events that was seen in HERS (Hulley *et al.*, 1998).

Postmenopausal hormone therapy and risk of stroke.

J A Simon, J Hsia, J A Cauley, *et al. Circulation* 2001; **103**: 638.

BACKGROUND. Observational studies have shown that postmenopausal hormone therapy may increase, decrease, or have no effect on the risk of stroke. To date, no clinical trial has examined these questions. To investigate the relation between oestrogen plus progestin therapy and risk of stroke among postmenopausal women, data collected from the HERS project, a secondary CHD prevention trial, was analysed.

INTERPRETATION. Hormone therapy with conjugated equine oestrogen and progestin had no significant effect on the risk for stroke among postmenopausal women with coronary disease. In this study 2763 postmenopausal women were randomly assigned to receive conjugated oestrogen plus progestin, or placebo. The primary outcome measures were stroke incidence and stroke death during a mean follow up of about 4 years. A total of 149 women (5% of the population) had one or more strokes, of which 85% were of ischaemic origin, resulting in 26 deaths. First, there was no early increase in risk of stroke in the hormone-treated group but, overall, hormone replacement therapy had no impact on the risk of stroke or transient ischaemic attack.

Comment

This substudy among the HERS participants showed that 82 women in the HRT group had strokes compared with 67 women in the placebo group. This difference does not statistically significant and was taken as some reassurance that HRT was not associated with an increased risk of thrombotic events.

Observational studies

Primary prevention of coronary heart disease in women through diet and lifestyle.

M J Stampfer, F B Hu, J E Manson, E B Rimm, W C Willett. *N Engl J Med* 2000; **3436**: 16–22.

BACKGROUND. Many life-style-related risk factors for CHD have been identified, but little is known about their effect on the risk of disease when they are considered together.

INTERPRETATION. Among women, adherence to life-style guidelines involving diet, exercise, and abstinence from smoking is associated with a very low risk of CHD. This was a report on 84 129 women participating in the Nurses' Health Study. During 14 years of follow-up, 1128 major coronary events (296 deaths) were documented and the analysis assessed those diet and life-style factors associated with low and high risk.

Women in the low-risk category (3% of the total population) had a relative risk of coronary events of 0.17 as compared with all the other women. In the study cohort, 82% of coronary events could be attributed to the lack of adherence to the low-risk life-style pattern.

Trends in the incidence of coronary heart disease and changes in diet and lifestyle in women.

F Hu, M Stampfer, J Manson, *et al. N Engl J Med* 2000; **343**: 530–7.

BACKGROUND. **Previous studies have found concurrent declines in BP, serum cholesterol levels and the incidence of and mortality from coronary disease. However, the effects of changes in diet and life-styles on trends in coronary disease are largely unknown.**

INTERPRETATION. Reduction in smoking, improvement in diet and an increase in postmenopausal hormone use accounted for much of the decline in the incidence of coronary disease in this group of women. An increasing prevalence of obesity, however, appears to have slowed the decline in the incidence of coronary disease. This was a report of 85 941 healthy women who were 34–59 years old and who were followed from 1980 to 1994 in the Nurses' Health Study. Diet and life-style variables were assessed at baseline and updated throughout follow up during which time, after adjustment for the effect of age, the incidence of coronary disease declined by 31%. The proportion of postmenopausal women using HRT increased by almost twofold and while smoking declined by 41% the prevalence of overweight (body mass index > 25 kg/m^2) increased by 38%. It was calculated that the reduction in smoking explained a 13% decline in the incidence of coronary disease; the improvement of diet explained a 16% decline; and the increased use of HRT explained a 9% decline. In contrast, the increase in body mass index explained an 8% increase in the incidence of coronary disease.

Comment

These two reports from the Nurses' Health Study are confirmatory in nature, although they shed no new light on the factors implicated in the development of atherosclerotic disease. Thus, the dietary and life-style recommendations, if adhered to, carry predicted reductions in the incidence of coronary disease: by 13% through smoking cessation, by 16% through adherence to a diet with a low fat and glycaemic load, etc. and by 9% in association with HRT.

HRT and Alzheimer's disease

Cognitive decline in women in relation to non-protein-bound oestradiol concentrations.

K Yaffe, L Lui, D Grady, *et al. Lancet* 2000; **356**: 708–12.

BACKGROUND. Previous studies have found no association between serum concentrations of total oestradiol and cognitive function, but these measurements may not reflect concentrations of hormone available to the brain. The hypothesis was tested that concentrations of non-protein bound (free) and loosely bound (bioavailable) sex hormones are associated with cognitive function in older women.

INTERPRETATION. Women with high serum concentrations of non-protein bound and bioavailable oestradiol, but not testosterone, were less likely to develop cognitive impairment than women with low concentrations. This finding supports the hypothesis that higher concentrations of endogenous oestrogen prevent cognitive decline.

Postmenopausal estrogen replacement therapy and the risk of Alzheimer's disease.

S Seshadri, G L Zornberg, L Derby, *et al. Arch Neurol* 2001; **58**: 435–40.

BACKGROUND. Previous studies have examined the relation between postmenopausal ERT and the risk of Alzheimer's disease. The findings have been inconsistent, as some studies have been interpreted as showing a protective effect while others have reported no effect.

INTERPRETATION. The use of ERT in women after the onset of menopause was not associated with a reduced risk of developing Alzheimer's disease.

Cognitive function in postmenopausal women treated with raloxifene.

K Yaffe, K Krueger, S Sarkar, *et al. N Engl J Med* 2001: **344**(16): 1207–13.

BACKGROUND. In postmenopausal women, oestrogen may have a beneficial effect on cognitive function or reduce the risk of decline in cognitive function. Whether raloxifene, a selective oestrogen-receptor modulator, might have similar actions is not known.

INTERPRETATION. Raloxifene treatment for 3 years does not affect overall cognitive scores in postmenopausal women with osteoporosis.

Conclusion

While the evidence might not yet be considered to be definitive, on balance HRT has no significant impact in either age-related cognitive decline or, ultimately, the development of Alzheimer's disease.

HRT: practical issues

Ethnic differences in use of hormone replacement therapy: community based survey.

T J Harris, D G Cook, P D Wicks, F P Cappuccio. *Br Med J* 2000; **319**: 610–11.

BACKGROUND. Hormone replacement therapy is widely promoted to prevent cardiovascular disease and osteoporosis, and relieve menopausal symptoms; however, concern exists that much of the cardiovascular effects may be due to its selection by healthy women. Little is known about its use by women from different ethnic groups in the UK.

INTERPRETATION. The differences in use of hormone replacement reported here have not to our knowledge been described before in the UK. This population-based survey were carried out in South London in women aged 40–59 years. The response rate was 60% and 802 of the 941 women were of Afro-Caribbean or South-East Asian descent. The salient result was that 25% of white women were using HRT and this was significantly more than the 15% in the Afro-Caribbean women and the 10% in the South-East Asian women.

Comment

These authors identified an important issue, which, potentially, might be a source of bias in observational studies, i.e. ethnic or cultural differences between those women who use HRT and those who do not. However, they also convey a potentially more important message that the process of assessing women for HRT provides an opportunity for health promotion in general, including the assessment of conventional cardiovascular risk factors and discussion about cervical and breast cancer screening. Irrespective of the need for HRT, opportunities for such discussion with women from ethnic minority groups may be missed, as it is also recognized that the uptake of other preventive health measures is lower, for example, in South-East Asian women.

Hormone replacement therapy.

Clinical Synthesis Panel on HRT. *Lancet* 1999; **345**: 152–5.

BACKGROUND. On 23–25 June 1999, a conference was held at the European Institute of Oncology, Milan, Italy, with the aim of synthesizing the clinical data on HRT.

INTERPRETATION. Although there is considerable evidence about the health effects of long-term use of HRT, on average the balance between the risk and benefits is not overwhelming in either direction. For many women the benefits of long-term HRT use will outweigh the risks; for others the risks outweigh the benefits. The use of HRT has to be tailored to the needs and desires of the individual.

Comment

This is a thoughtful and well-referenced summary of the arguments relating to clinical issues. The conclusions are balanced and reasonable and the principal summarizing recommendations are shown in Tables 6.2 and 6.3.

Table 6.2 Cardiovascular disease

- Although a cause and effect relation is not proved, evidence that HRT lowers the risk of CHD in women without a history of this disease is sufficiently strong to consider this potential benefit when deciding whether to use HRT.
- HRT raises the risk of venous thromboembolism, but the absolute risk is small in women without predisposing conditions

Source: Clinical Synthesis Panel on HRT (1999).

Table 6.3 HRT and the risk of cancer

- HRT is associated with a slight increase in the risk of breast cancer that is restricted to current and recent users, the risk increasing with increasing duration of use. This effect wears off within 5 years of stopping use. Among 1000 women who use HRT continuously for 10 years starting at age 50, it is estimated that there will be an additional six breast cancers raising the incidence from a background of 45 cases to 51 cases. Progestagens do not seem to diminish the excess risk associated with oestrogen. Use of HRT for a few years should not lead to an appreciable risk of breast cancer.
- The excess risk of endometrial cancer due to oestrogen HRT use can be substantially reduced by concurrent progestagen therapy during at least 12 days in each month. Progestagens are sometimes poorly tolerated. Doctors should inform their patients of the importance of adherence and should check adherence with progestagen therapy while oestrogen is being taken. Failure to take progestagen with oestrogen can raise the risk of endometrial cancer.
- The breast and endometrial cancers that are diagnosed in HRT users are less aggressive clinically than those in never users.
- Current and recent use of HRT may be associated with a decreased risk of colorectal cancer.

Source: Clinical Synthesis Panel on HRT (1999).

The Women's Health Initiative Memory Study (WHIMS): a trial of the effect of estrogen therapy in preventing and slowing the progression of dementia.

S Schumaker, B A Reboussin, M A Espeland, *et al. Control Clin Trials* 1998; **19**: 604–21.

B A C K G R O U N D . **Evidence from animal, human, cross-sectional, case–control and prospective studies indicate that HRT is promising treatment to delay the onset of symptoms of dementia.**

I N T E R P R E T A T I O N . WHIMS is designed to provide more than 80% statistical power to detect a 40% reduction in the rate of all-cause dementia, an effect that could have profound public health implications for older women's health and functioning.

Comment

This study has been positioned at the conclusion of this chapter to illustrate that this type of prospective outcome study is conspicuously sparse in the current literature on HRT. Objective evidence of this nature is essential for defining the future role of HRT, and its overall safety.

Conclusion

Epidemiological studies have consistently shown an association between HRT/ERT and lower rates of cardiovascular morbidity and mortality. This is illustrated by the results of a recent meta-analysis of 20 observational studies showing that women taking HRT, usually unopposed oestrogen treatment, had a relative risk of 0.5 for developing CAD, relative to non-users. The results of these observational studies are not supported by prospective randomized outcome studies and some doubts therefore remain. At its most simplistic, those women who are motivated to request HRT, and who have no contraindication to its use, are likely to have an overall healthier life-style. Although statistical adjustments have taken account of all known confounding factors in the observational studies it remains possible that the findings were biased.

There remain many unanswered questions about the use of HRT primarily because of the lack of well designed prospective clinical studies. With respect to cardiovascular disease there are several mechanisms by which HRT might be beneficial and modest but positive changes have been demonstrated in relation to BP, vascular compliance, endothelial function and lipid parameters. Unfortunately, concerns remain because the first prospective randomized study of HRT produced a mixed picture suggesting that HRT might actually be harmful if initiated in patients who had increased cardiovascular risk by virtue of their pre-existing cardiac disease.

Overall, however, the balance of evidence suggests that HRT is likely to be beneficial for delaying the progression of atherosclerotic cardiovascular disease and it may therefore be an appropriate treatment for primary prevention as part of a lifestyle package that addresses cardiovascular risk reduction. There remain some concerns, however, about initiating HRT in women with established CHD. The results of further studies (ideally, prospective outcome studies) are awaited with interest to allow clarification of many important practical issues.

References

1. Lobo RA. The role of progestogens in hormone replacement therapy. *Am J Obstet Gynecol* 1992; **168**: 1997–2004.
2. Sismondi P, Biglia N, Gioi M, Campognoli C. Hormone replacement therapy and breast cancer. *Eur Menop J* 1996; **3**: 227–31.

Part III

Hypertension: emerging concepts

7

Essential hypertension: the search for specific genetic markers

Introduction

The completion of the Human Genome Mapping project earlier this year provides a landmark in the understanding of complex human disorders that have a genetic basis. Although still in 'draft' format, the information provides a major advance. Surprisingly, the total number of genes identified is rather less than earlier estimates (about 30 000), although this number is likely to increase. At present the specific genetic cause of disease has been identified for only a small number of monogenic disorders using the technique of positional cloning. These disorders include Huntington's chorea, familial cardiomyopathy and cystic fibrosis. Interestingly, some hypertensive disorders fall into this category and include glucocorticoid remedial aldosteronism and Liddle's syndrome. These are discussed below, and provide some possible clues into more common forms of hypertension. However, it is acknowledged that understanding the genetic basis of complex polygenic disorders, such as essential hypertension, which reflect an interaction between environmental factors and genetic predisposition, is a difficult problem.

Human essential hypertension is a complex, multifactorial polygenic disorder that arises as a consequence of the interaction of environmental risk factors and genetic susceptibility. There is a substantial body of evidence that suggests that, as well as the major life-style-dictated environmental factors of obesity and sodium intake, *in utero* environment is also important in determining the programming of several physiological systems involved in the subsequent risk of adult cardiovascular disease [1-3]. This environmental susceptibility interacts with genetic risk, which is estimated to account for 30–40% of the variance in blood pressure (BP) within a population. The aim of current genetic studies is, therefore, to identify the genes that predispose to this genetic susceptibility. This, in turn, will aid our understanding of the underlying pathophysiological basis of hypertension and provide stratification of risk and prognosis based on an individual's genotype.

Approaches to the identification of causal genes

Several complementary approaches can be used in the identification of the genes that give rise to essential hypertension. Clearly, information from animal studies provides possible candidates that can be tested. Additionally, understanding of physiological mechanisms that contribute to cardiovascular regulation provides fertile ground for testing hypothesis about the canditature of specific genes. Areas of relevance are identified below. In this regard, the Human Genome Project has provided a major advance with better characterization of the extent of variability in genes. For example, single nucleotide polymorphisms are frequent (at least one per thousand nucleotides), and allow comparison of common genetic variants to be made between hypertensive patients and controls.

The simplest genetic analysis exploits association analysis, where patients with hypertension are compared with control subjects. In this type of study, variation in a candidate gene is compared between cases and controls. However, with this type of study a number of criteria should be met before a particular DNA change can be linked to a disease trait. In particular, the polymorphism should result in a functional alteration in gene product, and the number of individuals demonstrating a specific association between genotype and phenotype should be large enough to be convincing. In addition, the hypothesis must be biologically plausible and the phenotypes easily distinguished. Notwithstanding these concerns and the limitations of candidate gene studies, such investigations have been informative in identifying potential loci and mechanisms that may underlie the genetic basis of high BP.

More sophisticated types of analysis have been employed to examine the genetic basis of complex disorders. Of these, the most commonly used approach has been a modified form of linkage analysis in which the inheritance of alleles at given loci are studied in affected siblings with the disorder. Where the sharing of alleles in siblings deviates from that predicted by Mendelian principles, the gene is implicated in the disorder.

This approach is statistically complex, and is relatively weak, requiring very large numbers. Nonetheless, it offers a considerable advantage in allowing a large number of loci to be studied in populations; in this manner, a genome-wide search can be carried out using anonymous markers distributed throughout the genome that identify variation in order that candidate regions that might be associated with hypertension can be defined.

Finally, recent proposals have suggested that a modified form of association analysis, in which family members (parents) provide the control population for alleles of candidate genes have been made. With this type of approach (transmission disequilibrium testing [TDT]) the inheritance of alleles at given candidate genes is examined in affected individuals and the frequency of alleles compared with that in the parental population. Where there appears to be preferential transmission of a given allele along with the disease phenotype, the role of the gene in development of the disorder is inferred. At present the value of this approach remains to be demonstrated in major complex disorders. Again, this particular approach is of greatest value in examining specific candidates that one suspected from known physiology or pathology.

In summary, therefore, the various approaches identified for studying the genes involved in complex disorders should be seen as complementary rather than alternatives. In many instances candidate regions will be identified by family linkage studies (affected sibling pairs) and the precise role confirmed by large-scale association studies either using a case/control or family association paradigm. At present, many studies have focused on candidates associated with known physiological mechanisms and these will be considered in greater detail below.

Candidate studies have included genes involved in systems associated with renal sodium balance, including the renin/angiotensin system and renal tubular sodium pumps and genes involved in vascular contractility, including adrenoreceptors and endothelial nitric oxide (NO) synthase.

Renin–angiotensin–aldosterone system

Angiotensinogen

The angiotensinogen (AGT) gene encodes the protein that is cleaved by renin to yield angiotensin I (see Fig. 7.1). Initial studies in families with a predisposition to developing high BP suggested that AGT levels were higher in those with a strong family history of the disorder, drawing attention to the locus |4|. Linkage studies confirmed an association between the AGT gene locus and hypertension, and to date 10 biallelic polymorphisms have been identified at this locus.

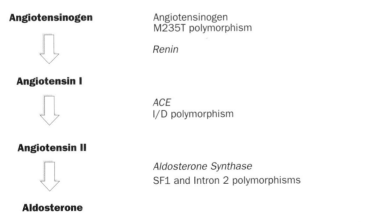

Fig 7.1 Renin–angiotensin–aldosterone system and common polymorphisms.

The polymorphic variant that has generated most interest is characterized by the mutation encoding threonine instead of methionine at amino acid position 235 (M235T). This is in turn associated with variation in plasma levels of AGT, with homozygotes for the M235 variant having the lowest levels and homozygotes for the 235T variant demonstrating the highest. Functionally, it appears that the M235T variant is in tight linkage with a proposed causal mutation in the promoter region of the gene, which is thought to affect basal transcription rates.

Evaluation of the angiotensinogen locus in human essential hypertension.

E Brand, N Chatelain, B Keavney, *et al. Hypertension* 1998; **31**: 725–9.

BACKGROUND. Different family and case–control studies support genetic linkage and association at the human AGT locus with essential hypertension. To extend these previous observations, a European collaborative study of nine centres was set up to create a large resource of affected sibling pairs.

INTERPRETATION. Although several arguments from association studies suggest a role of the AGT gene in essential hypertension, this large family study did not replicate the initial linkage reported in smaller studies. The results highlight the difficulty of identifying susceptibility genes by linkage analysis in complex diseases.

This large, multicentre, European collaborative study aimed to ascertain if there was support, from genetic linkage analysis, for an association of the AGT locus with essential hypertension. The cohort consisted of 350 families, comprising 630 affected sibling pairs. Linkage analysis with AGT microsatellites in hypertensive sibships failed to find any significant difference between the allele frequency in each group and overall estimated allele frequency. Further analysis, after adjusting for severity of BP, age of onset and body mass index, in isolation or in combination, again failed to find any evidence of linkage of the AGT locus with essential hypertension.

Comment

This type of study assesses the inheritance pattern of alleles within sibling pairs. Where a large number of affected sibling pairs with hypertension (or any other complex disorder) can be assembled, the inheritance by descent of a particular allele can be examined. Simple genetic principles dictate that siblings share, on average, no more than 50% of a single allele by descent; where the proportion of sharing is significantly increased from this, the allele is implicated in the inheritance of the phenotype. The main limitation of the affected sibling pair approach is that, although relatively simple in design, it is not particularly powerful and for this reason, large numbers of siblings are necessary to identify loci that carry, in themselves, relatively weak relative risks.

The European study detailed above utilizes this design, and the power of the study is such that, had the AGT M235T polymorphism influenced BP regulation, it would have been detected. However, in view of its negative findings, this study casts doubt on the importance of the AGT locus in essential hypertension.

Angiotensin-converting enzyme (ACE)

Studies of rodent hypertension identified a Quantitative Trait Locus (QTL) for hypertension on rat chromosome 10, and this QTL was found to contain the gene encoding ACE |5|. Subsequent sequencing of the human ACE gene, on chromosome 17, demonstrated a biallelic polymorphism within the gene. This polymorphism is characterized by the presence (insertion) or absence (deletion) of a 287 bp fragment in intron 16 of the gene, and Rigat *et al.* (1990) demonstrated that this polymorphism accounted for approximately 50% of the variance in serum and tissue ACE levels and activity |6|. Individuals homozygous for the deletion allele have twice the level of ACE of those homozygous for the insertion allele, with heterozygotes demonstrating intermediate levels. The most recent study assessing any association between the ACE polymorphism and hypertension has been the Framingham Heart Study.

Evidence for association and genetic linkage of the angiotensin-converting enzyme locus with hypertension and blood pressure in men but not women in the Framingham Heart Study.

C J O'Donnell, K Lindpainter, M G Larson, *et al. Circulation* 1998; **97**: 1766–72.

BACKGROUND. There is controversy regarding the association of the ACE insertion–deletion (ACE I/D) polymorphism with systemic hypertension and with BP. We investigated these relationships in a large population-based sample of men and women using association and linkage analyses.

INTERPRETATION. In our large, population-based sample, there is evidence for association and genetic linkage of the ACE locus with hypertension and with diastolic BP in men but not women. These data support the hypothesis that ACE, or a nearby gene, is a sex-specific candidate gene for hypertension. Confirmatory studies in other large population-based samples are warranted.

Background

The Framingham Heart Study started in 1948, with the initial cohort consisting of 5209 subjects. In 1971, a further 5124 cohort offspring and spouses were enrolled. Participants were invited to attend on a regular basis, and between 1987 and 1991, 3095 subjects (1445 males, 1650 females) were genotyped for the ACE I/D polymorphism and found to be eligible for the study.

Aim

The aim was to assess the association of the ACE I/D polymorphism and systemic hypertension and BP variation using association and linkage analysis (hypertension being defined as systolic BP > 140 mmHg or diastolic > 90 mmHg or current use of antihypertensive treatment).

Results

Association study: A sex-specific association of the ACE genotype and age-adjusted diastolic BP was noted in males only (see Table 7.1), with mean diastolic BPs of 81.6 ($\pm$ 0.5), 80.9 ($\pm$ 0.4) and 79.6 ($\pm$ 0.6) for the DD, DI and II genotypes, respectively ($P = 0.03$). This result was no longer statistically significant when adjusted for other covariants (body mass index, diabetes mellitus, cigarette smoking, alcohol consumption and ischaemic heart disease). No association was found for pulse pressure or systolic BP in males or diastolic or systolic BP or pulse pressure in females. Subgroup analysis of the hypertensive cohort (689 males, 705 females) indicated a similar sex-specific effect in males, with an odds ratio for hypertension of 1.67 (95% confidence interval [CI] 1.21–2.31) and 1.19 (95% CI 0.88–1.61) in the DD and DI groups, respectively, with the II group used as the reference. In this instance the odds ratios remained similar after adjusting for other covariants. Again, in the female cohort no relationship between ACE genotype and hypertension was noted.

Linkage analysis: A cohort of 1044 sibling pairs was available for the linkage study. The analyses provided support for linkage of the ACE I/D polymorphism with diastolic BP in male siblings only. There was no evidence for linkage with pulse pressure in males or with either variable in females.

Aldosterone synthase

Excess production of aldosterone, such as occurs in Conn's syndrome and glucocorticoid remediable aldosteronism, results in sodium retention, hypokalaemia and hypertension. Aldosterone synthase is the enzyme that regulates the terminal conversion of deoxycorticosterone to aldosterone in the zona glomerulosa of the

Table 7.1 Odds ratios for hypertension according to ACE genotype in men and women

Sex	ACE genotype	Odds ratio	95% CI
Male	DI	1.18	0.87–1.62
	DD	1.59	1.13–2.23
Female	DI	0.78	0.56–1.09
	DD	1.00	0.70–1.44

The II genotype is the reference group. CI = confidence interval.
Source: O'Donnell *et al.* (1998).

adrenal cortex. Polymorphisms associated with the aldosterone synthase gene again make attractive candidates in essential hypertension. Polymorphisms identified to date include a single nucleotide variation, (C→T), in the 5′ promoter region at position −344, known as the steroidogenic factor-1 binding site (SF-1) |7|. This polymorphism alters the binding of a steroidogenic factor, and potentially may change expression of the gene within the zona glomerulosa. It is of interest that this polymorphism is in tight linkage disequilibrium with another variation that results in conversion of intron 2 of the aldosterone synthase gene to the intron of the immediately adjacent gene encoding corticosteroid 11β-hydroxylase |7|.

Recent studies have examined the relevance of these polymorphisms in relation to aldosterone excretion, BP and left ventricular mass and function.

Aldosterone excretion rate and blood pressure in essential hypertension are related to polymorphic differences in the aldosterone synthase gene (*CYP11B2*).
E Davies, C D Holloway, M C Ingram, *et al. Hypertension* 1999; **33**: 703–7.

B A C K G R O U N D . Significant correlation of body sodium and potassium with BP may suggest a role for aldosterone in essential hypertension. In patients with this disease, the ratio of plasma renin to plasma aldosterone may be lower than in control subjects and plasma aldosterone levels may be more sensitive to angiotensin II infusion. Because essential hypertension is partly genetic, it is possible that altered control of aldosterone synthase gene expression or translation may be responsible.

I N T E R P R E T A T I O N . Urinary aldosterone excretion rate may be a useful intermediate phenotype linking these genotypes to raised BP. However, no causal relationship has yet been established, and it is possible that the polymorphisms may be in linkage with other causative mutations.

Comment

This well-matched case–control study examined the frequencies of two linked polymorphisms, one in the SF-1 binding site and the other an intronic conversion (IC) of the aldosterone synthase gene, in 138 hypertensives and 200 normotensive controls. The cases had significantly higher BP, at 154.3 (± 22)/95.8 (± 10.9) mmHg compared with 123.8 (± 15)/76.8 (± 8.7) mmHg in controls. Other baseline parameters, including age and sex, were individually matched.

Genetic analysis of the general population for the SF-1 binding site polymorphism indicated population frequencies for the C allele of 0.49 and 0.51 for the T allele. The allele frequencies for the IC site were 0.48 for the wild type and 0.52 for the conversion allele. There was evidence of significant linkage between the polymorphisms, with three common haplotypes observed, T/conversion (0.38), T/wild (0.13) and C/wild (0.45). In the case–control populations, both polymorphisms were in Hardy–Weinberg equilibrium in the control group, as was the IC in the

Table 7.2 Genotype and allele frequencies of the SF-1 and intronic conversion polymorphisms of the aldosterone synthase gene in hypertensive and normotensive groups

	Genotype (%)			Allele (%)	
SF-1 site	**CC**	**CT**	**TT**	**C**	**T**
Cases	8	65	27 $\Big\}$	40	60 $\Big\}$
			P=0.042		P=0.009
Controls	20	53	26	47	53
Intronic site	**WT 11**	**12**	**Con 22**	**Wild**	**Con**
Cases	20	49	32 $\Big\}$	44	56 $\Big\}$
			P=0.02		P=0.016
Controls	33	49	18	58	42

Source: Davies *et al.* (1999).

hypertensive cohort. However, the SF-1 binding site polymorphism failed to demonstrate Hardy–Weinberg equilibrium ($P = 0.0007$), with evidence of an excess of TT homozygotes ($P = 0.042$) and T allele overall ($P = 0.009$) (see Table 7.2).

In a further study of 486 subjects from the North Glasgow MONICA (Monitoring Trends and Determinants of Cardiovascular Disease) population, SF-1 and IC genotypes were compared with tetrahydroaldosterone (THALDO) excretion rate. Despite both polymorphisms being in Hardy–Weinberg equilibrium, the THALDO levels were significantly higher in those individuals with the T allele of the SF-1 binding site and conversion allele of the IC site ($P = 0.021$), suggesting that urinary aldosterone excretion rates can provide an intermediate phenotype linking genotype and hypertension.

Sodium handling

Renal

Adducin

Adducin is a membrane cytoskeletal protein that regulates the activity of Na$^+$K$^+$-ATPase and subsequent sodium transport. Abnormalities of renal sodium reabsorption may be important in the initiation and maintenance of hypertension, and therefore the genes involved in renal sodium handling are of interest in this regard. The adducin gene was initially implicated in hypertension when a mutation in rat α-adducin was found to account for 50% of a major hypertensive effect in the Milan strain of rat |**8**|. In human, a specific point mutation at amino acid 460 in the α-adducin gene results in the substitution of tryptophan for glycine.

The significance of this polymorphism has been assessed in various different ethnic cohorts.

Human α-adducin gene, blood pressure, and sodium metabolism.

A Kamitani, Z Y H Wong, R Fraser, *et al. Hypertension* 1998; **32**: 138–43.

BACKGROUND. The adducin genes contribute significantly to population variation in rat BP and cell membrane sodium transport. The 460Trp mutation of the human α-adducin gene has been associated with hypertension, in particular hypertension sensitive to sodium restriction.

INTERPRETATION. These findings suggest that in this study's Scottish population, the α-adducin 460Trp polymorphism is not related to BP and does not affect whole body or cellular sodium metabolism.

Comment

This population-based association study was performed to examine the relationship of the α-adducin 460Trp polymorphism on BP variation and whole-body and cellular sodium metabolism in a Scottish cohort. A 'four corner' approach was used to select young adults with a contrasting genetic predisposition to high BP. From 603 families, 151 offspring and 224 patients with BP in either the upper or lower 30% of the population were genotyped for the 460Trp α-adducin polymorphism. The influence of the polymorphism on sodium metabolism was also assessed with estimates of total exchange sodium and water, as well as cellular sodium and potassium concentrations in 79 of the offspring cohort.

No difference was detected in genotype or allele frequencies in the offspring or parents with high or low BP. The overall frequency of the 460Trp allele was 24% and 29% in the high- and low-pressure groups, respectively. Additional analysis of total exchangeable and intracellular sodium and components of the renin–angiotensin system in the offspring cohort failed to find any relationship with the 460Trp mutation.

α-adducin and angiotensin 1-converting enzyme polymorphisms in essential hypertension.

C J Clark, E Davies, N H Anderson, *et al. Hypertension* 2000; **36**: 990–4.

BACKGROUND. The role of adducin and ACE as possible cardiovascular genetic determinants has previously been discussed. However, it is possible that particular genotypes may exert interactive effects, a concept that is addressed in this paper.

INTERPRETATION. Neither ACE nor adducin genotype was associated with hypertension in this case/control study. No evidence of interaction between the genetic variants was seen.

Comment

This study uses a case–control approach to examine the adducin and ACE loci in subjects with hypertension and in matched cases. Any potential interaction (epistasis) between the two loci was also examined. No evidence of an influence of either adducin or ACE, on their own, was found when cases were compared with controls. In addition, no evidence of an association between the adducin and the ACE locus was found. The same authors had previously shown involvement of the aldosterone synthase locus in hypertension in this patient group. No interaction between this gene and either adducin or ACE was noted.

Although some studies have reported positive findings for adducin, there are large numbers of negative case–control studies involving this locus. Small case/control studies such as this, are probably insufficiently powered to demonstrate a minor effect of ACE or adducin on BP. None the less, the data in relation to these loci suggest that its influence, if any, on hypertension is small. The epistasic interaction of genes in developing hypertension is a complex area and will need to be examined in future studies in greater detail.

Endothelial function

Nitric oxide

Essential hypertension is associated with vascular endothelial dysfunction. Therefore, alterations in genes encoding proteins that regulate endothelial NO production are of interest as potential candidate genes in essential hypertension. The enzyme responsible for the generation of endothelial NO is endothelial nitric oxide synthase (eNOS). Several lines of evidence exist to implicate eNOS in hypertension. For example, NO production is reported to be reduced in essential hypertension; inhibition of NOS elevates BP in healthy humans, while studies of mice homozygous for the knockout of the eNOS gene show that they have a BP 15 mmHg higher than that of control mice. The gene encoding eNOS is located on human chromosome 7, and to date five polymorphic variants have been identified. Only one, a single nucleotide polymorphism on exon 7, results in an amino acid substitution (an aspartate for glutamine at amino acid residue 298; Glu[298]Asp). Two recent trials have assessed the importance of this polymorphism of the eNOS gene for hypertension.

Endothelial nitric oxide synthase gene is positively associated with essential hypertension.
Y Miyamoto, Y Saito, N Kajiyama, et al. Hypertension 1998; **32**: 3–8.

BACKGROUND. Essential hypertension has a genetic basis. Accumulating evidence, including findings of elevation of arterial BP in mice lacking the eNOS gene, strongly suggests that alteration in NO metabolism is implicated in hypertension.

INTERPRETATION. It was concluded that the Glu^{298}Asp mis-sense variant was significantly associated with essential hypertension, which suggests that it is a genetic susceptibility factor for essential hypertension.

Comment

This was a genetic association study of two independent Japanese populations, in which 218 hypertensives and 240 controls were recruited from one centre and 187 hypertensives and 223 controls from another. Not surprisingly, the hypertensive cohort had a higher baseline left ventricular mass index, plasma atrial naturetic peptide, brain naturetic peptide and uric acid levels. All other baseline characteristics, including age, body mass index, cholesterol and serum creatinine, were similar.

The Glu^{298}Asp mis-sense variant demonstrated a significant effect of genotype on hypertension, with an odds ratio of 2.3 (95% CI 1.4–3.9, $P = 0.0015$). The allele frequencies of the Glu^{298}Asp variant were 5.0% in normotensives and 10.3% in hypertensives. No significant gender difference was noted.

Lack of evidence for association between the endothelial nitric oxide synthase gene and hypertension.
N Kato, T Sugiyama, H Morita, *et al. Hypertension* 1999; **33**: 933–6.

BACKGROUND. Significant association between Glu^{298}Asp polymorphism of the *eNOS* gene and essential hypertension was recently reported in Japanese populations, with the ^{298}Asp variant showing a higher prevalence in hypertensive patients (10.3–12.0%) than in normotensive subjects (5.0–5.8%). In contrast, another study demonstrated that the ^{298}Glu variant was significantly associated with hypertension in a Caucasian population.

INTERPRETATION. Taken together, these results do not support the previous observation that the molecular variant of the *eNOS* gene may confer the principal susceptibility for essential hypertension, but rather suggest the existence of sampling variation.

Comment

This association study of a larger Japanese cohort of 1062 (549 hypertensives, 513 controls) subjects aimed to establish whether there was an association between the Glu^{298}Asp variant of the *eNOS* gene and essential hypertension. Statistical analysis was performed in two ways. First, a case–control study assessing allele frequencies between hypertensives and controls was examined, and secondly an analysis of variance was performed in which BP was considered as a continuous variable across the entire population. Both types of analysis failed to demonstrate any association.

The frequency of the Glu^{298}Asp variant was 8.4% and 8.2% in cases and controls, respectively.

The results from several studies assessing the Glu^{298}Asp variant of the *eNOS* gene have been inconclusive. The inherent weakness of small association studies means that we will still have to wait for a more detailed linkage analysis that is powerful enough for the task before this locus can be conclusively excluded.

Association analyses of endothelial nitric oxide synthase gene polymorphisms in essential hypertension.

A V Benjafield, B J Morris. *Am J Hypertens* 2000; **13**: 994–8.

BACKGROUND. NO produced by vascular endothelium is a potent regulator of cardiovascular homeostasis; decreased NO production has been reported in hypertensive patients. A polymorphism in a coding region of the *eNOS* provides an attractive candidate that might alter NO availability.

INTERPRETATION. No association was observed between the *eNOS* polymorphism and hypertension; one allele of the gene did, however, appear to track with body mass index.

Comment

Previous studies have examined the role of the *eNOS* gene in hypertension. In this particular study a well characterized group of patients with hypertension, all of whom had a strongly positive family history, were compared with normotensive subjects who had no family history. This particular population has been well characterized in previous studies and is likely to be of considerable value in identifying important candidate genes. In this analysis, two polymorphisms associated with *eNOS* were examined.

No allele was seen more frequently in hypertensive subjects compared with normotensives. Nonetheless, there was an apparent association with one polymorphism that leads to an amino acid change in *eNOS* and body mass index. While the mechanism of this association is obscure, and its significance uncertain, the data are of some interest given the suggestions that obesity acts as an independent risk factor for vascular dysfunction. Nonetheless, there is no support, from this study, that genetic variation at the *eNOS* locus is primarily associated with essential hypertension.

Endothelin-1 and endothelin A and B receptors

Endothelin-1 (ET1) is a potent vasoconstrictor produced by cleavage from its 38 amino acid precursor by endothelin-converting enzyme. ET1 exerts its effects by binding to the endothelin A (ETA) and B (ETB) receptors on vascular smooth muscle cells, and is thought to contribute to basal vascular tone. Therefore, the genes encoding ET1 and the ETA and B receptors again make attractive candidate genes for hypertension. To date, only one study, the Etude Cas-Témoins sur l'Infarctus du Myocarde (ECTIM) study, has examined the relationship between polymorphisms of the endothelin receptors and BP.

Polymorphisms of the endothelin-A and -B receptor genes in relation to blood pressure and myocardial infarction.

The Etude Cas-Témoins sur l'Infarctus du Myocarde (ECTIM) Study. V Nicaud, O Poirier, Behague, *et al. Am J Hypertens* 1999; **12**: 304–10.

BACKGROUND. ET-1 is a potent vasoconstrictor that also has mitogenic properties, stimulating the synthesis and secretion of several vasoactive molecules. There is much evidence to suggest that ET-1 might be involved in the pathogenesis of hypertension, atherosclerosis and ischaemic heart disease. ET-1 exerts its effects through at least two receptors, ETA and ETB, which are encoded by different genes and have separate tissue distributions and biological properties. The objective of this study was to identify polymorphisms of the ETA and ETB receptor genes and to study their association with myocardial infarction (MI) and BP.

INTERPRETATION. These results do not support an involvement of the endothelin receptor genes in a predisposition to MI or the determination of BP levels, but suggest that a polymorphism of the ETA receptor gene might influence the pulse pressure. This result will have to be confirmed in other studies.

Comment

The ECTIM study, as detailed above, also examined the genes encoding the ETA and ETB receptors and their relationship, if any, with BP. From this multicentre study, comparing 652 patients having survived an MI and 773 controls, six and three polymorphisms of the gene encoding the ETA and ETB receptors were identified, respectively. Associations between these polymorphisms, BP and MI were studied. The allele distribution for these numerous polymorphisms was similar between cases and controls, and measurements of mean systolic and diastolic BP did not vary between genotypes. One polymorphism (C→T) in exon 8 of the ETA gene was associated with pulse pressure; however, the clinical significance of this finding is unclear. Once again large multicentre studies will be required to clarify the role of this locus in essential hypertension.

Adrenergic receptors

Adrenoreceptors are G-protein coupled receptors that transduce signals for catecholamines; α_1-adrenoreceptors are vasoconstrictor, while β_2-adrenoreceptors, in the vasculature, are vasodilator. These receptors provide, for that reason, attractive candidates that might be involved in hypertension. In the last few years, a number of studies have been published that implicate, in particular, the β_2-adrenoreceptor as a potential key regulator of vascular function.

Association analysis of β_2 adrenoceptor polymorphisms with hypertension in black African population.

G Candy, N Samai, G Norton, *et al. J Hypertens* 2000, **18**: 167–72.

β_2 adrenergic receptor polymorphisms at codon 16, cardiovascular phenotypes and essential hypertension in whites and African Americans.

V Herrmann, R Buscher, M M Go, *et al. Am J Hypertens* 2000; **13**: 1021–6.

BACKGROUND. The β_2-adrenoreceptor subserves vasodilatation in vascular tissue. Previous studies have suggested that this locus might be involved in hypertension; polymorphisms in relation to the β_2-adrenoreceptor have been described that alter amino acid sequence. These two papers examine the association of the same polymorphism in codon 16 in hypertensive populations.

Comment

The study by Candy *et al.* focuses on subjects of black South African origin. Careful BP measurements were carried out and normal tensives and hypertensives compared. No association was found between the common polymorphism in codon 16 and BP or left ventricular mass; a possible finding of interest was an association between the polymorphism and body mass index in hypertensive subjects, although this was not seen in normotensives. The significance of this result is uncertain. In passing, it is of interest that the allelic frequencies in this population are different to caucasian populations. This illustrates the need for careful control for ethnicity in any case/control study.

The examination by Herrmann *et al.* looks at the same polymorphism in hypertensive and control subjects. The hypertensives were defined as either of white or African origin based on grandparental ancestry. A weakness of the study is, however, the relatively low numbers in each group. Of interest is that in this particular study no major difference in the allele frequency was detected in either population. Furthermore, no association between the polymorphism in codes 16 and hypertension was noted.

In summary, neither of these studies lends support for the notion that the β_2-adrenoreceptor gene is a key candidate in essential hypertension. In both studies, phenotyping was very carefully performed and the results must be regarded as robust.

Family linkage studies

Large-scale linkage analysis in hypertension are now coming to fruition. Many of these have employed an affected sibling pair design. It needs to be acknowledged that the power of these studies is relatively weak, and negative findings do not, necessarily, exclude particular regions as being involved in hypertension. Nonetheless, such studies do allow the use of genome-wide searches that avoid the need for candidate gene analysis. The advantage of this approach is that genes that otherwise might not be regarded as conventional candidates may be identified. It is likely that a number of other large-scale studies employing this design will be published over the next few years.

Evidence for a gene influencing blood pressure on chromosome 17

Genome scan linkage results for longitudinal blood pressure phenotypes in subjects from the Framingham Heart Study.

D Levy, A L DeStefano, M G Larson, *et al.* 2000; **36**(4): 469–70.

BACKGROUND. Linkage approaches use the co-transmission of phenotype and genotype within related individuals to summate protruder genetic loci. The approach requires large numbers of subjects to offer sufficient power to identify or exclude regions. Studies can either focus on preselected individuals, or use a genome-wide approach with a large number of anonymous markers.

Comment

The study of Levy *et al.* utilizes the Framingham population and uses a linkage type approach to identify a candidate region on chromosome 17. Here, change in BP with time within families could be examined and the heritability of BP phenotypes in this longitudinal manner studied. These data show that long-term BP phenotypes were significantly heritable for both systolic and diastolic pressure. Thereafter, the investigators carried out a genome-wide scan. Suggestive regions of linkage were found on chromosomes 5, 9 and 10 but the most strong support for linkage was found with chromosome 17 with LOD scores of > 3. These are highly significant findings and strongly suggest that this region harbours an important gene involved in BP regulation.

The nature of the gene that might be present with this region remains to be demonstrated. However, the human chromosome 17 contains within it a region that is syntenic with a quantitative trait locus on rat chromosome 10 that is also linked with high BP. This region contains genes that regulate the endothelial sodium channel, the chloride/bicarbonate exchanger and is also close to the ACE gene locus.

Thus, this is an important study that provides evidence that a family approach with a genome-wide analysis can, potentially, identify important genes involved in hypertension.

Genome-wide linkage analysis of systolic and diastolic blood pressure. The Quebec family study.
T Rice, T Rankinen, M A Province, *et al. Circulation* 2000; **102**: 1956–63.

A genome-wide search for susceptibility loci to human essential hypertension.
P Sharma, J Fatibene, F Ferraro, *et al. Hypertension* 2000; **35**: 1291–6.

Comment

The studies of Rice *et al.* and Sharma *et al.* both report genome-wide scans carried out in subjects with hypertension. The study by Rice *et al.* is based on the Quebec family study and includes 679 individuals. In this study, however, subjects were not selected on the basis of hypertension and BP was treated as a continuous variable. Suggestive evidence of linkage to BP was said to be found for regions on chromosome 19 and 22. However, the LOD scores for these regions were not high (all but one were less than 2), and the real significance of this finding remains uncertain. By convention, studies require LOD scores of > 3 to be regarded as supportive of linkage of a genotype with phenotype.

The paper by Sharma *et al.* examined siblings with hypertension (effectively 169 sibships). Using a genome-wide scan, a possible region of linkage was found on chromosome 11 but this was not supported by a more rigorous analysis. However, this is a small study; estimates of the number of sibling pairs necessary to have sufficient power to identify loci would suggest that this needs to be one order of magnitude less than that reported here. Thus, although no other regions were identified in this analysis, the study is unable to exclude, effectively, any particular regions of the genome.

In summary, these two studies identify the need for large carefully constructed collections of family linkage studies. The Quebec study examined BP as a continuous variable; while this is appropriate, a study of much greater size would be necessary to have sufficient power to identify responsible loci influencing BP regulation. The study by Sharma *et al.* is also insufficiently large and illustrates the need for careful collections of suitable populations in which this type of approach can be utilized.

Association of the Human Y chromosome with high blood pressure in the general population.

J A Ellis, M Stebbing, S B. Harrap. *Hypertension* 2000; **36**: 731–3.

BACKGROUND. Men have higher BP than women, and it is possible that this reflects a genetic effect. Few studies in humans have examined the role of the Y chromosome in BP variability.

Comment

This is an interesting study that has examined the relationship between BP and a marker associated with the Y chromosome in male subjects. Evidence suggests that a polymorphism of the Y chromosome is associated with variation in diastolic BP within the population. No change was noted for systolic BP.

This study is of interest, and illustrates the need to consider sex chromosomes in aspects of BP regulation. These would not, generally, be included in genome-wide searches. This finding may, however, explain some of the reasons for the known difference in BP between men and women in the population.

Conclusion

The current status of studies into the genetics of cardiovascular disease can be considered to be unsatisfactory, as at present there are many contradictory reports on a relatively limited number of candidate genes. The most appropriate way to identify important loci would be to perform large-scale, suitably powered studies that could provide comprehensive coverage of the human genome using a genome-wide search. This type of approach is now being carried out in large-scale studies both nationally and internationally. New technological developments may be vital in this regard. For example, recent availability of DNA 'chip' technology allows the rapid and high-throughput screening of large numbers of samples for single nucleotide polymorphisms, which are frequent within the human genome. Indeed, very recent papers have used this approach to study potential genes involved in cardiovascular regulation, and have shown that such polymorphisms are frequent and alter protein sequence. The functional importance of this variability remains unclear, but the availability of this dense genetic information holds considerable promise for future identification of the important genes involved in hypertension. However, until such data are available, it would seem hazardous to speculate about the relative importance of existing candidates. The information from these large-scale studies and the dividend from the Human Genome Mapping project may well identify new and hitherto unsuspected loci, which may be important in cardiovascular disease and may lead, in time, to new methods of drug development and targeting of patients at high risk.

References

1. Fall CH, Osmond C, Barker DJ, Clark PM, Hales CN, Stirling Y, Meade TW. Fetal and infant growth and cardiovascular risk factors in women [see comments]. *BMJ* 1995; **310**(6977): 428–32.

2. Barker DJ, Osmond C, Golding J, Kuh D, Wadsworth ME. Growth *in utero*, blood pressure in childhood and adult life, and mortality from cardiovascular disease. *BMJ* 1989; **298**(6673): 564–7.

3. Barker DJ, Osmond C, Simmonds SJ, Wield GA. The relation of small head circumference and thinness at birth to death from cardiovascular disease in adult life. *BMJ* 1993; **306**(6875): 422–6.

4. Walker WG, Whelton PK, Saito H, Russell RP, Hermann J. Relation between blood pressure and renin, renin substrate, angiotensin II, aldosterone and urinary sodium and potassium in 574 ambulatory subjects. *Hypertension* 1979; **1**(3): 287–91.

5. Hilbert P, Lindpaintner K, Beckmann JS, Serikawa T, Soubrier F, Dubay C, Cartwright P, De Gouyon B, Julier C, Takahasi S, *et al*. Chromosomal mapping of two genetic loci associated with blood-pressure regulation in hereditary hypertensive rats. *Nature* 1991; **353**: 521–9.

6. Rigat B, Hubert C, Alhenc-Gelas F, Cambien F, Corvol P, Soubrier F. An insertion/deletion polymorphism in the angiotensin I-converting enzyme gene accounting for half the variance of serum enzyme levels. *J Clin Invest* 1990; **86**(4): 1343–6.

7. White PC, Slutsker L. Haplotype analysis of *CYP11B2*. *Endocr Res* 1995; **21**(1–2): 437–42.

8. Salardi S, Saccardo B, Borsani G, Modica R, Ferrandi M, Tripodi MG, Soria M, Ferrari P, Baralle FE, Sidoli A, *et al*. Erythrocyte adducin differential properties in the normotensive and hypertensive rats of the Milan strain. Characterization of spleen adducin m-RNA. *Am J Hypertens* 1989; **2**(4): 229–37.

8

Insulin resistance, hypertension and endothelial function

Introduction

The association between hypertension and hyperinsulinaemia is widely acknowledged, although the full clinical significance still requires detailed clarification. Nevertheless, in essential hypertension abnormalities of insulin-mediated glucose metabolism have been invoked to explain aspects of pathogenesis, complications and the responses to treatment. There remain controversies, however, with recent evidence both for and against 'the insulin hypothesis'. The following questions might be posed to explore the clinical relevance of insulin resistance, hyperinsulinaemia and the interrelationships with hypertension, vascular endothelial function and responses to drug treatment:

1. Is insulin resistance associated with hypertension?

2. Do high insulin levels increase blood pressure?

3. (a) Does insulin have a vascular action?
   (b) Could blunting of insulin's vasodilator action cause hypertension?

4. (a) Could vascular endothelial dysfunction associated with hypertension cause insulin resistance?
   (b) Could primary insulin resistance result in endothelial dysfunction and promotion of hypertension?

5. Could an adverse lipid environment be the common antecedent linking insulin resistance and endothelial dysfunction/hypertension?

6. Could chronic inflammation play a role in the aetiology of insulin resistance and endothelial dysfunction/hypertension?

7. Do insulin-sensitizing drugs lower blood pressure?

8. What are the principal clinical issues?

Insulin resistance and hypertension

Studies using the hyperinsulinaemic euglycaemic clamp technique [1] have demonstrated that hyperinsulinaemia occurs in hypertension as a compensatory response to a reduction in insulin-mediated glucose uptake in skeletal muscle ('insulin resistance') |2,3|. The known major determinants of insulin sensitivity are age, weight and body fat distribution; but it should be noted that there is a threefold variation in insulin sensitivity amongst subjects matched for these variables |4|. Insulin resistance is absent in secondary hypertension |5| but present in normotensive offspring of essential hypertensive patients |6,7|, suggesting that it may be of pathophysiological relevance in this context.

Insulin resistance, hyperinsulinemia, and blood pressure: role of age and obesity.

E Ferrannini, A Natali, B Capaldo, M Lohtovirta, S Jacob, H Yki-Jarvinen. *Hypertension* 1997; **30**: 1144–9.

BACKGROUND. In population surveys, blood pressure (BP) and plasma insulin concentration are related variables, but the association is confounded by age and obesity. Whether insulin resistance is independently associated with higher BP in normal subjects is debated. The authors analysed the database of the European Group for the Study of Insulin Resistance, made up of non-diabetic men and women from 20 centres, in whom insulin sensitivity was measured by the euglycaemic insulin clamp.

INTERPRETATION. In normotensive, non-diabetic Europeans, insulin sensitivity and age are significant, mutually independent correlates of BP, whereas body mass is not. The relation of BP to both insulin action and circulating insulin levels is compatible with distinct influences on BP by insulin resistance or compensatory hyperinsulinaemia.

It has been suggested that the relationship between insulin resistance and BP may be confounded by obesity, as Body Mass Index (BMI) has a strong negative correlation with insulin sensitivity |8|. However, in the above paper by Ferrannini and colleagues, it was shown, using pooled analysis of insulin sensitivity data from 333 subjects from various European centres, that both systolic and diastolic BP have a negative relationship with insulin sensitivity even after adjustment for age, gender, BMI and fasting serum insulin concentration, i.e. the association between BMI and BP may be mediated by insulin sensitivity. From this analysis, the authors estimated that in terms of cardiovascular risk a 30% reduction in insulin sensitivity was equivalent to a 1.4 mmHg rise in BP. Although this may not seem large at first glance, at a population level a rise of this order could result in a 17% relative increase in incidence of cerebrovascular disease and a 10% increase in incidence of ischaemic heart disease |9|.

Comment

Overall, it appears that insulin resistance is independently associated with BP levels.

Hyperinsulinaemia and blood pressure

An elevation in serum insulin concentrations in patients with essential hypertension was first noted over 30 years ago |**10**|, and a number of cross-sectional epidemiological studies have supported an association between insulin levels and BP |**11,12**|. Whether hyperinsulinaemia is a cause, a consequence or an epiphenomenon in hypertension is hotly debated, but the relationship is certainly not direct and simple. For example, chronic artificial elevation of serum insulin concentrations increases BP in rats |**13**|, but has no effect in dogs |**14**|. Patients with insulinomas do not tend to have hypertension |**15**|. Nevertheless, prospective studies have shown that individuals with hyperinsulinaemia have a higher risk of going on to develop both hypertension |**16,17**| and coronary events |**18**|.

Insulin resistance and the effect of insulin on blood pressure in essential hypertension.
T Heise, K Magnusson, L Heinemann, P T Sawicki. *Hypertension* 1998; **32**: 243–8.

BACKGROUND. The aim of this study was to investigate the effect of 2 weeks of insulin administration on BP and simultaneously to measure insulin sensitivity and insulin-induced vasodilation in obese hypertensive patients.

INTERPRETATION. Insulin infusion increased limb blood flow significantly in the healthy controls, but not in obese insulin-resistant hypertensive subjects. Obese hypertensive patients are resistant to the effects of insulin with regard to both glucose uptake and vasodilation. Administration of insulin exerts a small BP-lowering effect in these patients. These data strongly argue against the postulated pressor action of insulin in essential hypertension.

Comment

In the above well-designed study by Heise and colleagues, it was shown that administration of insulin to insulin-resistant non-diabetic obese hypertensives had, if anything, a BP-lowering effect, i.e. insulin has vasodilator properties. These data support the notion that the link between insulin action and BP is more closely related to insulin resistance (i.e. at a tissue or cellular level) than to high levels of circulating insulin.

Vascular effects of insulin

Does insulin have a vascular action?

It is now generally accepted that systemic hyperinsulinaemia results in significant limb vasodilation |**19–22**|, although the physiological relevance of insulin as a vasodilator has been questioned |23|. It has been suggested that changes in blood flow may be occurring via central mechanisms rather than as a result of direct stimulation of insulin in limb vascular beds, a concept that has been supported by studies demonstrating little or no vasodilation in response to intra-arterial insulin infusion |24,25|.

The vasodilating effect of insulin is dependent on local glucose uptake: a double-blind, placebo-controlled study.

S Ueda, J R Petrie, S J Cleland, H L Elliott, J M C Connell. *J Clin Endocrinol Metab* 1998; **83**: 2126–31.

BACKGROUND. During systematic hyperinsulinaemia in man, skeletal muscle vasodilation has consistently been demonstrated. However, most studies that have examined the vascular effect of local hyperinsulinaemia have reported either no effect or only weak vasodilation. The present studies were designed in a double-blind, placebo-controlled manner to evaluate the direct (local) vascular effect of insulin alone and in association with physiological concentrations of D-glucose.

INTERPRETATION. These data suggest that local uptake of D-glucose by insulin-sensitive tissues is an important determinant of insulin-mediated vasodilation.

The above study set out to test the hypothesis that insulin-mediated glucose uptake is a key step in the mechanism of insulin-mediated vasodilation. The authors concluded that local glucose uptake was an important determinant of insulin's vascular effect, a result that might explain conflicting results between local and systemic studies: when insulin is infused systemically, 20% glucose is co-infused to prevent hypoglycaemia, whereas this is unnecessary in intra-arterial studies. This result has led the authors |26| and others |27| to propose that the underlying mechanisms of insulin's metabolic and vascular actions are functionally coupled, which might help to explain some of the observed associations among defects in insulin action, endothelial dysfunction and hypertension.

Comment

What mechanisms underlie the relationship between insulin and BP? Firstly, as has been shown above, the hormone has depressor peripheral vasodilator actions mainly in skeletal muscle vascular beds. Secondly, it has pressor effects mainly via stimulation of the sympathetic nervous system |19| and enhancement of renal sodium absorption |28,29|. The net physiological effect is a balance of pressor and depressor effects, and maintenance of BP. In pathophysiological states such as obesity, the balance may be disrupted by enhanced sympathetic activation in response to hyperinsulinaemia |30|, together with 'blunting' of insulin-mediated vasodilation (vascular insulin resistance) |31|.

Hypertension and impaired responsiveness to insulin

Insulin resistance in essential hypertension is characterized by impaired insulin stimulation of blood flow in skeletal muscle.

H Laine, M J Knuuti, U Ruotsalainen, *et al. Hypertension* 1998; **16**: 211–9.

BACKGROUND. The objective of this study was to determine whether insulin-stimulated blood flow in patients with mild essential hypertension is altered.

INTERPRETATION. The ability of insulin to stimulate blood flow in patients with mild essential hypertension is impaired.

Comment

In the above study by Laine and colleagues, the technique of positron emission tomography was used to measure limb blood flow and muscle glucose uptake in lean patients with mild essential hypertension. They concluded that there was, indeed, evidence to suggest that insulin-stimulated muscle blood flow is impaired in hypertension. This result concurs with previous reports of a negative correlation between insulin-induced vasodilation and BP using less sensitive techniques for measurement of flow |**20,32**|. In these studies supraphysiological doses of insulin were used to detect the relationship, and it has not so far been possible to confirm their findings using more physiological doses over shorter periods |**19,33**|. There-fore, it remains unclear whether blunting of insulin-mediated vasodilation con-tributes to hypertension in insulin-resistant states via increased peripheral vascular resistance.

Conclusion

Taken together, the results of these two studies indicate that the metabolic and vascular effects of insulin are mechanistically related. However, it remains unclear which is the primary defect: thus does a blunted vasodilation response to insulin contribute to the development of hypertension or does increased peripheral vascu-lar resistance create an insulin-resistant state?

Vascular endothelial dysfunction, hypertension and insulin resistance

Is vascular endothelial function associated with insulin resistance in hypertension?

 Insulin action is associated with endothelial function in hypertension and type 2 diabetes.
S J Cleland, J R Petrie, M Small, H L Elliott, J M Connell. *Hypertension* 2000; **35**(1 Pt 2): 507–11.

B A C K G R O U N D . **This study was designed to characterize more fully the relations between insulin action and endothelial function in male patients with essential hypertension or type 2 diabetes along with healthy control subjects matched for age, body mass index, and lipid profile.**

I N T E R P R E T A T I O N . In all three groups there were significant associations between (1) insulin sensitivity and insulin-mediated vasodilation (r = 0. 46, P <0.05) (2) insulin sensitivity and basal vascular nitric oxide production (r = 0.44, P <0.05) (3) insulin-mediated vasodilation and and basal vascular nitric oxide production (r = 0.52, P <0.01).

Comment

This study supports the concept of functional coupling between insulin action (both metabolic and vascular) and basal endothelial nitric oxide production in humans. These physiological associations are apparent in health and also in conditions of insulin resistance such as essential hypertension and type 2 diabetes.

Could vascular endothelial dysfunction associated with hypertension cause insulin resistance?

One common feature that has been proposed to account for the link between insulin resistance and BP is vascular endothelial dysfunction. Defects in basal and stimulated endothelial function have been demonstrated in some groups of patients with essential hypertension |**34–36**| and also in other insulin-resistant conditions such as obesity |**37**| and type II diabetes |**38,39**|. In healthy volunteers, whole-body insulin sensitivity has been shown to correlate with basal endothelial nitric oxide production |**40**|. In addition, insulin appears to cause vasodilation, at least in part, by stimulation of endothelial nitric oxide production |**41–43**|, and insulin-mediated vasodilation has been shown to correlate positively with insulin-stimulated glucose uptake |**26,27,44**|. Decreased blood flow to nutritive capillary beds could conceivably result in insulin resistance via a reduction in substrate delivery to target tissues |**20,44**|. Hence, primary endothelial dysfunction could contribute to high BP while at the same time causing blunting of insulin-mediated vasodilation and impaired insulin-mediated glucose uptake.

Vasodilation with sodium nitroprusside does not improve insulin action in essential hypertension.

A Natali, A Q Galvan, N Pecori, G Sanna, E Toschi, E Ferrannini.
Hypertension 1998; **31**: 632–6.

BACKGROUND. The vasodilation induced by systemic insulin infusion is mediated by nitric oxide and is impaired both in obese subjects and in patients with essential hypertension. Whether this vascular defect explains the metabolic resistance in insulin action is uncertain.

INTERPRETATION. The authors conclude that in overweight male patients with essential hypertension, increasing forearm perfusion with sodium nitroprusside does not attenuate the insulin resistance of forearm tissue.

Comment

If endothelial dysfunction blunts insulin-mediated vasodilation, one would predict that increasing blood flow to skeletal muscle vascular beds using vasodilators such as adenosine, bradykinin or sodium nitroprusside would result in an increase in glucose uptake. The above study by Natali and colleagues does not support this hypothesis. Despite local limb vasodilation with sodium nitroprusside, they were unable to demonstrate any improvements in insulin-mediated glucose uptake in a group of overweight male hypertensives. This negative finding is supported by two previous studies |**45,46**|, and the conclusion must be that primary endothelial dysfunction with associated blunting of insulin-mediated vasodilation is unlikely to be a significant determinant of insulin resistance.

Could primary insulin resistance result in endothelial dysfunction and promotion of hypertension?

Characterization of selective resistance to insulin signalling in the vasculature of obese zucker (*fa/fa*) rats.

Z Y Jiang, Y-W Lin, A Clemont, *et al. J Clin Invest* 1999; **104**: 447–57.

BACKGROUND. Both insulin resistance and hyperinsulinaemia have been reported to be independent risk factors for cardiovascular disease. However, little is known regarding insulin signalling in the vascular tissue in insulin-resistant states. In this report, insulin signalling on the phosphatidylinositol 3-kinase (PI 3-kinase) and mitogen-activated protein (MAP) kinase pathways were compared in vascular tissues of lean and obese Zucker (fa/fa) rats in both *ex vivo* and *in vivo* studies.

INTERPRETATION. To our knowledge, these data provided the first direct measurements of insulin signalling in the vascular tissue, and documented a selective resistance to PI 3-kinase (but not to MAP kinase pathways) in the vascular tissue of obese Zucker rats.

A more compelling explanation for the relationship between insulin sensitivity, essential hypertension and endothelial function is suggested by experiments in cultured endothelial cells in which enzymes central to intracellular glucose metabolism were blocked, resulting in abolition of insulin-stimulated nitric oxide production |47|. Furthermore, it has been demonstrated recently that mice which are deficient in IRS-1, the major substrate of the insulin receptor and a functionally important step in the insulin-signalling pathway, also appear to have impaired endothelium-dependent vascular relaxation |48|. Thus primary insulin resistance in endothelial cells may contribute to vascular dysfunction, hypertension and its cardiovascular complications.

Comment

The above study by Jiang and colleagues provides the most convincing evidence to date that defects in the insulin-signalling pathway persist in vascular tissues of an insulin-resistant animal model. Thus primary 'vascular insulin resistance' may lead to relative endothelial dysfunction and promotion of hypertension. Results from vascular endothelial cell insulin receptor 'knock-out' studies are awaited with interest.

Regulation of endothelial constitutive nitric oxide synthase gene expression in endothelial cells and in vivo: a specific vascular action of insulin.

K Kuboki, Z Y Jiang, N Takahara, *et al. Circulation* 2000; **101**(6): 676–81.

BACKGROUND. The vasodilatory effect of insulin can be acute or increase with time from 1 to 7 hours, suggesting that insulin may enhance the expression of endothelial nitric oxide synthase (eNOS) in endothelial cells. The objective of the present study was to characterize the extent and signaling pathways by which insulin regulates the expression of eNOS in endothelial cells and vascular tissues.

INTERPRETATION. Insulin can regulate the expression of the eNOS gene, mediated by the activation of PI-3 kinase, in endothelial cells and microvessels. Thus, insulin may chronically modulate vascular tone. The activation of Protein Kinase C in the vascular tissues as in insulin resistance and diabetes may inhibit PI-3 kinase activity and eNOS expression and may lead to endothelial dysfunction in these pathological states.

Comment

There is now evidence that insulin can upregulate genes involved in control of vascular tone and endothelial function as well as acutely stimulating enzyme activity. This implies a more chronic modulatory vascular role for insulin. This too appears to be blunted in conditions of insulin resistance.

Insulin resistance, endothelial dysfunction, hypertension and the lipid environment

While it seems likely that defects in insulin action and endothelial dysfunction are causally associated, it is possible that both are influenced independently by a common antecedent. One of the strongest candidates for this 'third factor' is the 'atherogenic lipid profile', which has been shown to be associated with both insulin resistance and vascular endothelial dysfunction.

Elevated circulating free fatty acid levels impair endothelium-dependent vasodilation.

H O Steinberg, M Tarshoby, R Monestel, *et al. J Clin Invest* 1997; **100**: 1230–9.

B A C K G R O U N D . **The authors have recently shown that insulin-resistant obese subjects exhibit impaired endothelial function. Here, they test the hypothesis that elevation of circulating free fatty acids (FFA) to levels seen in insulin-resistant subjects can impair endothelial function. They studied leg blood flow responses to graded intrafemoral artery infusions of the endothelial-dependent vasodilator methacholine chloride or the endothelium-independent vasodilator sodium nitroprusside during the infusion of saline and circulating FFA levels exogenously via a low- or high-dose infusion of Intralipid plus heparin or endogenously by an infusion of somatostatin (SRIF) to produce insulinopenia in groups of lean healthy humans.**

I N T E R P R E T A T I O N . In conclusion, elevated circulating FFA levels cause endothelial dysfunction, and impaired endothelial function in insulin-resistant humans may be secondary to the elevated FFA concentrations observed in these parts.

Comment

In the above study, Steinberg and colleagues demonstrated that infusion of FFA caused acute endothelial dysfunction in insulin-resistant subjects. Interestingly, co-infusion of insulin restored endothelial function, suggesting a direct effect of insulin in promoting endothelial nitric oxide production.

Free fatty acid elevation impairs insulin-mediated vasodilation and nitric oxide production.

H O Steinberg, G Paradisi, G Hook, K Crowder, J Cronin, A D Baron. *Diabetes* 2000; **49**(7): 1231–8.

B A C K G R O U N D . **The effect and time course of FFA elevation on insulin-mediated vasodilation and the relationship of FFA elevation to changes in insulin-mediated** glucose uptake was studied. In addition, the effect of FFA on blood flow responses to nitric oxide synthase inhibition was studied.

INTERPRETATION. Long FFA infusion decreased rates of whole-body glucose uptake, insulin-mediated increases in leg blood flow, and insulin-induced increases in NOx flux. Importantly, throughout all groups, FFA-induced changes in whole-body glucose uptake correlated significantly with FFA-induced changes in insulin-mediated increases in LBF ($r = 0.706$, $P < 0.001$), which indicates coupling of metabolic and vascular effects. Short FFA elevation blunted the leg blood flow response to nitric oxide synthase inhibition, indicating that FFA elevation interferes with shear stress-induced NO production. Thus, impairment of shear stress-induced vasodilation and insulin-mediated vasodilation by FFA elevation occurs with different time courses, and impairment of insulin-mediated vasodilation occurs only if glucose metabolism is concomitantly reduced.

Comment

FFA-induced reduction in NO production may contribute to the higher incidence of hypertension and macrovascular disease in insulin-resistant patients.

The role of chronic inflammation in the aetiology of insulin resistance and endothelial dysfunction/ hypertension

Recently, it has been proposed that low-grade chronic inflammation may play a key role in the process of vascular endothelial dysfunction and atherosclerosis. In the following study on blood samples from over 100 healthy volunteers, C-reactive protein levels were significantly related not only to markers of endothelial activation, but also to surrogate measurements of insulin resistance and obesity. Furthermore, it was suggested that cytokines causing metabolic and vascular dysfunction could be released from centrally distributed adipose tissue, thus explaining the observed coexistence of insulin resistance, endothelial dysfunction and hypertension in centrally obese patients.

C-reactive protein in healthy subjects: association with obesity, insulin resistance, and endothelial dysfunction; a potential role for cytokines originating from adipose tissue?

J S Yudkin, C D A Stehouwer, J J Emeis, S W Coppack. *Arterioscler Thromb Vasc Biol* 1999; **19**: 972–8.

BACKGROUND. C-reactive protein, a hepatic acute phase protein largely regulated by circulating levels of interleukin-6, predicts coronary heart disease incidence in healthy subjects. The authors have shown that subcutaneous adipose tissue secretes interleukin-6 *in vivo*. This study sought associations of levels of C-reactive protein and interleukin-6 with measures of obesity and of chronic infection as their putative determinants. It also related levels of C-reactive protein and interleukin-6 to markers of the insulin resistance syndrome and of endothelial dysfunction.

INTERPRETATION. These data suggest that adipose tissue is an important determinant of a low-level, chronic inflammatory state as reflected by levels of interleukin-6, tumour necrosis factor-alpha and C-reactive protein, and that infection with *H. pylori*, *C. pneumoniae* and cytomegalovirus is not. Moreover, these data support the concept that such a low-level, chronic inflammatory state may induce insulin resistance and endothelial dysfunction, and thus link the latter phenomena with obesity and cardiovascular disease.

Comment

This is an interesting and plausible hypothesis. However, causal relationships cannot be proved from cross-sectional correlation studies, and further prospective research is required in this interesting area.

TNF-α inhibits flow and insulin signaling leading to NO production in aortic endothelial cells.

F Kim, B Gallis, M A Corson. *Am J Physiol Cell Physiol* 2001; **280**(5): C1057–65.

BACKGROUND. Endothelial cells release nitric oxide (NO) acutely in response to increased "flow" or fluid shear stress (FSS), and the increase in NO production is correlated with enhanced phosphorylation and activation of endothelial nitric oxide synthase (eNOS). Both vascular endothelial growth factor and FSS activate endothelial protein kinase B (PKB) by way of incompletely understood pathway(s), and, in turn, PKB phosphorylates eNOS at Ser-1179, causing its activation.

INTERPRETATION. In this study, either FSS or insulin stimulated IRS-1 resulted in increased IRS-1-associated phosphatidylinositol 3-kinase activity, phosphorylation of PKB Ser-473, phosphorylation of eNOS Ser-1179, and NO production. Brief pretreatment of bovine aortic endothelial cells with tumour necrosis factor-alpha (TNF-α) inhibited the above described FSS- or insulin-stimulated protein phosphorylation events and almost totally inhibited FSS- or insulin-stimulated NO production. These data indicate that FSS and insulin regulate eNOS phosphorylation and NO production by overlapping mechanisms.

Comment

This study suggests one potential mechanism for the development of endothelial dysfunction in disease states with alterations in insulin regulation and increased TNF-α levels.

Effect of insulin-sensitizing drugs on blood pressure

Vasodilatory effects of troglitazone improve blood pressure at rest and during mental stress in type 2 diabetes mellitus.

B H Sung, H L Izzo Jr, P Dandona, M F Wilson. *Hypertension* 1999; **34**: 83–8.

BACKGROUND. The present study examined the haemodynamic mechanisms of BP lowering by troglitazone in patients with type 2 diabetes mellitus (DM) at rest and during a mental arithmetic test. Twenty-two patients with DM with normal to high-normal BP and 12 controls matched for age, gender, glucose tolerance and BP were studied.

INTERPRETATION. Improved insulin resistance rather than improved glycaemic control is associated with lower resting and stress BP values in patients with DM. A reduction in vascular resistance may be a primary haemodynamic mechanism of the manner in which troglitazone lowers BP. Insulin sensitizers may offer potential therapeutic advantage in subjects with DM with elevated BP.

Comment

Insulin-sensitizing agents, such as the thiazolidinedione derivatives ('glitazones') |49|, appear to exert their effects via peroxisome proliferator-activated receptor gamma on post-receptor binding steps in the transduction of the insulin response |50|. Studies in man examining other primary endpoints have serendipitously reported significant reductions in BP |51,52|. In the above study by Sung and colleagues, BP, both at rest and during a mental arithmetic test, was significantly reduced by troglitazone treatment, but not by glyburide, in a group of type II diabetic patients. This effect occurred in association with decreased peripheral resistance. Therefore, it appears that troglitazone influences metabolic and vascular pathways in parallel. Current research is attempting to elicit the intracellular mechanisms involved in these effects and, in doing so, may provide valuable insights into the physiological mechanisms responsible for the apparent coupling between insulin's metabolic and vascular actions and their relationship with vascular endothelial function.

Dominant negative mutations in human PPAR associated with severe insulin resistance, diabetes mellitus and hypertension.

I Barroso, M Gurnell, V E Crowley, *et al. Nature* 1999; **402**(6764): 880–3.

BACKGROUND. Thiazolidinediones are a new class of antidiabetic agent that improve insulin sensitivity and reduce plasma glucose and blood pressure in subjects with type 2 diabetes. Although these agents can bind and activate an orphan nuclear receptor, peroxisome proliferator-activated receptor γ (PPARγ), there is no direct evidence to conclusively implicate this receptor in the regulation of mammalian glucose homeostasis. Two different heterozygous mutations in the ligand-binding domain of PPARγ are reported in three subjects with severe insulin resistance.

INTERPRETATION. In the PPARγ crystal structure, the mutations destabilize helix 12 which mediates transactivation. Consistent with this, both receptor mutants are markedly transcriptionally impaired and, moreover, are able to inhibit the action of coexpressed wild-type PPARγ in a dominant negative manner. In addition to insulin resistance, all three subjects developed type 2 diabetes mellitus and hypertension at an unusually early age.

Comment

These findings represent the first germline loss-of-function mutations in PPARγ and provide compelling genetic evidence that this receptor is important in the control of insulin sensitivity, glucose homeostasis and blood pressure in man.

Improved endothelial function with metformin in type 2 diabetes mellitus.

K J Mather, S Verma, T J Anderson. *J Am Coll Cardiol* 2001; **37**(5): 1344–50.

BACKGROUND. Abnormalities in vascular endothelial function are well recognized among patients with type 2 (insulin-resistant) diabetes mellitus. Insulin resistance itself may be central to the pathogenesis of endothelial dysfunction. The effects of metformin, an antidiabetic agent that improves insulin sensitivity, on endothelial function have not been reported. Subjects with diet-treated type 2 diabetes but without the confounding collection of cardiovascular risk factors seen in the metabolic syndrome were treated with metformin 500 mg twice daily ($n = 29$) or placebo ($n = 15$) for 12 weeks.

INTERPRETATION. Subjects who received metformin demonstrated statistically significant improvement in acetylcholine-stimulated forearm blood flow compared with controls. There was a significant improvement in insulin resistance with metformin and by stepwise multivariate analysis insulin resistance was the sole predictor of endothelium-dependent blood flow following treatment.

Comment

Metformin treatment improved both insulin resistance and endothelial function, with a strong statistical link between these variables. This supports the concept of the central role of insulin resistance in the pathogenesis of endothelial dysfunction in type 2 diabetes mellitus. This has important implications for the investigation and treatment of vascular disease in patients with type 2 diabetes.

Insulin resistance and cardiovascular disease: the clinical issues

Lifestyle issues and specific drug treatments

Prevention of type 2 diabetes mellitus by changes in lifestyle among subjects with impaired glucose tolerance.

J Tuomilehto, J Lindstrom, J G Eriksson, *et al. N Engl J Med* 2001; **344**(18): 1343–50.

BACKGROUND. Type 2 diabetes mellitus is increasingly common, primarily because of increases in the prevalence of a sedentary lifestyle and obesity. Whether type 2 diabetes can be prevented by interventions that affect the lifestyles of subjects at high risk for the disease is not known. Middle-aged, overweight subjects (*n* = 522) with impaired glucose tolerance were randomly assigned to either the intervention group or the control group. Each subject in the intervention group received individualized counseling aimed at reducing weight, total intake of fat, and intake of saturated fat and increasing intake of fibre and physical activity. An oral glucose-tolerance test was performed annually; the diagnosis of diabetes was confirmed by a second test. The mean duration of follow-up was 3.2 years.

INTERPRETATION. The mean amount of weight lost between baseline and the end of year 1 was 4.2 kg in the intervention group and 0.8 kg in the control group. The cumulative incidence of diabetes after four years was 11% in the intervention group and 23% in the control group. During the trial, the risk of diabetes was reduced by 58% (*P* <0.001) in the intervention group. The reduction in the incidence of diabetes was directly associated with changes in lifestyle.

Comment

Having identified insulin resistance as a potential independent cardiovascular risk factor and having proposed lifestyle intervention and insulin-sensitizing drugs as potential risk-reduction strategies, it can be argued that the issue of insulin resistance still remains of academic interest rather than realistic clinical relevance. Although weight loss and aerobic exercise have been shown to improve insulin sensitivity, it is recognized that attempts in routine clinical practice to investigate major lifestyle changes are usually disappointing |**53**|. However, this study is the first to demonstrate convincingly that type 2 diabetes can be prevented by changes in the lifestyles of high-risk subjects.

Practical management issues

It is becoming clear that insulin-resistant subjects (i.e. these at high cardiovascular risk) benefit more from traditional cardiovascular risk-reduction management: therefore, it may be that the main clinical relevance of identifying insulin resistance is to target those individuals who warrant more aggressive cardiovascular risk reduction. For example, recent studies of type 2 diabetes subgroups in a number of BP-lowering trials have revealed a two- to three-fold increase in relative risk reduction for cardiovascular events |54–56| irrespective of the class of antihypertensive agent used. Furthermore, aiming for a target diastolic BP of < 80 mmHg compared with <90 mmHg resulted in a 50% further reduction in cardiovascular event rate in type II diabetic patients |55|, emphasizing the importance of aggressive risk reduction. In addition, it has long been known that diabetic patients benefit more than their non-diabetic counterparts from thrombolysis following myocardial infarction, as well as from cessation of smoking in terms of reduction of cardiovascular morbidity and mortality.

Antihypertensive drugs and insulin resistance

The reported deleterious metabolic effects of 'older' antihypertensive agents (β-blockers and diuretics) have been implicated by some in the shortfall in the reductions achieved (compared with those predicted) in mortality from coronary heart disease in treated hypertensive populations |57|.

Additionally, influential reports of improved insulin sensitivity during angiotensin converting enzyme (ACE) inhibitor drug treatment have led to the proposal of a variety of mechanisms by which the renin–angiotensin system might influence insulin responsiveness. However, many of these apparently positive studies have used uncontrolled and/or flawed study designs, or indirect measures of insulin sensitivity, or have been conducted in subjects receiving potentially confounding medications |58|. One of the most widely cited and well-publicized studies in this area reported an improvement in insulin sensitivity in non-diabetic patients with hypertension randomized to captopril treatment versus hydrochlorothiazide |59|. The original oft-quoted study by Pollare *et al.* was designed as a cross-over study to compare captopril with hydrochlorothiazide, and did not include a direct comparison with placebo. However, data in the second treatment period were unsuitable for analysis, owing to a carry-over effect, and the results were presented separately for the two groups as comparisons with the baseline placebo period. The captopril group ($n=23$) at the start of treatment had similar measured insulin sensitivity to that of the diuretic-treated group ($n=27$) at the end of treatment. This suggests the possibility that the reported treatment effect may simply represent regression towards the mean. Despite these shortcomings, this trial has been extremely influential in support of the perception that ACE inhibitors improve insulin sensitivity.

The landmark UK Prospective Diabetes Study has recently emphasized the benefits of antihypertensive treatment in type 2 diabetes, reporting similar efficacy of captopril and atenolol on diabetic complications in these patients. Furthermore, a recent study using the euglycaemic clamp technique has demonstrated that captopril does not effect insulin sensitivity in non-diabetic patients with essential hypertension |60|. Therefore, it can be concluded that there is, as yet, no compelling evidence for beneficial metabolic effects of ACE inhibitors over other classes of antihypertensive drugs. Instead, the clinical emphasis remains with 'tight' BP control with effective hypertensive drugs, alone and in combination.

Conclusion

Insulin resistance is associated with hypertension in man. In addition to its well-known metabolic actions, insulin causes vasodilation, which is dependent of both endothelial nitric oxide production and cellular glucose uptake. Insulin's metabolic and vascular actions appear to have a common physiological mechanism. Hence blunting of insulin-mediated vasodilation and subsequent increased peripheral vascular resistance could explain the observed association between insulin resistance and hypertension. There are three possible explanations for the observed association between insulin action and vascular endothelial function: (1) primary endothelial dysfunction may cause a reduction in blood flow to insulin-sensitive tissues, resulting in relative insulin resistance; (2) primary defects in the insulin-signalling pathway in vascular tissues may cause vascular dysfunction in parallel with metabolic insulin resistance; or (3) a 'third factor' may be influencing both insulin-mediated glucose uptake and endothelial function—potential candidates include lipid profile and cytokines. Treatment with thiazolidinediones in man enhances insulin sensitivity and lowers BP. Further elucidation of the intracellular mechanisms involved in the insulin-signalling pathway may reveal new therapeutic targets in cardiovascular and metabolic disorders.

References

1. DeFronzo RA, Tobin JD, Andres R. Glucose clamp technique: a method for quantifying insulin secretion and resistance. *Am J Physiol* 1979; **237**: E214–23.

2. Ferrannini E, Buzzigoli G, Bonadonna R, Giorico MA, Oleggini M, Graziadei L, *et al.* Insulin resistance in essential hypertension. *N Engl J Med* 1987; **317**: 350–7.

3. Lind L, Berne C, Lithell H. Prevalence of insulin resistance in essential hypertension. *J Hypertens* 1995; **13**: 1457–62.

4. Hollenbeck G, Reaven GM. Variations in insulin-stimulated glucose uptake in healthy individuals with normal glucose tolerance. *J Clin Endocrinol Metab* 1987; **64**: 1169–73.

5. Shamiss A, Carroll J, Rosenthal T. Insulin resistance in secondary hypertension. *Am J Hypertens* 1992; **5**: 26–8.

6. Beatty OL, Harper R, Sheridan B, Atkinson AB, Bell PM. Insulin resistance in offspring of hypertensive parents. *Br Med J* 1993; **307**: 92–6.

7. Endre T, Mattiasson I, Lennart Hulthen U, Lindgarde F, Berglund G. Insulin resistance is coupled to low physical fitness in normotensive men with a family history of hypertension. *J Hypertens* 1994; **12**: 81–8.

8. Jarrett RJ. In defence of insulin: a critique of syndrome X. *Lancet* 1992; **340**: 469–71.

9. MacMahon S, Peto R, Cutler J, Collins R, Sorlie P, Neaton J, Abbott R, Godwin J, Dyer A, Stamler J. Blood pressure, stroke and coronary artery disease. Part 1: Prolonged differences in blood pressure: prospective observational studies corrected for the regression dilution bias. *Lancet* 1990; **335**: 765–74.

10. Welborn TA, Breckenridge A, Dollery CT, Rubenstein AH, Russell Fraser T. Serum insulin in essential hypertension and in peripheral vascular disease. *Lancet* 1966; **1**: 1336–7.

11. Modan M, Halkin H, Almog S, Lusky A, Eshkol A, Shefi M, Shitrit A. Hyperinsulinaemia. A link between hypertension, obesity and glucose intolerance. *J Clin Invest* 1985; **75**: 809–17.

12. Feskens EJM, Tuomilehto J, Stengard JH, Pekkanen J, Nissinen A, Kromhout D. Hypertension and overweight associated with hyperinsulinaemia and glucose tolerance: a longitudinal study of the Finnish and Dutch cohorts of the Seven Countries Study. *Diabetologia* 1995; **38**: 839–47.

13. Brands MW, Mizelle HL, Gaillard DA, Hildebrandt DA, Hall JE. The haemodynamic response to chronic hyperinsulinaemia in conscious dogs. *Am J Hypertens* 1991; **4**: 164–8.

14. Brands MW, Hildebrandt DA, Mizelle HL, Hall JE. Sustained hyperinsulinaemia increases arterial pressure in conscious rats. *Am J Physiol* 1991; **260**: R764–8.

15. Fujita N, Baba T, Tomiyami T, Kodama T, Kako N. Hyperinsulinaemia and blood pressure in patients with insulinoma. *Br Med J* 1992; **304**: 1157.

16. Haffner SM, Valdez RA, Hazuda HP, Mitchell BD, Morales PA, Stern MP. Prospective analysis of the insulin-resistance syndrome (syndrome X). *Diabetes* 1992; **41**: 715–22.

17. Bao W, Srinivasan S, Berenson G. Persistent elevation of plasma insulin levels is associated with increased cardiovascular risk in children and young adults. *Circulation* 1996; **93**: 54–9.

18. Despres JP, Lamarche B, Mauriege P, Cantin B, Dagenais GR, Moorjani S, Lupien PJ. Hyperinsulinaemia as an independent risk factor for ischaemic heart disease. *N Engl J Med* 1996; **334**: 952–7.

19. Anderson EA, Hoffman RP, Balon TW, Sinkey CA, Mark AL. Hyperinsulinemia produces both sympathetic neural activation and vasodilation in normal humans. *J Clin Invest* 1991; **87**: 2246–52.

20. Baron AD. Cardiovascular actions of insulin in humans. Implications for insulin sensitivity and vascular tone. *Bailliere's Clin Endocrinol Metab* 1993; **7**: 961–87.

21. Natali A, Taddei S, Galvan AQ, Camastra S, Baldi S, Frascerra S, Virdis A, Sudano I, Salvetti A, Ferrannini E. Insulin sensitivity, vascular reactivity and clamp-induced vasodilatation in essential hypertension. *Circulation* 1997; **96**: 849–55.

22. Utriainen T, Nuutila P, Takala T, Vicini P, Ruotsalainen U, Ronnemaa T, Tolvanen T, Raitakari M, Haaparanta M, Kirvela O, Cobelli C, Yki-Jarvinen H. Intact insulin

stimulation of skeletal muscle blood flow, its heterogeneity and redistribution, but not of glucose uptake in non-insulin-dependent diabetes mellitus. *J Clin Invest* 1997; **100**: 777–85.

23. Yki-Jarvinen H, Utriainen T. Insulin-induced vasodilatation: physiology or pharmacology? *Diabetologia* 1998; **41**: 369–79.

24. Sakai K, Imaizumi T, Masaki H, Takeshita A. Intra-arterial infusion of insulin attenuates vasoreactivity in human forearm. *Hypertension* 1993; **22**: 67–73.

25. Natali A, Buzzigoli G, Taddi S, Sanatoro D, Cerri M, Pedrinelli R, Ferrannini E. Effects of insulin on hemodynamics and metabolism in human forearm. *Diabetes* 1990; **39**: 490–500.

26. Cleland SJ, Petrie JR, Ueda S, Elliott HL, Connell JMC. Insulin-mediated vasodilation and glucose uptake are functionally linked in humans. *Hypertension* 1999; **33**(Suppl 2): 554–8.

27. Feldman RD, Hramiak IM, Finegood DT, Behme MT. Parallel regulation of the local vascular and systemic metabolic effects of insulin. *J Clin Endocrinol Metab* 1995; **80**: 1556–9.

28. DeFronzo RA, Cooke CR, Andres R, Faloona GR, David PJ. The effect of insulin on renal handling of sodium, potassium, calcium and phosphate in man. *J Clin Invest* 1975; **55**: 845–55.

29. Ferrannini E, Natali A. Insulin resistance and hypertension: connections with sodium metabolism. *Am J Kidney Dis* 1993; **21**(Suppl 2): 37–42.

30. Scherrer U, Randin D, Tappy L, Vollenweider P, Jequier E, Nicod P. Body fat and sympathetic nerve activity in healthy subjects. *Circulation* 1994; **89**: 2634–40.

31. Laakso M, Edelman SV, Brechtel G, Baron AD. Decreased effect of insulin to stimulate skeletal muscle blood flow in obese man: a novel mechanism for insulin resistance. *J Clin Invest* 1990; **85**: 1844–52.

32. Feldman RD, Bierbrier GS. Insulin-mediated vasodilation: impairment with increased blood pressure and body mass. *Lancet* 1993; **342**: 707–9.

33. Hunter SJ, Harper R, Ennis CN, Sheridan B, Atkinson AB, Bell PM. Skeletal muscle blood flow is not a determinant of insulin resistance in essential hypertension. *J Hypertens* 1997; **15**: 73–7.

34. Calver A, Collier J, Moncada S, Vallance P. Effect of local intra-arterial N(G)-monomethyl-L-arginine on patients with hypertension: the nitric oxide dilator mechanism appears abnormal. *J Hypertens* 1992; **10**: 1025–31.

35. Panza JA, Casino PR, Kilcoyne CM, Quyyumi AA. Role of endothelium-derived nitric oxide in the abnormal endothelium-dependent vascular relaxation of patients with essential hypertension. *Circulation* 1993; **87**: 1468–74.

36. Cockcroft JR, Chowienczyk PJ, Benjamin N, Ritter JM. Preserved endothelium-dependent vasodilatation in patients with essential hypertension. *N Engl J Med* 1994; **330**: 1036–40.

37. Steinberg HO, Chaker H, Leaming R, Johnson A, Brechtel G, Baron AD. Obesity/insulin resistance is associated with endothelial dysfunction. *J Clin Invest* 1996; **97**: 2601–10.

38. McVeigh E, Brennan GM, Johnston GD, McDermott BJ, McGrath LT, Henry WR, Andrews JW, Hayes JR. Impaired endothelium-dependent and independent vasodilation in patients with type 2 (non-insulin-dependent) diabetes mellitus. *Diabetologia* 1992; **35**: 771–6.

39. Williams SB, Cusco JA, Roddy M, Johnstone MT, Creager MA. Impaired nitric oxide-mediated vasodilation in patients with non-insulin-dependent diabetes mellitus. *J Am Coll Cardiol* 1996; **27**: 567–74.

40. Petrie J, Ueda S, Webb DJ, Elliott HL, Connell JMC. Endothelial nitric oxide production and insulin sensitivity: a physiological link with implications for pathogenesis of cardiovascular disease. *Circulation* 1996; **93**: 1331–3.

41. Scherrer U, Randin D, Vollenweider P, Vollenweider L, Nicod P. Nitric oxide release accounts for insulin's vascular effects in humans. *J Clin Invest* 1994; **94**: 2511–15.

42. Steinberg HO, Brechtel G, Johnson A, Fineberg N, Baron AD. Insulin-mediated skeletal muscle vasodilation is nitric oxide dependent: a novel action of insulin to increase nitric oxide release. *J Clin Invest* 1994; **94**: 1172–9.

43. Cleland SJ, Petrie JR, Ueda S, Elliott HL, Connell JMC. Insulin vasodilatation is abolished by both L-NMMA and angiotensin II. *J Hypertens* 1997; **15**(Suppl 4): S71 (Abstract).

44. Baron AD, Steinberg HO, Chaker H, Leaming R, Johnson A, Brechtel G. Insulin-mediated skeletal muscle vasodilation contributes to both insulin sensitivity and responsiveness in lean humans. *J Clin Invest* 1995; **96**: 786–92.

45. Natali A, Bonadonna R, Santoro D, Galvan AQ, Baldi S, Frascerra S, Palombo C, Ghione S, Ferrannini E. Insulin resistance and vasodilation in essential hypertension: studies with adenosine. *J Clin Invest* 1994; **94**: 1570–6.

46. Nuutila P, Raitakari M, Laine H, Kirvela O, Takala T, Utriainen T, Makimattila S, Pitkanen OP, Ruotsalainen U, Iida H, Knuuti J, Yki-Jarvinen H. Role of blood flow in regulating insulin-stimulated glucose uptake in humans: studies using bradykinin, [^{15}O]water, and [^{18}F]fluoro-deoxy-glucose and positron emission tomography. *J Clin Invest* 1996; **97**: 1741–7.

47. Zeng G, Quon MJ. Insulin-stimulated production of nitric oxide is inhibited by wortmannin. *J Clin Invest* 1996; **98**: 894–8.

48. Abe H, Yamada N, Kamata K, Kuwaki T, Shimada M, Osuga J, Shionoiri F, Yahagi N, Kadowaki T, Tamemoto H, Ishibashi S, Yazaki Y, Makuuchi M. Hypertension, hypertriglyceridemia, and impaired endothelium-dependent vascular relaxation in mice lacking insulin receptor substrate-1. *J Clin Invest* 1998; **101**: 1784–8.

49. Petrie JR, Small M, Connell JMC. 'Glitazones', a prospect for non-insulin-dependent diabetes. *Lancet* 1997; **349**: 70–1.

50. Kotchen TA. Attenuation of hypertension by insulin-sensitizing agents. *Hypertension* 1996; **28**: 219–23.

51. Nolan JJ, Ludvik B, Beersden P, Joyce M, Olefsky J. Improvement in glucose tolerance and insulin resistance in obese subjects treated with troglitazone. *N Engl J Med* 1994; **331**: 1188–93.

52. Ogihara T, Rakugi H, Ikegami H, Mikami H, Masuo K. Enhancement of insulin sensitivity by troglitazone lowers blood pressure in diabetic hypertensives. *Am J Hypertens* 1995; **8**: 316–20.

53. NIH Technology Assessment Conference Panel. Methods for voluntary weight loss and control. *Ann Intern Med* 1993; **119**: 764–70.

54. Curb JD, Pressel SL, Cutler JA, Savage PJ, Applegate WB, Black H, Camel G, Davis BR, Frost PH, Gonzalez N, Guthrie G, Oberman A, Rutan GH, Stamler J. Effect of diuretic-based antihypertensive treatment on cardiovascular disease risk in older diabetic patients with isolated systolic hypertension. *JAMA* 1996; **276**: 1886–92.

55. Hansson L, Zanchetti I, Carruthers SG, Dahlof B, Elmfeldt D, Julius S, Menard J, Rahn KH, Wedel H, Westerling S. Effects of intensive blood pressure lowering and low-dose aspirin in patients with hypertension. Principal results of the Hypertension Optimal Treatment (HOT) randomised trial. *Lancet* 1998; **35**: 1755–62.

56. UK Prospective Diabetes Study Group. Efficacy of atenolol and captopril in reducing risk of macrovascular and microvascular complications in type 2 diabetes. *Br Med J* 1998; **317**: 713–20.

57. Collins R, Peto R, MacMahon S, Herbert P, Fiebach NH, Eberlein KA, Godwin J, Oizilbash N, Taylor JO, Hennekens CH. Blood pressure, stroke and coronary heart disease. Part 2. Short-term reductions in blood pressure: overview of randomised drug trials in their epidemiological context. *Lancet* 1990; **335**: 827–38.

58. Donnelly R. Angiotensin-converting enzyme inhibitors and insulin sensitivity: metabolic effects in hypertension, diabetes and heart failure. *J Cardiovasc Pharmacol* 1992; **20**(Suppl 1): S38–S44.

59. Pollare TG, Lithell H, Berne C. A comparison of the effects of hydrochlorothiazide and captopril on glucose and lipid metabolism in patients with hypertension. *N Engl J Med* 1989; **321**: 672–86.

60. Wiggam MI, Hunter SJ, Atkinson AB, Ennis CN, Henry JS, Browne JN, Sheridan B, Bell PM. Captopril does not improve insulin action in essential hypertension: a double blind placebo-controlled study. *J Hypertens* 1998; **16**: 103–9.

9

Mineralocorticoid hypertension: from recent research to clinical developments

Introduction

High blood pressure associated with excessive renal sodium reabsorption in the distal renal tubule, expansion of the extracellular fluid compartment and increased body sodium content, leading to suppression of synthesis and release of renin, is defined as mineralocorticoid hypertension (for a review, see Stewart 1999 |**1**|). Mineralocorticoid hypertension results from excessive activation of the epithelial sodium channel, which is normally regulated by the mineralocorticoid receptor. Recently, detailed understanding of the various biochemical and molecular mechanisms that result in a common clinical phenotype has shed light on the basic mechanisms involved in blood pressure and volume homeostasis. In turn, this has identified important candidate mechanisms that might contribute to the development of essential hypertension. In this regard, it is important to note that the majority of studies on the genetic basis of human essential hypertension have focused on candidate genes encoding components of the renin–angiotensin–aldosterone system or on genes involved in renal sodium retention. For example, some, but not all, studies have supported the involvement of the angiotensinogen locus in human essential hypertension |**2–4**|. In addition, the gene encoding human aldosterone synthase (*CYP11B2*) has been reported, in several studies in the last 12 months, to be associated with high blood pressure and increased urinary aldosterone excretion.

Evaluation of the angiotensin locus in human essential hypertension.

E Brand, N Chatelain, B Keavney, *et al. Hypertension* 1998; **31**: 725–9.

BACKGROUND. Different family and case–control studies support genetic linkage and association at the human angiotensinogen (AGT) locus with essential hypertension. To extend these previous observations, a European collaborative study of nine centres was set up to create a large resource of affected sibling pairs.

METHODS AND RESULTS. **The AGT locus was studied using a highly polymorphic dinucleotide repeat in the 3'-flanking region of the gene in 350 European families, comprising 630 affected sibling pairs. Statistical analyses using two different methods did not show any evidence for linkage either in the whole panel or in family subsets selected for severity or early onset of disease.**

INTERPRETATION. Although several arguments from association studies suggest a role of the AGT gene in essential hypertension, this large family study did not replicate the initial linkage reported in smaller studies. Our results highlight the difficulty of identifying susceptibility genes by linkage analysis in complex diseases.

Comment

The role of the AGT locus in hypertension has been the subject of a number of studies over the last year. In this investigation, a large sibling pair collection from across Europe was investigated and showed no evidence for linkage of the AGT locus with hypertension. This study suggests that previous investigations may have shown false-positive results due to small numbers, and illustrates the importance of performing appropriately powered studies in the investigation of the genetic basis of hypertension.

Structural analysis and evaluation of the aldosterone synthase gene in hypertension.

E Brand, N Chatelain, P Mulatero, *et al. Hypertension* 1998; **32**: 198–204.

BACKGROUND. **Anomalies in either of the tightly linked genes encoding the enzymes *CYP11B1* (11 beta-hydroxylase) or *CYP11B2* (aldosterone synthase) can lead to important changes in arterial pressure and are responsible for several monogenically inherited forms of hypertension. Mutations in these genes or their regulatory regions could thus contribute to genetic variation in susceptibility to essential hypertension. To test this hypothesis, the authors performed two complementary studies of the *CYP11B1/CYP11B2* locus in essential hypertension.**

METHODS AND RESULTS. **After characterizing a DNA contig containing the *CYP11B1* gene and mapping the gene in the Centre d'Etudes du Polymorphisme Humain reference panel of families, a linkage study was performed with 292 hypertensive sibling pairs and a highly informative microsatellite marker near *CYP11B1*. Also analysed were the association of two frequent bi-allelic polymorphisms of the *CYP11B2* gene, one in the promoter at position –344 (–344C/T) and the other a common gene conversion in intron 2, with hypertension in 380 hypertensive patients and 293 normotensive individuals. Statistical analyses did not show significant linkage of the *CYP11B1* microsatellite marker to hypertension.**

INTERPRETATION. No positive association with hypertension was found with the gene conversion in intron 2, but a positive association with hypertension was found with the

–344T allele. The hypertensive and normotensive samples differed significantly in both
genotype (P=0.023) and allele frequencies (P=0.010). Our data suggest a modest
contribution of the *CYP11B2* gene to essential hypertension.

Aldosterone excretion rate and blood pressure in essential hypertension are related to polymorphic differences in the aldosterone synthase gene *(CYP11B2)*.

E Davies, C D Holloway, M C Ingram, *et al. Hypertension* 1999; **33**:
703–7.

BACKGROUND. Significant correlation of body sodium and potassium with blood
pressure (BP) may suggest a role for aldosterone in essential hypertension. In patients
with this disease, the ratio of plasma renin to plasma aldosterone may be lower than in
control subjects, and plasma aldosterone levels may be more sensitive to angiotensin
II infusion. Because essential hypertension is partly genetic, it is possible that altered
control of aldosterone synthase gene expression or translation may be responsible.
We compared the frequency of two linked polymorphisms, one in the steroidogenic
factor-1 (SF-1) binding site and the other an intronic conversion (IC), in groups of
hypertensive and normotensive subjects. In a larger population, the relationship of
aldosterone excretion rate to these polymorphisms was also evaluated.

METHODS AND RESULTS. In 138 hypertensive subjects, there was a highly
significant excess of TT homozygosity (SF-1) over CC homozygosity compared with a
group of individually matched normotensive control subjects. The T allele was
significantly more frequent than the C allele in the hypertensive group compared with
the control group. Similarly, there was a highly significant relative excess of the
conversion allele over the 'wild-type' allele and of conversion homozygosity over wild-
type homozygosity in the hypertensive group compared with the control group. In 486
subjects sampled from the North Glasgow Monitoring of Trends and Determinants in
Cardiovascular Disease (MONICA) population, SF-1 and IC genotypes were compared
with tetrahydroaldosterone excretion rate. Subjects with the SF-1 genotypes TT or TC
had significantly higher excretion rates than those with the CC genotype. The T allele
was associated with higher excretion rates than the C allele. However, no significant
differences were found in excretion rate between subjects of different IC genotype.

INTERPRETATION. Urinary aldosterone excretion rate may be a useful intermediate
phenotype linking these genotypes to raised BP. However, no causal relationship has yet
been established, and it is possible that the polymorphisms may be in linkage with other
causative mutations.

Comment

These two studies have examined the association of a polymorphism associated
with the gene encoding aldosterone synthase (see Fig. 9.1) with hypertension. In
both studies, a case–control approach showed a positive finding with the same
polymorphism and essential hypertension. In the first study (Brand *et al.*), a separate

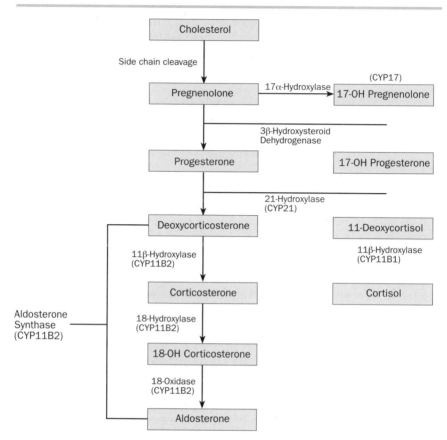

Fig. 9.1 The conversions carried out by aldosterone synthase (zona glomerulosa) and 11β-hydroxylase (zona fasciculata) are shown.

linkage study using hypertensive sibling pairs failed to show any association of a microsatellite marker around this locus with hypertension. However, linkage studies of this type may be less powerful than case–control analyses, and the positive findings with the polymorphism in the 5-promoter region of the aldosterone synthase gene do suggest that this is a real effect. Furthermore, in the second paper, this genetic variant was associated with increased aldosterone metabolite levels in urine. Thus there is a plausible physiological explanation (increased aldosterone production) for the association between this genetic change and hypertension.

Primary aldosteronism (PA) is the most common form of mineralocorticoid excess. By definition, the syndrome occurs as a result of excessive and inappropriate aldosterone production. Solitary benign adenomas of the adrenal cortex (Conn's adenomas) account for 70% of patients with PA, while the majority of the remainder have bilateral adrenal hyperplasia (described in greater detail below). In a very small number of patients, an autosomal dominant form of aldosterone excess (glucocorticoid remediable aldosteronism: GRA) is present. Again, this is described in detail below. Other forms of mineralocorticoid hypertension include constitutive activation of the epithelial sodium channel (Liddle's syndrome) and altered corticosteroid metabolism, in which cortisol acts as a mineralocorticoid hormone (syndrome of apparent mineralocorticoid excess). Again, these are discussed in greater detail below.

Normal physiology of the renin–angiotensin–aldosterone system

In order to understand recent developments in mineralocorticoid hypertension it is necessary to review, briefly, the physiological regulation of the renin–angiotensin–aldosterone system. Aldosterone is produced in the zona glomerulosa cells of the adrenal cortex from cholesterol, in a series of biochemical reactions that involve sequential hydroxylation and dehydrogenation steps. These are summarized in Fig. 9.1. The unique components of the pathway in aldosterone formation are in the 18-hydroxylation of corticosterone followed by a dehydration to yield aldosterone. These steps are catalysed by the enzyme, aldosterone synthase. Expression of this enzyme is regulated by angiotensin II and extracellular potassium concentration |**4**|.

Aldosterone secretion is normally regulated by changes in body sodium status through the activity of the renin–angiotensin system (for a review, see Fraser 1988 |**5**|). Loss of sodium (or volume depletion) stimulates the system; this results in synthesis and release of renin by the juxta-glomerular apparatus of the kidney. In turn, renin, through generation of angiotensin I and its subsequent conversion to angiotensin II determines aldosterone release. Potassium also stimulates aldosterone secretion in an interactive way with angiotensin II. Thus the sensitivity of aldosterone to angiotensin II stimulation is determined by prevailing potassium levels. The pituitary hormone ACTH acutely stimulates aldosterone secretion from the adrenal cortex, but after chronic administration, aldosterone synthesis and release is suppressed.

The adrenal cortex produces relatively small amounts of aldosterone (up to 150 μg daily), and this is very much less than the amount of cortisol secreted (over 100-fold less). A paradox that remained ill understood for many years was the fact that cortisol and aldosterone showed similar binding affinity for the mineralocorticoid receptor *in vitro*. This led to a conceptual difficulty in identifying a means by which aldosterone could act as a specific mineralocorticoid hormone in the presence of much higher cortisol concentration. However, it is now clear that the mineralocorticoid receptor is protected from activation by cortisol by the enzyme 11β-hydroxysteroid dehydrogenase (type 2), which converts cortisol to the inactive metabolite cortisone, thus allowing aldosterone to occupy the receptor |**6**|. In circumstances where this enzyme is inhibited pharmacologically or is inactive owing to genetic mutations, cortisol acts as a mineralocorticoid (syndrome of apparent mineralocorticoid excess) [7] and this is reviewed below.

Mineralocorticoid receptors are present in the distal renal tubule, vascular smooth muscle cells, heart, distal colon, salivary gland and central nervous system. In the kidney, occupation of the receptor leads to increased activity of the epithelial sodium channel on the luminal membrane. This heterotrimeric protein, composed of three subunits (α, β and γ), transports sodium from the lumen of the tubule into the cell [8].

The exchanger is coupled to an intracellular protein (Nedd4), whose function appears to be to terminate activity of the exchanger. Mineralocorticoid receptor occupancy also increases synthesis of the energy-dependent sodium–potassium transporter, so that the net effect of excess aldosterone action in the kidney is to increase transport of sodium from the lumen of the renal tubule into the bloodstream in exchange for potassium and hydrogen.

The role of the mineralocorticoid receptor in other tissues in relation to cardiovascular regulation is less clear. Nonetheless, recent evidence shows that mineralocorticoid action on the heart increases cardiac fibrosis [9] and that this can be blocked by specific aldosterone antagonists [10]. In blood vessels, aldosterone causes increased catecholamine and angiotensin-II-induced vasoconstriction. Finally, activation of mineralocorticoid receptors in the central nervous system has a direct effect to raise BP through activation of central sympathetic outflow [11]. In addition, these receptors regulate sodium and water homeostasis by modifying ingestive behaviour.

Clinical forms of mineralocorticoid hypertension

Liddle's syndrome

This rare form of hypertension was first identified in 1963 by Liddle, who described a family with high BP and low renin but low, rather than high, aldosterone levels [12]. Although Liddle recognized that the defect lay in the renal tubule, progress in identifying the cause of the hypertension was not made until cloning of the mineralocorticoid-dependent epithelial sodium channels in the renal tubule was achieved. In all cases of Liddle's syndrome thus described, activating mutations affecting either the β or γ subunits are present [8,13]. (These subunits are encoded by two genes on chromosome 16 in man.) In each instance, the mutations lead to loss of the intracellular cytoplasmic tail of the subunit, which is thought to act as an anchor site for the Nedd4 protein described above. Given that interaction of the subunits with Nedd4 represents a likely mechanism for channel inactivation, the mutations result in constitutive overactivity of the sodium channel.

Defective regulation of the epithelial Na$^+$ channel by Nedd4 in Liddle's syndrome.

H Abriel, J Loffig, J F Rebhun, J H Pratt, *et al. J Clin Invest* 1999; **103**: 667–73.

BACKGROUND. Liddle's syndrome is an inherited form of hypertension linked to mutations in the epithelial sodium channel (ESC). ENaC is composed of three subunits (α, β, γ), each containing a COOH-terminal PY motif (xPPxY). Mutations causing Liddle's syndrome alter or delete the PY motifs of β- or γ-ENaC. The authors recently demonstrated that the ubiquitin–protein ligase Nedd4 binds these PY motifs, and that ENaC is regulated by ubiquitination.

METHODS AND RESULTS. This study investigates, using the *Xenopus* oocyte system, whether Nedd4 affects ENaC function. Overexpression of wild-type Nedd4, together with ENaC, inhibited channel activity, whereas a catalytically inactive Nedd4 stimulated it, probably by acting as a competitive antagonist to endogenous Nedd4. These effects were dependent on the PY motifs, because no Nedd4-mediated changes in channel activity were observed in ENaC lacking them. The effect of Nedd4 on ENaC missing only one PY motif (of β-ENaC), as originally described in patients with Liddle's syndrome, was intermediate. Changes were due entirely to alterations in ENaC numbers at the plasma membrane, as determined by surface binding and immunofluorescence.

INTERPRETATION. These results demonstrate that Nedd4 is a negative regulator of ESC, and suggest that the loss of Nedd4 binding sites in ENaC observed in Liddle's syndrome may explain the increase in channel number at the cell surface, increased sodium reabsorption by the distal nephron, and hence the hypertension.

Comment

Liddle's syndrome is associated with a mutation in the ESC—this mutation causes loss of a cytoplasmic tail in the protein of the channel. In this paper, Abriel and colleagues demonstrate that an intracellular protein binds to the cytoplasmic tail of the channel to regulate its activity. Thus the mutation in Liddle's syndrome that leads to loss of this cytoplasmic tail results in failure of the intracellular protein (Nedd4) to bind. In turn, this results in constitutive overactivity of the channel. There is, therefore, a clear biological mechanism which accounts for the increased sodium channel activity in Liddle's syndrome, and the relationship between genetic variation, protein structural change and ultimate biological functional outcome is clear.

Liddle's syndrome responds clinically to treatment with amiloride, which specifically blocks the ESC. As aldosterone levels are not high, the aldosterone receptor antagonist, spironolactone, is ineffective in this circumstance.

Although it is rare, one important feature of Liddle's syndrome is the possible candidate role it highlights for the ESC in hypertensive subjects. Baker and colleagues have described an association between a mutation in the ESC and hypertension in Afro-Caribbean subjects. Although other reports have not yet confirmed this observation, excessive renal tubular sodium reabsorption through this means provides an attractive pathophysiological mechanism for other more common types of hypertension.

Association of hypertension with T594M mutation in β subunit of epithelial sodium channels in black people resident in London.

E H Baker, Y B Dong, G A Sagnella, *et al. Lancet* 1998; **351**: 1388–92.

BACKGROUND. Liddle's syndrome is a rare inherited form of hypertension in which mutations of the epithelial sodium channel (ESC) result in increased renal sodium reabsorption. Essential hypertension in black patients also shows clinical features of sodium retention, so we screened black people for the T594M mutation, the most commonly identified sodium-channel mutation.

METHODS AND RESULTS. In a case–control study, 206 hypertensive (mean age 48.0 [SD 11.8] years, men:women 80:126) and 142 normotensive (48.7 [7.4] years; 61:81) black people who lived in London, UK, were screened for T594M. Part of the last exon of the ESC beta-subunit from genomic DNA was amplified by polymerase chain reaction (PCR). The T594M variant was detected by single-strand conformational polymorphism analysis of PCR products and confirmed by DNA sequencing. The results showed that 17 (8.3%) of 206 hypertensive participants compared with three (2.1%) of 142 normotensive participants possessed the T594M variant (odds ratio [OR]=4.17 [95% confidence interval (CI) 1.12–18.25], P=0.029). A high proportion of participants with the T594M variant were women (15 of 17 hypertensive participants and all three normotensive participants), whereas women constituted a lower proportion of the individuals screened (61.2% hypertensive, 57.7% normotensive). However, the association between the T594M variant and hypertension persisted after adjustment for sex and Body-Mass Index (Mantel-Haenszel OR=5.52 [1.40–30.61], P=0.012). Plasma renin activity was significantly lower in 13 hypertensive participants with the T594M variant (median=0.19 ng/ml/h) than in 39 untreated hypertensive individuals without the variant (median=0.45 ng/ml/h), P=0.009).

INTERPRETATION. Among black London people the T594M sodium-channel beta-subunit mutation occurs more frequently in people with hypertension than those without. The T594M variant may increase sodium-channel activity, and could raise BP in affected people by increasing renal tubular sodium reabsorption. These findings suggest that the T594M mutation could be the most common secondary cause of essential hypertension in black people identified to date.

Comment

In this case–control study of black people in London, the frequency of a polymorphism (T594M) in the codon region of the gene for the β-subunit of the ESC was examined. This genetic variation changes a threonine for a methionine residue.

Activating mutations of this gene cause the rare monogenic form of hypertension, Liddle's syndrome.

The mutant allele was present more frequently in hypertensive subjects (8.3%) than normotensives (2.1%). There was a slightly lower plasma renin activity in the hypertensives with the mutation than in those with only the wild-type allele. The hypertensive group is well matched with the controls, apart from weight—the hypertensives were significantly heavier.

Case–control studies are open to criticism, as it can be difficult to ensure that the two groups are derived from the same population. Thus differences in the distribution of a genetic marker between cases and controls might represent heterogeneity of population, rather than a true association with disease. In this study the matching seems to be carefully performed. For case–control association studies, a positive association suggests that the causal gene is very close (in genetic terms) to the marker studied, owing to the large number of genetic recombinations that occur in a sample derived from a free-breeding population. Thus this result suggests that the β-subunit of the ESC is an important candidate gene for hypertension. In genetic studies, it is important to establish a plausible biological link between genotype and ultimate phenotype (high BP in this instance). In this paper, there was a small reduction in plasma renin activity in subjects bearing the mutant allele, suggesting that this was associated with excessive renal sodium retention. However, it should be noted that numbers were small, and no difference was seen in normotensive patients.

Finally, despite the positive nature of this study, only a minority of hypertensive subjects carried the mutant allele, and its contribution to essential hypertension must be small. The importance of this study lies in the link that it provides between a monogenic disorder—Liddle's syndrome—and a common clinical phenotype—essential hypertension, with a plausible biochemical intermediate phenotype (low renin activity).

Syndrome of apparent mineralocorticoid excess

As was detailed above, cortisol can, potentially, act as a mineralocorticoid receptor agonist. Indeed, when present in very high concentrations, cortisol displays classical mineralocorticoid effects: when healthy volunteers are given high doses of hydrocortisone, they retain sodium avidly, lose potassium and become hypertensive [14]. Similarly, subjects with ectopic ACTH syndrome show classical features of mineralocorticoid hypertension, with profound hypokalaemia. Under more usual physiological circumstances, however, the mineralocorticoid receptor is protected from the effects of cortisol by the type 2 11β-hydroxysteroid dehydrogenase enzyme, which converts cortisol to cortisone [14]. The type 2 enzyme is found in the kidney, large bowel and salivary gland; it is also present in placenta, brain and vascular endothelium (for a review, see Albiston *et al.* [15]).

The syndrome in which cortisol can act as a mineralocorticoid owing to inactivation of this enzyme was first described in children in 1979 [16]. However, the role of 11β-hydroxysteroid dehydrogenase in this syndrome was not appreciated until 1988, when Stewart and colleagues described abnormalities in cortisol to cortisone conversion in an adult with severe hypertension |7|. Since then, a number of kindreds showing autosomal-recessive inheritance of this defect have been described. In most instances, heterozygote subjects are apparently normal. The syndrome responds to inhibition of cortisol production by dexamethasone; alternatively, spironolactone or amiloride can be effective.

As with other rare monogenic forms of hypertension, the syndrome of apparent mineralocorticoid excess offers a potential candidate mechanism that may be involved in essential hypertension. Given that heterozygote subjects (with loss of one allele encoding 11β-hydroxysteroid dehydrogenase) have no phenotypic abnormality, it seems unlikely that minor mutations at this locus will have major consequences for cortisol metabolism and, hence, the development of hypertension. Nonetheless, there have been reports of associations between polymorphisms at the 11β-HSD2 locus and hypertension in subjects with sodium sensitivity, and more detailed investigation of this is necessary |17|. An alternative mechanism by which this system may be involved in hypertension may be in the presence of inhibitors of 11β-hydroxysteroid dehydrogenase function. Thus the active derivative of liquorice, glycyrrhetinic acid, causes hypertension and sodium retention through inhibition of 11β-hydroxysteroid dehydrogenase type 2 activity |18|.

Impact of dietary Na⁺ on glycyrrhetinic acid-like factors (kidney 11β-HSD2-GALFS) in human essential hypertension.

D J Morris, Y H Lo, W R Litchfield, G H Williams. *Hypertension* 1998; **31**: 469–72.

BACKGROUND. Previous studies by these authors have shown that human urine contains glycyrrhetinic acid-like factors (GALFs) that possess inhibitory activity against kidney 11β-hydroxysteroid dehydrogenase isoform 2 (HSD2). The present studies were undertaken to determine the impact of dietary sodium intake on the levels of kidney 11β-(HSD2)-GALFs.

METHODS AND RESULTS. The excretion of kidney 11β-(HSD2)-GALFs in 24-hour urine samples of 30 unmedicated subjects (10 normotensive and 10 high/normal-renin and 10 low-renin essential hypertensive subjects) on both 200- and 10-mmol sodium diets was studied. No differences in the urinary levels of kidney 11β-(HSD2)-GALFs were observed among the three groups on the high-sodium diet. However, with a low-sodium diet, the levels of kidney 11β-(HSD2)-GALFs were significantly increased in hypertensive subjects but not in normal subjects. Levels increased from 8.3 ± 1.4 to 17.3 ± 2.9 and 6.7 ± 1.3 to 10.6 ± 1.4 carbenoxolone sodium units/d in high/normal-renin (*P*=0.01) and low-renin hypertensive subjects (*P*=0.07), respectively; normal subjects changed from 8.0 ± 1.9 to 10.6 ± 2.4.

INTERPRETATION. The levels of kidney 11β-(HSD2)-GALFs were significantly higher in the high/normal-renin hypertensive subjects than in either the control normotensive subjects or the low-renin hypertensive subjects when challenged with the low-sodium diet

($P{<}0.05$ by Wilcoxon rank-sum test). The greater response of the high/normal-renin essential hypertensive subjects indicated that they may utilize kidney 11β-(HSD2)-GALFs when challenged with a low-sodium diet, whereas the low-renin essential hypertensive subjects do not.

Comment

Studies showing an association between 11β-hydroxysteroid dehydrogenase activity, altered sodium balance and hypertension have largely focused on the rare genetic syndromes that lead to loss of 11β-HSD2 activity (syndrome of apparent mineralo-corticoid excess). However, this paper suggests that in essential hypertension, inhibitors of the enzyme may also give rise to reduced function. In turn, this would result in decreased cortisol to cortisone conversion, and excessive binding of corti-sol to the mineralocorticoid receptor. In the paper of Morris *et al.*, a bio-assay was used to examine the presence of inhibitors of the enzyme in the urine of patients with hypertension in comparison to normal controls. The study was carried out during high- and low-sodium intakes, and hypertensive subjects were divided into those with high- or low-renin activity. The main finding of the study was that patients with high renin activity showed a significantly greater increase in the in-hibitor of the enzyme when changing from a low to a high salt intake in comparison to low-renin patients or control subjects. As the increase in enzyme inhibitor activity during low-sodium intake might be regarded as an appropriate homeostatic re-sponse to allow increased cortisol availability to the mineralocorticoid receptor, the significance of the greater increase in high-renin hypertensive patients is uncertain. Nonetheless, the paper does identify an interesting biological mechanism that may help regulate renal sodium retention during altered salt intake, and provides another potential biological function that may, when functioning abnormally, contribute to development of volume-dependent hypertension.

It is possible that endogenous inhibitors of this enzyme exist—there are recent reports of increased concentration of these type of inhibitors in hypertensive sub-jects |**19**|. Again, more detailed studies of this phenomenon in larger groups of patients with hypertension are required.

Other non-aldosterone-dependent forms of mineralocorticoid hypertension

Rarely, other steroid hormones can cause mineralocorticoid hypertension. Of these, the commonest is deoxycorticosterone, which is a precursor steroid pro-duced by the adrenal cortex (see Fig. 9.1). Some subjects with adrenal carcinomas produce deoxycorticosterone to excess. Although the hormone has weaker affinity for the mineralocorticoid receptor than aldosterone, deoxycorticosterone can cause hypertension with suppression of renin. The other situations in which deoxy-corticosterone is present in excess are the syndromes of 11β-hydroxylase deficiency and 17α-hydroxylase deficiency. These conditions are, however, excessively rare, and the reader is referred to a review for a more detailed description |**5**|.

Deficiency of 11β-hydroxylase does, however, illustrate one important feature which is relevant to essential hypertension. The enzyme is the key control step in the zona fasciculata, which converts deoxycortisol to cortisol, and deoxycorticosterone to corticosterone (see Fig. 9.1). In the rare autosomal recessive condition of enzyme deficiency, complete lack of this activity leads to major build-up of deoxycorticosterone. Deficiency of cortisol leads to excessive ACTH stimulation of the gland, and the syndrome responds to treatment with dexamethasone. As with the other rare forms of hypertension, however, it is clear that lesser abnormalities might lead to mild forms of deoxycorticosterone excess, which could contribute to the development of more common forms of hypertension. At present, few studies have examined this in great detail. There are, however, reports of increased deoxycorticosterone levels in the plasma of patients with hypertension, both in the basal situation and after ACTH stimulation |20|. Thus this rare circumstance again illustrates a potential candidate mechanism by which high BP might occur through a mineralocorticoid-dependent mechanism.

Mineralocorticoid hypertension due to aldosterone excess

Primary aldosteronism

Glucocorticoid remediable aldosteronism (GRA)

GRA is a rare, autosomal dominantly inherited form of primary aldosteronism (PA). It occurs as a result of the presence of a chimeric gene, comprising the 5′ regions from 11β-hydroxylase (*CYP11B1*), which contain the ACTH-responsive elements, attached to the 3′ coding regions of aldosterone synthase (*CYP11B2*) |21|. This gene, whose expression is regulated by ACTH, leads to production of aldosterone synthase in the zona fasciculata. The chimeric gene occurs as a result of unequal recombination between *CYP11B1* and *CYP11B2* during meiosis. Subjects with GRA have aldosterone excess, with variable severity of hypertension, often from a young age. Aldosterone excess (and BP) respond to administration of an aldosterone receptor antagonist, such as spironolactone, or treatment with amiloride. Aldosterone production can also be suppressed with a glucocorticoid such as dexamethasone, and this provides an alternative form of treatment.

Intracranial aneurysm and hemorrhagic stroke in glucocorticoid remediable aldosterone.
W R Litchfield, B F Anderson, R J Weiss, R P Lifton, R G Dluhy.
Hypertension 1998; **31**: 445–50.

BACKGROUND. There are anecdotal reports of early cerebrovascular complications occurring in patients with GRA. The issue has never been systematically evaluated.

This study retrospectively reviewed the International Registry for GRA to see if there was an association between cerebrovascular complications and GRA.

METHODS AND RESULTS. The authors searched the records of 376 patients from 27 genetically proven GRA pedigrees for premature death or cerebrovascular complications. Each case was subsequently verified through the referring physician or autopsy reports. The number of complications occurring in patients with proven GRA was compared to GRA-negative subjects from the same pedigrees. There were 18 cerebrovascular events in 15 patients with proven GRA ($n=167$) and none in the GRA-negative group ($n=194$; $P<0.001$). There were an additional 15 events in 15 subjects that were suspected of having GRA based on clinical history. Seventy per cent of events were hemorrhagic strokes; the overall case fatality rate was 61%. The mean ($\pm$ SD) age at the time of the initial event was 31.7 $\pm$ 11.3 years. In total, 48% of all GRA pedigrees and 18% of all GRA patients had cerebrovascular complications, which is similar to the frequency of aneurysm in adult polycystic kidney disease. GRA is associated with high morbidity and mortality from early onset of hemorrhagic stroke and ruptured intracranial aneurysms.

INTERPRETATION. Screening for intracranial aneurysm with magnetic resonance angiography is advised for patients with genetically proven GRA.

Comment

Glucocorticoid remediable aldosteronism is a rare genetic cause of hypertension caused by excessive aldosterone production from the adrenal gland. In this paper, the authors report an apparent high rate of cerebrovascular events in patients with GRA (of these, most were due to cerebral haemorrhages due to intracranial aneurysm), and recommend that patients with proven GRA be prospectively screened for the presence of aneurysms.

While the finding is of interest, the patient population studied here is highly selected and may be subject to reporting bias. Thus detailed investigation to look for a cause of hypertension may be more likely in families that present with severe early-onset disease associated with cerebral haemorrhage. In order to be certain that there was a true increased risk of intracranial aneurysm associated with GRA, a more thorough screening programme would be necessary, comparing family members with or without the genetic defect. Nonetheless, it is certainly prudent to ensure that patients with GRA have optimal BP control.

GRA can be readily diagnosed by genetic means (either by a Southern blotting technique to identify a unique restriction fragment or by a recently reported reliable polymerase chain reaction method that provides a simple and rapid means of screening families at risk).

Rapid diagnosis and identification of cross-over sites in patients with glucocorticoid remediable aldosteronism.

A A MacConnachie, K F Kelly, A McNamara, *et al. J Clin Endocrinol Metab* 1998; **83**: 4328–31.

BACKGROUND. Glucocorticoid remediable aldosteronism (GRA) is an autosomal dominant cause of PA and high blood pressure resulting from a chimeric 11 beta-hydroxylase/aldosterone synthase gene. Abnormal expression of aldosterone synthase causes PA, which can be inhibited by glucocorticoids. Diagnosis of GRA has depended on the identification of a restriction enzyme product in genomic DNA of affected individuals. Recently, a two-tube-long polymerase chain reaction (PCR) method was described that allowed diagnosis of GRA in a kindred group in Australia. A similar long PCR method confirmed the diagnosis of GRA in members of five northeastern Scotland families previously identified by Southern blotting, and detected affected members of five GRA families previously identified in Glasgow. A multiplex PCR protocol is described here that allows the control aldosterone synthase amplification and chimeric gene amplification to be carried out in the same tube.

METHODS AND RESULTS. We describe the regions of cross-over in each of 10 kindreds identified in Scotland. To identify cross-over regions in each of the kindreds, the chimeric long PCR product was cloned and sequenced.

INTERPRETATION. Five cross-over sites were identified ranging from intron 2 to exon 4, indicating the reliability of the method in identifying chimeric genes resulting from different sites of cross-over.

Comment

The diagnosis of GRA has hitherto relied on demonstration of primary aldosterone excess by biochemical means, followed by a demonstration that aldosterone can be effectively suppressed by administration of a glucocorticoid. This test can give rise to false-positive results. Following the identification of the genetic cause of the disorder by Lifton, diagnosis can be made using Southern blotting, but this is a time-consuming procedure. The above paper reports a rapid and reliable long PCR-based technique which allows the diagnosis of GRA to be made in a single step. No cases of GRA were missed using this technique. In the future, diagnosis of GRA (once suspected) may be best made using a molecular approach such as this rather than cumbersome biochemical methods.

Common forms of primary aldosteronism

Since the first description by Conn in 1965 of PA there has been controversy about many aspects of this form of hypertension. The most common forms are aldosterone producing adenoma with most of the remainder being ascribed to bilateral adrenal hyperplasia or idiopathic hyperaldosteronism. Estimates of prevalence of PA range from 2 to 15% of hypertensive patients |22–24|. This issue is central to the debate on screening and to the importance of PA as a cause of hypertension. PA has previously been thought to be a relatively benign form of hypertension, although it is now increasingly recognized that aldosterone may exert deleterious effects on the cardiovascular system both via and independent of its effects on BP.

Screening for primary aldosteronism with a logistic multivariate discriminant analysis.

G R Rossi, E Rossi, E Pavan, *et al. Clin Endocrinol* 1998; **49**: 713–23.

BACKGROUND. Primary aldosteronism (PA) is the most common endocrine cause of curable hypertension, but no single test unequivocally identifies it. Accordingly, the authors investigated the usefulness of a logistic multivariate discriminant analysis (MDA) approach for PA screening.

METHODS AND RESULTS. Generation of a logistic MDA function based on retrospective analysis of biochemical tests in a large cohort of referred patients with or without confirmed Conn's adenoma (CA) was followed by prospective validation of the model. The authors investigated 574 selected hypertensives: 206 (32 with and 174 without CA) retrospectively, 48 (with a 13% prevalence of CA) prospectively for the validation of the model, and 320 referred hypertensives (with a 3.4% prevalence of CA) similarly evaluated. Patients were referred to a specialized centre for hypertension (4th Clinica Medica–University of Padua) and to the Department of Internal Medicine of a regional hospital (Reggio Emilia).

Measurements. In all patients we measured several demographic and biochemical variables and performed a captopril test. A stepwise analysis of variance, based on a model fitted with several different variables, identified baseline (sALDO) and captopril-suppressed plasma aldosterone (cALDO), supine plasma renin activity (sPRA) and potassium as the most informative. Therefore, two models of logistic MDA with sPRA, potassium, and either sALDO (model A) or cALDO (model B) were developed and used. Receiver–operator curve analysis was also performed to assess the optimal cut-off values.

The model B MDA provided the best performance, and identified CA with 100% sensitivity and 81% accuracy. When used prospectively it showed 100% sensitivity, both in the Padua (88% accuracy) and in the Reggio Emilia series (90% accuracy). However, at both institutions most patients with idiopathic hyperaldosteronism (IHA) were also detected.

INTERPRETATION. Thus, although developed from patients with confirmed CA, a strategy based on MDA can be used prospectively for accurate screening for PA. Furthermore, it was proven to be accurate and applicable to patients tested with similar modalities at a different institution. Although this approach did not provide a clear-cut discrimination of CA from IHA, it may avoid unnecessary and costly further testing in patients with a low probability of PA.

Comment

This paper addresses the prevalence of PA in a hypertensive population and assesses the best methods of screening for the disorder. The first paper sets the scene for the second, and represents a very large (3900 subjects) screen of hypertensive patients for PA in a prospective manner. Measurements were made of renin in plasma, and of urinary aldosterone (and its major metabolites): 257 cases of PA were detected (6.6%), of whom 146 (3.9% of total) had adenomas.

In the second paper, an Italian group first examined retrospectively a population with high prevalence of aldosterone-producing adenomas (32 of 206) using mathematical modelling techniques to identify the best screening and diagnostic methods. They then used this to study, prospectively, an unselected hypertensive population to assess the utility of the methodology. They identified that a combination of supine plasma renin, serum potassium and aldosterone measurement after administration of captopril provided the best combination of tests, with a positive predictive value, in the retrospective study, of 40%. In the more realistic prospective study the accuracy of the tests was 90%, and the positive predictive value 26%. The prevalence of adenomas in this latter population was 3.6%, a value remarkably similar to that identified in the exhaustive screen of 3900 subjects detailed above.

Prevalence of primary aldosteronism

Recent reports have suggested a prevalence of up to 15% in the hypertensive population |24|. Studies reporting such a high prevalence of PA have been criticized because they have often been conducted in specialist hypertension clinics, which may be subject to referral bias. They have also been criticized because of the use of ratios of plasma aldosterone concentration to plasma renin activity as a screening test (ARR), which may be heavily influenced by the denominator. Thus in subjects with low plasma renin activity (PRA), such as is common the elderly or in black people, the ARR may be elevated when plasma aldosterone concentration (PAC) is normal or even low normal. Furthermore, elevated ARR has often been assumed to indicate PA and the lack of confirmatory tests of PA in studies reporting high prevalence rates has been criticized.

Most authors report plasma renin activity in ng/ml per hour; however, groups differ in the units used to denote aldosterone concentrations, both SI and conventional units being found in the literature. The conversion factor for conventional to SI is 27.7, thus aldosterone concentration of 20 ng/dl is equivalent to 550 pmol/l and an ARR in conventional units of 25 is equivalent to 700 in SI units. These factors must all be borne in mind when interpreting reports on prevalence rates for PA.

Prevalence of primary aldosteronism among Asian hypertensive patients in Singapore.
K-C Loh, E S Koay, M-C Khaw, S C Emmanuel, W F Young Jr.
J Clin Endocrinol Metab 2000; **85**(8): 2854–9.

B ACKGROUND. Debate continues about the prevalence of PA in the hypertensive population. The authors undertook a prevalence finding study in two large primary care hypertension clinics in Singapore.

M ETHODS AND RESULTS. Three hundred and fifty consecutive patients attending the primary care hypertension clinic were included in the study. Screening tests were performed without discontinuation of antihypertensive medication after sitting for 15 min. Sixty-three of 350 (18%) subjects had both ARR > 20 (560 using SI units) and PAC > 15 ng/dl (415 pmol/l); 56 of 63 subjects went on to have confirmatory testing in the form of a saline suppression test. PAC was measured following intravenous infusion of 2l of 0.9% saline over 2 h. Taking cut-off level as 10 ng/l (280 pmol/l) as positive confirmation of PA the estimated prevalence was 5.1%. Half of these subjects had an adrenal adenoma demonstrated on either computed tomography (CT) scan or adrenal vein sampling (estimated prevalence 2.3%) and only one-third were hypokalaemic. These subjects had worse BP control despite being on more antihypertensive medications than subjects with negative screening tests for primary hyperaldosteronism. Taking cut-off aldosterone concentrations of 5 ng/l (140 pmol/l) as failure to suppress the estimated prevalence of PA was 8.4%.

I NTERPRETATION. Eighteen per cent of subjects screened positive for possible PA, although this was confirmed in only 5.1–8.4% of patients depending on the cut-off value for failure to suppress aldosterone. Only the subjects who failed to suppress to below 10 ng/dl (280 pmol/l) went on to have CT scanning or AVS, therefore it is possible that their estimated prevalence of 2.3% for aldosterone producing adenoma may be an underestimate. The study also demonstrated that those subjects with a high ARR and failure to suppress aldosterone have more severe hypertension than those with normal ratios and that hypokalaemia is an insensitive indicator of PA.

Primary hyperaldosteronism in essential hypertensives: prevalence, biochemical profile and molecular biology.

C E Fardella, L Mosso, C Gomez-Sanchez, *et al. J Clin Endocrinol Metab* 2000; **85**: 1863–7.

B ACKGROUND. The prevalence of primary hyperaldosteronism has been hotly debated since it was first described by Conn. Glucocorticoid remediable hyperaldosteronism (GRA) is a rare, autosomally dominant form of primary hyperaldosteronism caused by an unequal crossing over between the CYP11B1 and CYP11B2 resulting in a chimeric gene, the product of which has aldosterone synthase activity regulated by ACTH. This study aimed to estimate the prevalence of both PA and GRA in a primary care hypertensive clinic population in Santiago, Chile.

M ETHODS AND RESULTS. Three hundred and five subjects attending a primary outpatient clinic hypertension programme, not known to have secondary hypertension, diabetes or renal disease were studied. Subjects were screened fasting, after sitting for 15 min. Fourteen per cent had ARR > 25 (equivalent to 700 in SI units). All subjects with high ARR went on to have suppression tests with 0.4 mg fludrocortisone and dietary supplementation with 110 mmol sodium per day for 4 days. Sixty-six per cent of those who screened positive failed to suppress PAC to less than 5 ng/dl, indicating a prevalence of PA in this Chilean population of 9.5%. All subjects with high ARR underwent dexamethasone suppression testing (dexamethasone 2 mg/day for 2 days). Thirty-four per cent suppressed to PAC < 4 ng/dl but only two people had had the chimeric gene for GRA. None of the subjects with PA were hypokalaemic. Only one had a demonstrable adenoma on CT scan, although five had bilateral adrenal hyperplasia.

INTERPRETATION. In a primary care setting approximately 15% of hypertensive patients have ARR > 25 (equivalent to 700 using alternative units). Approximately two-thirds of these subjects failed to suppress aldosterone to less than 5 ng/dl following fludrocortisone giving a prevalence of PA of 9.5%. The study again confirms that hypokalaemia is likely only to be present in the minority of subjects with PA. The study also confirms in a Chilean population that GRA is likely only to represent a small minority of subjects with PA. It is surprising that only one subject had a demonstrable adenoma on CT scan giving an estimated prevalence of APA of 0.3%.

High prevalence of primary hyperaldosteronism in the Tayside hypertension clinic population.

P O Lim, E Dow, G Brennan, R T Jung, T M MacDonald. *J Hum Hypertens* 2000; **14**: 311–15.

BACKGROUND. Ongoing debate about the prevalence of primary hyperaldosteronism among hypertensive patients.

METHODS AND RESULTS. Four hundred and sixty-five patients referred to a specialist hypertension assessment unit. Antihypertensive medication was discontinued for 7–10 days prior to assessment in subjects in whom there was no contraindication (60% of subjects). Blood samples for PRA and PAC were taken after sitting for 10 min. A number of subjects (16.5%) had ARR > 750 (equivalent to ratio of 27 using conventional units). Suppression tests were performed with 28 800 mg NaCl and 1.5 mg fludrocortisone were administered orally over a 4-day period. Ninety-one per cent failed to suppress aldosterone to less than 140 pmol/l (5 ng/dl) giving a confirmed prevalence of 9.2% for PA. The estimated prevalence of PA could be as high as 15% as fludrocortisone suppression was contraindicated in 41% of subjects with a raised ARR. No subject tested for the chimeric gene responsible for GSH. All subjects with a raised ARR had abdominal CT scanning, which identified an adenoma in five subjects, giving an estimated prevalence of APA of approximately 1%. Only two of 77 subjects with raised ARR had hypokalaemia.

INTERPRETATION. Confirmed prevalence of PA in this specialist BP clinic is 9.2%, although the estimated prevalence could be as high as 15%. The incidence of demonstrable adrenal adenoma on CT scan was low at 1%.

The positive predictive value of a raised ARR for non-suppression with aldosterone seen in this study is high at 91% compared with 50% and 66% for the studies that used lower values for ARR in screening, 560 and 700, respectively (Loh *et al.* 2000 and Fardella *et al.* 2000). This study again confirmed that the majority of subjects with PA will be normokalaemic and that GRA is likely to represent only the tiny minority of cases of PA.

Comment

Prevalence of aldosterone producing adenomas: The observed prevalence of aldosterone producing adenomas in these studies depended on the method of detection used. Studies in which CT scanning alone was used to detect APAs the prevalence was low, 0.3–1.0% (Loh *et al.* 2000 and Lim *et al.* 2000). Conversely, where CT and adrenal vein sampling were both used the prevalence of APAs was higher at 2.3% (Fardella *et al.* 2000). AVS is considered the gold standard for determining the aetiology of PA. A recent report found only 50% of APAs, as determined by adrenal vein sampling, had concordant findings on high resolution CT scanning (see Magill *et al.* 2001). Thus the true prevalence of APAs is likely to be 2–3% of hypertensive subjects.

Prevalence of primary hyperaldosteronism: Primary hyperaldosteronism not due to an APA has been considered to be due to bilateral adrenal hyperplasia, also referred to as idiopathic hyperaldosteronism. The above studies have answered many of the criticisms surrounding previous reports of high prevalence rates of primary hyperaldosteronism in that some have been conducted in a primary care setting |**25**| (see also Loh *et al.* 2000 and Fardella *et al.* 2000) and none have relied solely on ratios of plasma aldosterone concentrations to plasma renin activity to diagnose primary hyperaldosteronism.

There are none the less some existing difficulties in that the estimated prevalence of primary hyperaldosteronism depends on the cut-off levels used for its diagnosis. There is, therefore, a circular argument regarding the 'true' prevalence of hyperaldosteronism. Those studies using a looser definition of primary hyperaldosteronism detect a higher prevalence and vice versa.

Primary hyperaldosteronism is defined by a high PAC/PRA ratio together with non-suppressibility of aldosterone, although the absolute values are still controversial and there may be important methodological differences in measurement. Nonetheless primary hyperaldosteronism is likely to be present in 5–10% of unselected hypertensive subjects.

Prevalence of rarer familial forms of hyperaldosteronism: GRA is a rare autosomal dominant form of hyperaldosteronism described earlier in this chapter. Two of 305 hypertensive subjects in one study and none of 465 subjects in another study tested positive for the chimeric gene. These studies conform that it is likely to represent the tiny minority of hypertensive subjects and that subjects should only be screened if they have a positive family history of GRA or PA.

There are reports that some patients with PA due either to adenoma or bilateral adrenal hyperplasia can have a familial form of the disorder (referred to as familial hyperaldosteronism type 2) inherited in an autosomal dominant manner |**26**|. The molecular cause of this is uncertain: PA is reported in association with multiple endocrine neoplasia type 1, but this appears not to be the cause of the distinct form described above.

Adrenal pathology in primary aldosteronism

Aldosterone-producing tumours (Conn's adenomas) are benign. The tumour size is generally of 1–2 cm, and when its surface is cut, the tumour has a bright yellow appearance. The histological appearance shows the presence of zona fasciculata- and zona glomerulosa-type cells—there may be a relationship between the histological appearance of the tumour and the degree of responsiveness of aldosterone to angiotensin II in patients with PA, although this has little practical value.

There are few consistent reports of pathological findings in patients with non-tumorous bilateral adrenal hyperplasia. In some instances, diffuse hyperplasia of the zona glomerulosa has been described, and there are descriptions of multiple nodules being present within the gland. However, similar appearances are reported in post-mortem findings in patients with essential hypertension, and this raises the possibility that there may be no clear demarcation between patients with low renin essential hypertension and patients with bilateral adrenal hyperplasia with modest aldosterone excess |30|. Thus in both circumstances, renal levels are suppressed, aldosterone levels are inappropriate for the level of renin, and there may be pathological findings on examination of the adrenal gland. This, in turn, raises the question of the underlying cause of essential hypertension, and suggests that subtle changes in regulation of the renin–angiotensin–aldosterone system may take place in a substantial proportion of patients with this disorder.

Consequences of aldosterone excess

Aldosterone excess, in the acute phase, causes renal sodium and water retention and consequent volume expansion. This causes an increase in cardiac output. However patients with chronic PA do not show sustained increase in cardiac output, and high BP is likely to be maintained by other mechanisms. In this regard, the presence of aldosterone receptors in vascular smooth muscle cells and the central nervous system may be of relevance. Aldosterone promotes vasoconstriction and has central effects to raise BP. Thus maintenance of high BP in PA is likely to be complex.

PA was previously thought to be a relatively benign form of hypertension. However it is clear that high BP in this disorder can be severe and resistant to therapy (Loh *et al.* 2000, Fardella *et al.* 2000, and Lim *et al.* 2000). In addition, aldosterone excess has distinct effects on cardiovascular structure and function. Thus in experimental models aldosterone has been reported to cause changes in cardiac collagen content and histological appearance |9|. In addition a major role for aldosterone has been proposed in malignant nephrosclerosis and cerebrovascular lesions. It is of relevance that these changes are greatly exacerbated by a high sodium intake and can be prevented by use of aldosterone receptor blockers |10,28,29|.

The effects of aldosterone on renal structure in humans are not well reported. However, there is evidence from other forms of renal disease that aldosterone can be an important component in determining rate of progression |30|. Furthermore in animal studies, aldosterone excess causes very significant renal damage and, in addition, is a potent risk factor for the development of stroke. These abnormalities can be reversed by aldosterone receptor antagonism.

In human subjects studies of cardiac histological changes are not available. However, patients with PA are reported to have more severe left ventricular hypertrophy (LVH) than those with corresponding levels of BP due to essential hypertension |31|. Additionally, abnormal left ventricular motion is described, including abnormal diastolic relaxation.

Impact of aldosterone on left ventricular structure and function in young normotensive and mildly hypertensive subjects.

M P Schlaich, H P Schobel, K Hilgers, R E Schmieder. *Am J Cardiol* 2000; **85**: 1199–206.

BACKGROUND. LVH is an important cardiovascular risk factor. Factors known to be important in determining LVH include BP, age, sex, race and obesity but other factors may also be important. In rat models elevated circulating aldosterone is associated with myocardial fibrosis and with collagen accumulation in the ventricles. It is hypothesized that aldosterone excess leads to perivascular and interstitial fibrosis, resulting in increased myocardial stiffness and increased left ventricular mass. This study aimed to assess whether changes in aldosterone concentration after salt loading are related to myocardial functional and structural changes in essential hypertension.

METHODS AND RESULTS. Fifty-seven male students were assessed using 24-h ambulatory BP monitoring and classified as normotensive ($n = 26$, mean ambulatory BP 121/71) or mildly hypertensive ($n = 31$, mean ambulatory BP 132/78). All subjects had left ventricular mass assessed by echocardiography. Subjects had serum aldosterone, plasma renin activity and 24-h urinary sodium and aldosterone excretion rates measured before and after salt loading (6 g/day for 7 days). After salt loading urinary aldosterone concentration was correlated to left ventricular mass ($r = 0.45$, $P < 0.01$) for all subjects independent of BP. When analysed separately this was significant for mildly hypertensive subjects ($r = 0.46$, $P < 0.01$) but not in normotensive subjects. In addition the smaller the decrease in aldosterone concentration after salt loading the greater the left ventricular mass ($r = 0.35$, $P < 0.01$), again independent of BP. Urinary aldosterone concentration after salt loading was correlated with mid-wall fractional fibre shortening independently of BP ($r = 0.31$, $P < 0.02$).

INTERPRETATION. In young male subjects with mildly elevated BP inadequate suppression of aldosterone is related to left ventricular mass and function independently of BP. This supports the hypothesis that aldosterone has effects on left ventricular mass and function independently of BP.

Raised aldosterone to renin ratio predicts antihypertensive efficacy of spironolactone: a prospective cohort follow-up study.

P O Lim, R T Jung, T M MacDonald. *Br J Clin Pharmacol* 1999; **48**: 756–60.

BACKGROUND. Ratio of aldosterone to plasma renin activity (ARR) is used to screen hypertensive patients for primary hyperaldosteronism. Up to 15% of patients attending BP clinics may have ARR > 750 (> 27 using conventional units). The aim of the study was to assess the efficacy of spironolactone as an antihypertensive agent in this group.

METHODS AND RESULTS. Twenty-eight hypertensive patients who had ARR > 750 and failed to suppress aldosterone to < 140 pmol/l (5 ng/dl) following 28 800 mg NaCl and 1.5 mg fludrocortisone intake over a 4-day period were studied prospectively. Following 3 months of spironolactone, 46% (13 of 28) of subjects achieved BPs < 140/90 mmHg compared with 7% (two of 28) at baseline. The mean BP of the group decreased significantly from 161/91 mmHg to 146/83 mmHg following spironolactone treatment ($P < 0.01$) despite being on fewer antihypertensive medications (mean number of antihypertensive agents at baseline 2.3 compared with 1.8 at follow up, $P < 0.02$).

INTERPRETATION. Spironolactone is an effective antihypertensive agent in patients with a raised ARR who fail to suppress aldosterone in a fludrocortisone suppression test.

Comment

Schlaich *et al.* (2000) provides evidence for a link between aldosterone and left ventricular mass independently of BP. Importantly this relationship was only seen after a high salt intake (6 g/day). This complements animal models in which a high salt intake was necessary to mediate effects of aldosterone in causing interstitial and perivascular fibrosis. Clearly, the association of aldosterone dysregulation described in the above paper does not necessarily imply cause–effect relation of aldosterone with left ventricular mass. However, taken with animal work, it does support the hypothesis that aldosterone dysregulation could provide a link between high salt intake and LVH in hypertensive subjects independently of other factors.

Lim *et al.* (1999) above is a prospective cohort study of hypertensive subjects with a high aldosterone to plasma renin activity (> 750) who fail to suppress aldosterone following salt and fludrocortisone. The study describes an impressive BP response to spironolactone but is limited by its design. The absence of a control group of subjects with normal aldosterone to renin ratios and a control treatment make it impossible to ascribe a unique action to spironolactone in this subject group. This highlights the need for properly conducted randomized controlled trials of aldosterone receptor blockers in PA.

Diagnosis of primary aldosteronism

The diagnosis of PA is a two-step procedure. Firstly, aldosterone excess needs to be identified; thereafter, the cause needs to be studied. If PA affects up to 5% of hypertensive patients, half of whom may have an adenoma, it is worth considering which screening tests are appropriate or necessary in hypertensive populations.

Screening for primary aldosteronism

If the frequency of PA is as high as 15%, then screening programmes to detect the disorder would be reasonable in hypertensive clinics. However, this may be less persuasive an argument if the true prevalence is closer to 5%. Under these circumstances, looking for PA in subgroups of patients at particular risk would be a reasonable approach. For example, screening should be carried out in patients who are shown to be resistant to conventional antihypertensive drugs (in practice, those whose BP is not well controlled on two agents), patients who have a positive family history of PA and patients who are hypokalaemic. In this regard, however, it is noteworthy that frank hypokalaemia is now recognized to be present in less than 50% of patients with PA, and is not a reliable marker for the disorder |34|.

As was detailed above, simultaneous measurement of aldosterone and renin is the single best screening test for the disorder. It should be borne in mind, however, that plasma-renin activity measurements tend to be lower with age, particularly in patients with low-renin hypertension. As the denominator of the aldosterone:renin ratio, low plasma-renin activity measurements (in other words, values less than 1) can have a profound effect on the ratio, and lead to high levels of false-positive results. It is necessary, therefore, to set a fairly high cut-off for an aldosterone:renin ratio if large numbers of patients are not to be unnecessarily investigated. Under these circumstances, it would be pragmatic either simultaneously to use a threshold measurement of aldosterone, below which further investigations would not be appropriate, or to set a high threshold for the ratio. Given that aldosterone and renin assays vary from laboratory to laboratory, measurements and ranges need to be determined locally.

One advantage of the use of the aldosterone:renin ratio is the relatively robust nature of the measurement in relation to sodium intake and concurrent drug therapy. The majority of agents used to treat hypertension cause parallel changes in both aldosterone and renin. For this reason, few agents have a major distorting effect on the ratio, which facilitates its utility as a screening test. It is, of course, important to note that this is not the case when more detailed investigations are being carried out, where numerous drugs do suppress renin levels in patients with PA. In contrast, few agents can stimulate renin in patients with genuine aldosterone excess and a high renin measurement generally excludes PA.

When an abnormal aldosterone:renin ratio is present, the diagnosis of PA should be confirmed by other means. It is in those circumstances that patients should be asked to discontinue concurrent drug therapy, probably with the exception of α-blocking drugs.

Confirmatory tests for primary aldosteronism

Confirmation of the diagnosis should be made by careful measurements of aldosterone and renin—it is now accepted that a measurement made after recumbency (at least 30 minutes) or overnight rest while a patient is taking a normal sodium and potassium diet is appropriate. In normal subjects, renin and aldosterone rise after ambulation, while in patients with Conn's adenomas this is not normally the case: indeed, aldosterone levels generally fall, owing to an underlying ACTH-dependent diurnal rhythm. Thus a measurement of aldosterone and renin after 2 hours' ambulation is generally performed. Simultaneous measurement of cortisol allows one to make an indirect assessment of the concurrent effect of ACTH on aldosterone. When renin is low and aldosterone is high after recumbency, and where values are either unchanged or lower after 2 hours' ambulation, the diagnosis of PA is virtually certain, and the most likely cause is an aldosterone-producing adenoma.

Patients with bilateral adrenal hyperplasia (and a small subgroup of patients with aldosterone-producing adenomas) show responses of aldosterone to angiotensin II. In those circumstances, aldosterone can show a small rise after ambulation. However, this test, on its own, is not a sufficiently sensitive means of distinguishing between the presence or absence of a primary aldosterone-producing adenoma.

Measurement of urinary aldosterone excretion over a 24-hour period (either free aldosterone or aldosterone metabolite excretion) can be carried out. However, these measurements entail the need to make a 24-hour urine collection. Further tests to confirm the presence of PA are described below: in practice, a number of these are of little further value over the simple, carefully performed, baseline measurements of renin and aldosterone described above.

Saline infusion

The simplest test described is the infusion of normal saline (1.25 l over a 2-hour period). In normal subjects, plasma aldosterone levels are suppressed by this, while in patients with PA, levels remain elevated ($>$ 240 pmol/l) |**32**|.

Fludrocortisone suppression test

Administration of fludrocortisone (0.5 mg 4 times daily for 2 days) should invariably suppress aldosterone in normal subjects. In patients with PA, levels remain elevated. Although this is regarded as a definitive test, it may entail admission of patients to hospital, and carries with it a substantial risk of provoking severe hypokalaemia |**33**|.

Captopril test

This test involves administration of captopril (25 mg) with measurements of renin and aldosterone before and 2 hours after drug therapy is described. In normal subjects, this will suppress aldosterone levels, while in patients with Conn's adenomas, this is not the case. However, as noted above, aldosterone levels tend to fall during the day in patients with Conn's adenomas, and the captopril test has not been routinely assessed in a large number of patients, so that its true value remains uncertain.

In summary, confirmation of PA may best be made by careful measurements of aldosterone and renin in patients taking a normal dietary sodium intake and in whom drug therapy has been withdrawn.

Differential diagnosis of primary aldosteronism

In practice, the key differential diagnosis is to decide whether or not a patient has a single aldosterone-producing adenoma that might be removed surgically. It is, of course, worth considering whether patients might have rare inherited forms of PA such as GRA; positive family history and young age of onset would provide useful clues in this regard that should lead to the use of a genetic screening test.

Although aldosterone levels may be, on average, higher in patients with adenomas and in bilateral hyperplasia, this would be insufficient on its own to distinguish the two disorders. Other biochemical measurements, such as levels of 18-hydroxy-corticosterone and 18-hydroxycortisol are described as differentiating the two conditions [1], but these are not routinely performed. Similarly, although the dynamic tests described above may provide diagnostic pointers (with the notion that patients with aldosterone-producing adenomas do not show a rise in aldosterone on ambulation), this is not invariable, and should not be, on its own, relied on as a means of distinguishing between the two. For this reason, the simplest and best means of diagnosing a single aldosterone-producing adenoma is to image the adrenal glands and, if necessary, sample aldosterone levels in adrenal veins.

Definitive procedures to identify the presence of an aldosterone producing adenoma

Imaging of the adrenal glands can be carried out by CT or magnetic resonance imaging (MRI) scanning. Both techniques are useful in the identification of adrenal adenomas, although it should be noted that small lesions (in practice < 1 cm) may be below the limit of accurate resolution of either technique. For this reason, a negative adrenal scan does not exclude the presence of a small tumour.

In some patients with bilateral hyperplasia, CT scanning may show enlargement of the glands, with small nodules. However, it is important to note that the presence of non-functioning nodules within the adrenal is common. For this reason, it is not absolutely certain that patients with a demonstrable small lesion on CT scanning do indeed, have PA as a result. It is therefore common practice that adrenal vein sampling is carried out in situations of doubt, or where CT scanning is unhelpful. In these circumstances, simultaneous measurement of cortisol and aldosterone concentrations in both adrenal veins is appropriate. Cortisol measurements are necessary to correct for dilutional artefact and confirm the technical success of the procedure. A demonstration of a unilateral lesion is helpful in identifying patients who are best treated surgically.

Comparison of adrenal vein sampling and computed tomography in the differentiation of primary aldosteronism.

S B Magill, H Raff, J L Shaker, *et al. J Clin Endocrinol Metab* 2001; **86**(3): 1066–71.

BACKGROUND. Determination of aetiology of PA is important in selecting appropriate candidates for surgery. CT is limited by resolution and the common presence of non-functioning nodules within the adrenal glands. Adrenal vein sampling (AVS) is therefore considered to be the gold standard.

METHODS AND RESULTS. From 1987 to 1997, 62 patients with raised ARR (> 20) and increased urinary aldosterone excretion (> 38.8 nmol/day) after salt loading were studied; 38 had successful bilateral AVS and CT scanning using a GE 9800 scanner; 13 did not have AVS of whom two went straight to successful surgery because of unequivocal CT findings and the remainder elected to have medical management; 11 of the remaining 49 had incomplete catheterization. Aldosterone to cortisol ratios were calculated for both adrenals and IVC. A ratio of dominant to non-dominant of > 4 was considered diagnostic of APA. Fifteen of 38 had APAs on AVS. Of these only eight had concordant findings on CT, four had discordant findings and three had normal CT scans.

INTERPRETATION. Despite improvements in resolution CT scanning is an unreliable method to differentiate PA. In the vast majority of patients AVS will be necessary.

Treatment of primary aldosteronism

Surgical treatment

Surgical removal of an aldosterone-producing adenoma is normally the most appropriate treatment for patients with a unilateral lesion. However, before surgery is carried out, patients should be rendered normotensive by appropriate medical treatment. This is important, as use of an aldosterone receptor blocker or amiloride will also correct the major deficit in body potassium that would otherwise be present.

Recent surgical studies have demonstrated that laparoscopic adrenalectomy is a safe procedure that can reliably cure patients with PA |**34**|: the technique carries with it a low morbidity and entails a very short hospital stay for patients. Removal of Conn's adenomas cures hypertension in approximately two-thirds of patients and improves blood pressure control in the remainder.

Medical therapy

Medical therapy is appropriate for patients with bilateral adrenal hyperlasia, and in those patients with PA due to an adenoma where surgery is contraindicated. In those subjects, use of a mineralocorticoid receptor antagonist or amiloride is appropriate.

Spironolactone has been the most widely used mineralocorticoid receptor-blocking drug. It may need to be given in relatively high dose in patients with PA (up to 400 mg/day), and this may cause significant side-effects, particularly in male patients. These include gynaecomastia, diminished libido, impotence and dyspepsia. The newly developed receptor antagonist, eplerenone, is reportedly free of these side-effects, although large-scale studies demonstrating its use in PA are still awaited. An alternative to spironolactone is amiloride, which blocks the epithelial sodium channel. This effectively lowers blood pressure in PA; but, as with spironolactone, may need to be given in high doses (up to 60 mg/day).

In any medically treated patient it is important to monitor plasma potassium concentration. Plasma renin measurements may give some guide to the effectiveness of aldosterone blockade; where renin levels remain low, it is unlikely that effective aldosterone antagonism is being provided.

Summary

In the last few years, PA has been recognized as the most common cause of secondary hypertension. Recent screening studies have suggested that the prevalence may be as high as 15% in selected patient groups. Effective screening tests, using aldosterone:renin ratios, have now been described, and recent advances in therapy (laparoscopic surgery) and new drugs (novel aldosterone receptor antagonists) have provided alternative treatment options. In the context of essential hypertension, a better understanding of the physiology of regulation of the renin–angiotensin–aldosterone system and of the rare monogenic disorders that can cause mineralocorticoid hypertension have identified key mechanisms that may be relevant in the pathophysiology of common forms of hypertension and may, in the future, identify novel therapeutic targets.

References

1. Stewart PM. Mineralocorticoid hypertension. *Lancet* 1999; **353**: 1341–47.

2. Jeanemaitre X, Soubrier F, Kotelertster YV, Lifton RP, Williams CS, Charru A. Molecular basis of human hypertension: role of angiotensinogen. *Cell* 1992; **71**: 169–80.

3. Caulfield M, Lavender P, Newal-Price J, Farral M, Kamdar S, Daniel H. Linkage of the angiotensinogen gene locus to essential hypertension in African Caribbeans. *J Clin Invest* 1995; **96**: 687–92.

4. Mournet E, Dupont B, Bitek A, White PC. Characterization of two genes encoding human steroid 11β-hydroxylase (P-450 11β). *J Biol Chem* 1989; **264**: 20961–7.

5. Fraser R. Inborn errors of corticosteroid biosynthesis and metabolism: their effects on electrolyte metabolism. In: Robertson JIS (ed.): *Handbook of Hypertension*. Vol. 15: Clinical Hypertension. Amsterdam: Elsevier, 1988: 420–60.

6. Funder JW, Pearce PT, Smith R, Smith AL. Mineralocorticoid action: target tissue specificity is enzyme, not receptor, mediated. *Science* 1988; **242**: 583–5.

7. Edwards CRW, Stewart PM, Burt D, Brett L, McIntyre MA, Sutanto WS, de Kloet ER, Monder C. Localisation of 11β-hydroxysteroid dehydrogenase-tissue protector of the mineralocorticoid receptor. *Lancet* 1988; **2**: 986–9.

8. Shimkets RA, Warnock DG, Bostitis CM, Nelson-Williams C, Hansson JH, Schambelan M, Gill Jr JR, Ulick S, Milora RV, Findling JW, *et al.* Liddle's syndrome: heritable human hypertension caused by mutations in the β-subunit of the epithelial sodium channel. *Cell* 1994; **79**: 407–14.

9. Young M, Head G, Funder J. Determinants of cardiac fibrosis in experimental hyper-mineralocorticoid states. *Am J Physiol* 1995; **32**: E657–62.

10. Brilla CG, Matsubara LS, Weber KJ. Anti-aldosterone treatment and the prevention of myocardial fibrosis in primary and secondary hyperaldosteronism. *J Mol Cell Cardiol* 1993; **25**: 563–75.

11. Gomez-Sanchez EP. Intracerebroventricular infusion of aldosterone induces hypertension in rats. *Endocrinology* 1986; **118**: 819–23.

12. Liddle GW, Bledso T, Coppage WS. A familial renal disorder simulating primary aldosteronism but with negligible aldosterone secretion. *Trans Assoc Phys* 1983; **76**: 199–213.

13. Hansson JH, Nelson-Williams C, Suzuki H, Schild L, Shimkets R, Lu V, Canessa C, Iwasaki T, Rossier B, Lifton RP. Hypertension caused by a truncated epithelial sodium channel gamma subunit: genetic heterogeneity of Liddle syndrome. *Nat Genet* 1995; **11**: 76–82.

14. Connell JMC, Beastall GH, Davies DL, Buchanan K. Effect of low-dose dopamine infusion on insulin and glucagon-release in fasting normal man. *Horm Metab Res* 1986; **18**: 67–8.

15. Albiston AL, Obeyesekere VR, Smith RE, Krozowski ZS. Cloning and tissue distribution of the human 11β-hydroxysteroid dehydrogenase type 2 enzyme. *Mol Cell Endocrinol* 1994; **105**: R11–7.

16. Ulick S, Levine LS, Gunczler P, Zanconato G, Ramirez LC, Rauh W, Rosler A, Bradlow HL, New MI. A syndrome of apparent mineralocorticoid excess associated with defects in the peripheral metabolism of cortisol. *J Clin Endocrinol Metab* 1979; **49**: 757–64.

17. Watson B, Bergman SM, Myracle A, Callen DF, Acton RT, Warnock DG. Genetic association of 11β-hydroxysteroid dehydrogenase type 2 (*HSD11B2*) flanking microsatellites with essential hypertension in blacks. *Hypertension* 1996; **28**: 478–82.

18. Farese RV, Biglieri EG, Shackleton CHL, Ironary I, Gomez-Fontez R. Licorice-induced hypermineralocorticoidism. *N Engl J Med* 1991; **325**: 1223–7.

19. Takeda Y, Miyamori I, Iki K, Inaba S, Furukawa K, Hatakeyama H, Yoneda T, Takeda R. Endogenous renal 11 beta-hydroxysteroid dehydrogenase inhibitory factors in patients with low-renin essential hypertension. *Hypertension* 1996; **27**(2): 197–201.

20. De Simone G, Tommaselli AO, Rossi R, Valentino R, Lauria R, Scopacasa F, Lombardi G. Partial deficiency of adrenal 11β-hydroxylase: a possible cause of primary hypertension. *Hypertension* 1985; **7**: 204–10.

21. Lifton RP, Dluhy RG, Powers M, Rich GM, Gutkin M, Fallo F, Gill Jr JR, Feld L, Ganguly A, Laidlaw JC, *et al.* Hereditary hypertension caused by chimaeric gene duplications and ectopic expression of aldosterone synthase. *Nat Genet* 1992; **2**: 66–74.

22. Conn JW. Primary aldosteronism, a new clinical entity. *J Lab Clin Med* 1955; **45**: 3–17.

23. Hiramatsu K, Yamada T, Yukimura Y, Komiya I, Ichikawa K, Ishihara M, Nagata H, Izumiyama T. A screening test to identify aldosterone-producing adenoma by measuring plasma renin activity: results in hypertensive patients. *Arch Intern Med* 1981; **141**: 1589–93.

24. Gordon RD, Stowasser M, Klemm SA, Tunny TJ. High incidence of primary aldosteronism in 199 patients referred with hypertension. *Clin Exp Pharmacol Physiol* 1994; **21**: 315–8.

25. Lim PO, Rodgers P, Cardak K, Watson AS, MacDonald TM. Potentially high prevalence of primary aldosteronism in a primary care population. *Lancet* 1999; **353**: 40.

26. Strowasser M, Gordon RD, Tunny TJ, Klemm SA, Finn WL, Krek AL. Familial hyperaldosteronism type II: five families with a new variety of primary aldosteronism. *Clin Exp Pharmacol Physiol* 1992; **19**: 319–22.

27. Idiopathic aldosteronism: a diagnostic artefact? *Lancet* 1979; **2**: 1221–2.

28. Rocha R., Chander P. N., Khanna K., Zuckerman A. and Stier C.T. Role of aldosterone in renal vascular injury in stroke-prone hypertensive rats. *Hypertension* 1999; 33: 1-6

29. Rocha R., Chander P. N., Khanna K., Zuckerman A. and Stier C.T. Mineralocorticoid blockade reduced vascular injury in stroke-prone hypertensive rats. *Hypertension* 1998; 31: 451-458

30. Gordon RD, Stowasser M, Klemm SA, Tunny TJ. Primary aldosteronism and other forms of mineralocorticoid hypertension. In: Swales JD (ed.): *Textbook of Hypertension.* Oxford: Blackwell Scientific, pp. 865–92.

31. Rossi GP, Sacchetto A, Visentin P, Canali C, Graniero GR, Palatini P, Pessina AC. Changes in left ventricular anatomy and function in hypertension and primary aldosteronism. *Hypertension* 1996; **27**: 1039–45.

32. Holland OB, Brown H, Kuhnert L, Fairchild C, Risk M, Gomez-Sanchez CE. Further evaluation of saline infusion for the diagnosis of primary aldosteronism. *Hypertension* 1984; **6**: 717–23.

33. Gordon RD, Jackson RV, Strakosch CR, Tunny TJ, Rutherford JC, McCosker J, Moriarty W. Aldosterone-producing adenoma: fludrocortisone suppression and left adrenal vein catheterization in definitive diagnosis and management. *Aust NZ J Med* 1979; **57**: 676–82.

34. Takeda M, Go H, Imai T, Nishiyama T, Morishita H. Laparoscopic adrenalectomy for primary aldosteronism: report of initial ten cases. *Surgery* 1994; **115**: 621–5.

Part IV

Current practical issues

10

Selective angiotensin II receptor antagonists

Introduction

Pharmacological targeting of the renin–angiotensin–aldosterone system (RAAS) arguably constitutes one of the most significant therapeutic approaches to the management of cardiovascular diseases. The benefits of such an approach have been clearly established by angiotensin-converting enzyme (ACE) inhibitor treatments but similar benefits are anticipated from selective angiotensin II (AT_1) receptor antagonist drugs. These drugs are already licensed for the management of hypertension and their roles in the management of heart failure and in renal disorders are currently under investigation in a number of ongoing clinical trials. At present, selective AT_1 receptor antagonists are welcomed as additional or alternative first-line antihypertensive drugs but, with the current emphasis on 'tight' blood pressure (BP) control and its requirement for combination treatment regimens and long-term compliance, the good tolerability profile of this class may afford them a central role in antihypertensive drug treatment in the future.

Clinical pharmacology

The principal actions of angiotensin II are vasoconstriction of the resistance vessels and stimulation of aldosterone production and release. Angiotensin II also has a facilitatory role within the sympathetic nervous system. Several different angiotensin II receptor subtypes have been identified but the known cardiovascular functions are mediated via the AT_1 receptor (Fig. 10.1). An AT_2 receptor has also been clearly defined but its physiological role remains obscure. It has been hypothesized, for example, that the regulatory role of angiotensin II in cell growth and proliferation reflects a dynamic equilibrium between its growth promoting effects mediated via the AT_1 receptor and its antiproliferative effects mediated via the AT_2 receptor. More recent research has identified several further angiotensin II receptor subtypes but their functional roles remain obscure.

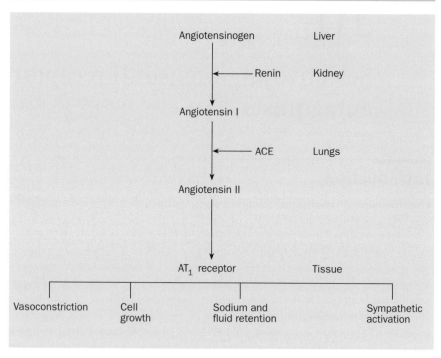

Fig. 10.1 Mediation of cardiovascular functions via the AT_1 receptor. ACE = angiotensin-converting enzyme.

AT_1 receptor blockade versus angiotensin-converting enzyme inhibition

There are several sites at which the RAAS might be inhibited or blocked but, in therapeutic terms, inhibition of ACE has to date proved to be the most successful (Fig. 10.2). However, ACE inhibition does not provide complete blockade of the RAAS because angiotensin II can be generated by non-ACE enzyme pathways, such as chymase, cathepsin and chymostatin-sensitive angiotensin II generating enzyme. Furthermore, ACE is also active in other metabolic pathways and, most notably, in the guise of kininase II it is responsible for the breakdown of vasoactive kinins, principally bradykinin. During ACE inhibitor treatment, therefore, the breakdown of kinins is inhibited: the resultant accumulation of kinins has been implicated in the causation of ACE inhibitor cough. As angiotensin II receptor antagonist drugs have no effect on kinin pathways there is no problem with cough as an adverse effect. Furthermore, as the angiotensin II receptor antagonists act directly on the AT_1 receptor, complete blockade of the RAAS is produced irrespective of the enzyme pathway by which the angiotensin II has been generated.

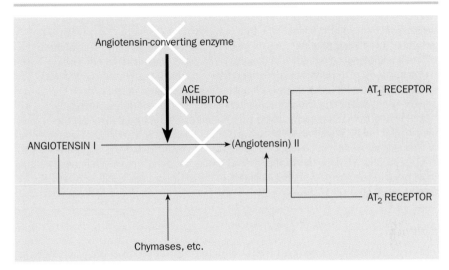

Fig. 10.2 Angiotensin II production effect of angiotensin-converting enzyme (ACE) inhibitor drugs.

Selective angiotensin II antagonist drugs

Since the development of the prototype agent, losartan, several further agents have become widely available: candesartan (cilexitil), eprosartan, irbesartan, telmisartan and valsartan. Although there are some differences in pharmacokinetics and specific pharmacological characteristics, all these agents (or their active metabolites) bind specifically to the AT_1 receptor. In general, the receptor-binding characteristics cannot be classified as 'competitive' according to classical pharmacological terminology but instead the binding characteristics provide a longer lasting antagonist effect such that 'non-competitive' or 'insurmountable' or 'irreversible' are terms that have become widely employed.

The selectivity of the action of angiotensin II receptor antagonists lends itself to clinical pharmacological studies in which the effectiveness of the receptor blockade can readily be quantified, typically by assessment of the responses to administered angiotensin II.

Angiotensin II receptor blockade in normotensive subjects: a direct comparison of three AT_1 receptor antagonists.

L Mazzolai, M Maillard, J Rossat, *et al. Hypertension* 1999; **33**: 850–5.

BACKGROUND. Use of angiotensin II AT_1 receptor antagonists for the treatment of hypertension is rapidly increasing, yet direct comparisons of the relative efficacy of antagonists to block the renin–angiotensin system in humans are lacking.

INTERPRETATION. This study thus demonstrates that the first administration of the recommended starting dose of irbesartan induces a greater and longer-lasting angiotensin II receptor blockade than that of valsartan and losartan in normotensive subjects. This clinical pharmacological study investigated the effectiveness of three different angiotensin II antagonists (losartan, valsartan and irbesartan) in a well designed study in 12 normotensive subjects. In a double blind, placebo-controlled, randomized, four-way cross study each subject received single doses of each angiotensin II antagonist and placebo and the effectiveness of the angiotensin II blockade was then assessed by three different methods: (a) by the extent of the inhibition of the BP response to the administration of exogenous angiotensin II; (b) by an *in vitro* angiotensin II receptor binding assay; and (c) by the reactive changes in plasma angiotensin II levels. Irbesartan appeared to produce the most marked blockade with the most effective and longest lasting inhibition of the BP response to administered angiotensin II (see Fig 10.3).

Comment

This is a very well designed and well conducted clinical pharmacological study that describes three different but related methodologies and their usefulness in evaluating the effectiveness of angiotensin II receptor antagonists drugs. However, as a discriminating methodology for determining duration of action and overall

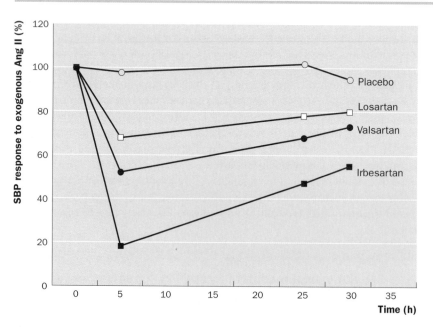

Fig. 10.3 Relative effectiveness of three angiotensin II (Ang II) antagonists in normotensive subjects. SBP = systolic blood pressure. Source: Mazzolai *et al.* (1999).

effectiveness it is necessary to study comparable doses under steady-state conditions. Unfortunately, for the clinician rather than the research worker, this single dose evaluation, with dosages that may not be comparable, does not provide any useful evidence for discriminating between these three drugs in terms of their therapeutic benefits.

Conclusion

There is a reasonably consistent body of evidence to suggest that losartan is not the most effective angiotensin receptor antagonist, but there is a confusion of evidence surrounding the relative effectiveness of the other drugs in this class. In fact, at present, there is no consistent and scientifically robust evidence base by which the other agents might be separated. For the present, eprosartan is probably not a contender (because of the paucity of information about its use as a once daily agent) but candesartan (cilexitil), irbesartan, telmisartan and valsartan can probably be considered to be equivalent.

Clinical trials with angiotensin II antagonist drugs

There is no doubt that angiotensin II receptor (AT_1) antagonists constitute an exciting and important new class of antihypertensive drug. There is little doubt that these drugs, as a class, constitute a clear advance by virtue of their very good tolerability, both symptomatic and metabolic, and particularly their lack of any obvious class-specific adverse effect. However, it has not always proved possible to demonstrate clearly that the antihypertensive efficacy is comparable with that of established agents. In this respect, the prototype drug, losartan, for which there is the greatest volume of information, has failed to demonstrate consistently that its BP-lowering effects are superior to those of established agents. Of greater concern are the reports that suggest that losartan may, in fact, be less potent than comparator agents both within its own class and across the different antihypertensive drug classes. Nevertheless, for any new agent, or any new class of drug, there remains a basic requirement that clinical usefulness be demonstrated at an early stage in terms of efficacy and tolerability. Thereafter, the requirement is for evidence of beneficial outcomes which, ideally, reflect improvements in cardiovascular morbidity and mortality or, at least, improvement in recognized surrogate markers of cardiovascular disease.

Hypertension

ABPM comparison of the antihypertensive profiles of the selective angiotensin II receptor antagonists telmisartan and losartan in patients with mild to moderate hypertension.

J M Mallion, J P Siche, Y Lacourcière, and the Telmisartan Blood Pressure Monitoring Group. *J Hum Hypertens* 1999; **13**: 657–64.

BACKGROUND. **The antihypertensive efficacy and tolerability profiles of the selective AT$_1$ receptor antagonists telmisartan and losartan were compared with placebo in a 6-week multinational, multicentre, randomized, double-blind, double-dummy, parallel study of 233 patients with mild to moderate hypertension, defined as clinic diastolic BP $\geq$ 95 and $\leq$ 114 mmHg, clinic systolic BP $\geq$ 140 and $\leq$ 200mmHg, and 24-h ambulatory diastolic BP $\geq$ 85 mmHg.**

INTERPRETATION. Telmisartan 40 mg and 80 mg once daily were effective and well tolerated in the treatment of mild to moderate hypertension, producing sustained 24-h BP control that compared favourably with losartan. This was a multicentre, randomized, double-blind, double-dummy, parallel group study of 223 patients who received 6 weeks of treatment with either placebo, or losartan 50 mg daily, or telmisartan 40 mg daily or telmisartan 80 mg daily. Overall, there were consistently greater BP reductions with the two different doses of telmisartan compared with losartan. In particular telmisartan 80 mg daily was consistently significantly more effective than losartan 50 mg across the measured parameters (see Tables 10.1 and 10.2).

Table 10.1 Comparison of telmisartan and losartan—reductions in blood pressure (from baseline: placebo-corrected)–1

	Losartan (50 mg)	Telmisartan (40 mg)	Telmisartan (80 mg)
Daytime (06.00–22.00)	*6.6/4.4*	*9.4/6.4*	**11.2/7.4**
Night-time (22.00–0600)	*5.1/3.7*	**9.6/6.8**	**11.2/7.4**
'Trough' (00.00–0600)	3.7/2.4	**8.4/5.5**	**9.9/5.8**
Morning (06.00–12.00)	*5.3/2.8*	*8.1/5.3**	**10.3/6.2**

*$P<$0.05 versus placebo; **$P<$0.05 versus placebo and losartan.
Source: Mallion *et al.* (1999).

Table 10.2 Comparison of telmisartan and losartan—reductions in blood pressure (from baseline: placebo-corrected)–2

	Losartan (50 mg)	Telmisartan (40 mg)	Telmisartan (80 mg)
Clinic BP	5.5/2.5	9.4/5.1	*11.1/6.2*
24-hour ABPM	6.2/4.1	*9.7/6.6*	*11.5/7.6*

*$P \leq$0.05 versus losartan. BP = blood pressure; ABPM = ambulatory blood pressure measurement.
Source: Mallion *et al.* (1999).

Comment

This well conducted study confirms the earlier concerns that losartan may not be the most effective agent within the class.

Efficacy and safety of telmisartan, a selective AT$_1$ receptor antagonist, compared with enalapril in elderly patients with primary hypertension.

B E Karlberg, L-E Lins, K Hermansson for the TEES Group. *J Hypertens* 1999; **17**: 293–302.

BACKGROUND. To assess the antihypertensive efficacy and safety of the novel AT$_1$ receptor antagonists, telmisartan, compared with that of enalapril in elderly patients with mild to moderate hypertension.

INTERPRETATION. These results demonstrate that telmisartan is well tolerated and is at least effective as enalapril in treating elderly patients with mild to moderate hypertension. This was a 26-week multicentre double blind, parallel group, dosage titration study involving 278 patients aged 65 years or more. Patients were randomly assigned to telmisartan across the dose range 20–40–80 mg or to enalapril 5–10–20 mg according to the supine diastolic BP response at trough. Both treatments lowered BP in a comparable and clinically meaningful manner with mean changes from baseline of 22.1/12.9 mmHg for telmisartan and 20.1/11.4 for enalapril. Both regimens were well tolerated; however, 16% of patients receiving enalapril reported cough compared with only 6.5% of those receiving telmisartan.

Comment

This conventional clinical trial illustrates again that comparable antihypertensive efficacy is more likely to be produced by one of the newer angiotensin II antagonists.

Comparison of the angiotensin II receptor antagonist irbesartan with atenolol for treatment of hypertension.

K O Stumpe, D Haworth, C Hoglund, *et al. Blood Pressure* 1998; **7**: 31–7.

BACKGROUND. In this multicentre, double-blind study, the antihypertensive efficacy and safety of irbesartan were compared with those of atenolol in patients with mild-to-moderate hypertension.

INTERPRETATION. In comparison with atenolol, irbesartan ≤ 150 mg provided at least equivalent BP control while demonstrating an excellent safety and tolerability profile. This study in 231 patients with mild-to-moderate hypertension was a routine comparative clinical trial in patients with seated diastolic BP in the range 95–110 mmHg. Treatments were initiated with irbesartan 75 mg or atenolol 50 mg daily and increased to 150 mg and 50 mg, respectively, according to the BP response with the option to then add hydrochlorothiazide and then nifedipine if seated diastolic BP remained above 90 mmHg. Overall, there were no significant differences in the antihypertensive effect of the two drug treatment regimens, although the BP reduction (from baseline) was slightly greater with irbesartan: by 1.9 mmHg for systolic BP and by 0.6 mmHg for diastolic BP. Adverse drug reports were similar but serious adverse events and discontinuations because of adverse events were slightly greater in the atenolol group at 9.1% *vs* 4.5%. These authors concluded that irbesartan provided at least equivalent BP control in comparison with atenolol while demonstrating an excellent safety and tolerability profile.

Comment

This routine clinical trial again illustrates the point that the newer angiotensin II antagonists appear better able to demonstrate antihypertensive comparability with representatives from other reference drug classes.

Angiotensin II type 1 (AT$_1$) in hypertensive women: candesartan cilexetil versus enalapril or hydrochlorothiazide.

K Malmqvist, T Kahan, M Dahl. *Am J Hypertens* 2000; **13**: 504–11.

BACKGROUND. Women have traditionally been treated with older types of antihypertensive drugs, mainly diuretics, often according to guidelines based on data from studies in men. Furthermore, women more frequently report side-effects from their medical treatment than do men, including dry cough found during ACE inhibitor treatment.

INTERPRETATION. Candesartan cilexetil 8–16 mm lowers systolic BP and diastolic BP more effectively than enalapril, with less risk for dry cough. Candesartan cilexetil 8–16 mg lowers systolic BP and diastolic BP more effectively than hydrochlorothiazide 12.5–25 mg, with less risk of hypokalaemia and hyperuricaemia. Quality of life was similar and well maintained in all treatment groups. The favourable effect on systolic BP with candesartan cilexetil is of particular interest as mean systolic BP is higher among postmenopausal women than in men of a similar age. This study in 429 women aged 40–69 years was a parallel group comparison of 12 weeks of treatment with candesartan (cilexetil) 8 or 16 mg, enalapril 10 or 20 mg or hydrochlorothiazide 12.5 or 25 mg. The BP reductions were significantly greater with candesartan compared with other treatments (Fig. 10.4). With candesartan BP was reduced by 19.0/11.1 compared with 13.5/9.0 with enalapril and 12.9/8.0 mmHg with hydrochlorothiazide.

Comment

The salient message is that candesartan is at least as effective as representative agents from alternative, established antihypertensive drugs.

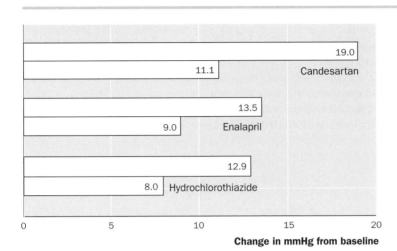

Fig. 10.4 Blood pressure reductions. Comparison of 12 weeks' treatment with candesartan, enalapril or hydrochlorothiazide. Source: Malmqvist *et al.* (2000).

Angiotensin II antagonists for hypertension: are there differences in efficacy?

P R Conlin, J D Spence, B Williams, *et al. J Hypertens* 2000; **13**: 418–26.

BACKGROUND. **We compared the antihypertensive efficacy of available drugs in the new angiotensin II antagonist class.**

INTERPRETATION. This comprehensive analysis shows comparable antihypertensive efficacy within the angiotensin II antagonist class, a near-flat angiotensin II antagonist dose–response when titrating from starting to maximum recommended dose, and substantial potentiation of the antihypertensive effect with the addition of HCTZ. The antihypertensive efficacy of losartan, valsartan, irbesartan and candesartan was evaluated from randomized controlled trials by performing a meta-analysis of 43 published randomized controlled trials. A total of 11 281 patients were assessed and the conclusion was drawn that the absolute weighted average reductions in systolic BP (between 10.4 and 11.8 mmHg) and in diastolic BP (between 8.2 and 8.9 mmHg) were comparable for all angiotensin II antagonist drugs. Responder rates, by conventional diastolic BP criteria were 48–55% for angiotensin II antagonist monotherapy and dose titration resulted in slightly greater BP reductions and an increase in responder rate to 53–63%. Combination treatments with hydrochlorothiazide also increased the responder rates in the range 56–70% with substantially greater reductions in systolic BP (between 16.1 and 20.6 mmHg) and in diastolic BP (between 9.9 and 13.6 mmHg).

Comment

This meta-analysis incorporates the published results from 43 randomized controlled trials whose designs, in general, were constrained for regulatory purposes and were of the 'equivalence' rather than the 'superiority' type. Despite the overall conclusion of the authors that there was comparability across the agents studied, it is interesting to note that the results reported for losartan are often inferior to the other agents. It is accepted that these differences are small and are not of statistical significance but the finding is relatively consistent. For example, starting dose monotherapy with losartan was associated with a 48% responder rate and an average BP reduction of 10.4/8.2 mmHg. The reported values for the other three agents are superior with the highest figures occurring with candesartan 8 mg and a responder rate of 55% in association with a mean reduction in seated BP of 11.8/8.9 mmHg.

Conclusion

These regulatory-style clinical trials are important for generating a database but seldom do they have real discriminatory power. However, the basic message remains unchanged: losartan appears to be the least effective agent within the class and the newer agents are more consistently able to demonstrate direct comparability with other reference drugs. But, which of the others—candesartan, irbesartan, telmisartan or valsartan—is the class leader?

Cardiac failure

The results of several major clinical outcome trials have clearly demonstrated the morbidity and mortality benefits associated with the use of ACE inhibitor drugs in patients with heart failure secondary to left ventricular dysfunction. With selective angiotensin II antagonists the first published study (Evaluation of Losartan in the Elderly Study, ELITE) suggested that losartan might be preferable to captopril particularly because of reductions in fatal myocardial infarction and sudden death. However, this possible benefit has not been substantiated in the follow-up study (ELITE II) and the preliminary results of clinical trials with other angiotensin II antagonists have not yet provided evidence that angiotensin II receptor blockade is superior to ACE inhibition in the management of cardiac failure.

Randomized trial of losartan versus captopril in patients over 65 with heart failure (Evaluation of Losartan in the Elderly Study, ELITE).
B Pitt, R Segal, F A Martinez, *et al. Lancet* 1997; **349**: 747–52.

BACKGROUND. To determine whether specific angiotensin II receptor blockade with losartan offers safety and efficacy advantages in the treatment of heart failure over ACE inhibition with captopril, the ELITE study compared losartan with captopril in older heart failure patients.

INTERPRETATION. In this study of elderly heart failure patients, treatment with losartan was associated with an unexpected lower mortality than that found with captopril. Although there was no difference in renal dysfunction, losartan was generally better tolerated than captopril and fewer patients discontinued losartan therapy. A further trial (ELITE II), evaluating the effects of losartan and captopril on mortality and morbidity in a larger number of patients with heart failure, is in progress. The ELITE trial enrolled 722 patients aged 75 years or more with NYHA class II–IV heart failure and randomized them to receive either losartan or captopril for approximately 1 year of treatment. The primary end-point was the tolerability assessment of renal function for which there was no difference between the two treatments. However, there was the unexpected finding of a statically significant reduction in all-cause mortality in the losartan group (17 deaths) compared with the captopril group (32 deaths).

Comment

This study produced an unexpected result in so far as all cause mortality was significantly reduced by losartan relative to captopril. However, the sample size, study design and declared outcome measures were not prospectively empowered to permit definitive conclusion.

Effects of losartan compared with captopril on mortality in patients with symptomatic heart failure: randomized trial—the Losartan Heart Failure Survival Study ELITE II.

B Pitt, P Poole-Wilson, R Segal, *et al. Lancet* 2000; **355**: 1582–7.

BACKGROUND. The ELITE study showed an association between the angiotensin II antagonist losartan and an unexpected survival benefit in elderly heart failure patients, compared with captopril, an ACE inhibitor. The ELITE II Losartan Heart Failure/Survival Study was done to confirm whether losartan is superior to captopril in improving survival and is better tolerated.

INTERPRETATION. Losartan was not superior to captopril in improving survival in elderly heart failure patients, but was significantly better tolerated. We believe that ACE inhibitors should be the initial treatment for heart failure, although angiotensin II receptor antagonists may be useful to block the renin angiotensin aldosterone system when ACE inhibitors are not tolerated. ELITE II was a double blind randomized controlled trial in 3152 patients aged 60 years or over with NYHA class 2–4 heart failure and a measured ejection fraction of 40% or less. Patients were randomly assigned to losartan up to 50 mg once daily or to captopril up to 50 mg three times daily. The salient finding were that there were no significant differences in all-cause mortality, 11.7 *vs* 10% average annual mortality rate for losartan *vs* captopril; or in sudden death or resuscitated arrests, 9 *vs* 7.3% respectively in the two groups. Overall, significantly fewer patients in the losartan group discontinued study treatment because of adverse effects, 9.7 *vs* 14.7%, although when allowance is made for the increased incidence of cough in the captopril treatment group, there was no significant difference in the discontinuation rate at 9.4 *vs* 12.0%.

Comment

For most observers, the result of this study was not unexpected in so far as it failed to confirm any suggestion of superiority of losartan treatment compared with captopril treatment in heart failure. This study had the particular advantage that it was statistically more powerful than ELITE I and the overall result of 'no difference' was therefore more reliable (but not unexpected). However, it is interesting to note that the trends in ELITE II favoured the captopril treatment and this tends to cast considerable doubt on the clinical relevance of the theoretical and potential advantages of losartan, which were advanced to support the unexpected finding in ELITE I. Alternatively, however, the simplest explanation may be the most plausible in so far as losartan 50 mg daily is unlikely to suppress the activity of the renin–angiotensin system to the same extent over 24 h as captopril 50 mg three times daily.

Comparison of candesartan, enalapril, and their combination in congestive heart failure. Randomised Evaluation of Strategies for Left Ventricular Dysfunction (RESOLVD) Pilot Study.

R S McKelvie, S Yusuf, D Pericak, *et al. Circulation* 1999; **100**: 1056–64.

BACKGROUND. We investigated the effects of candesartan (an angiotensin II antagonist) alone, enalapril alone, and their combination on exercise tolerance, ventricular function, quality of life, neurohormone levels and tolerability in congestive heart failure.

INTERPRETATION. Candesartan alone was as effective, safe and tolerable as enalapril. The combination of candesartan and enalapril was more beneficial for preventing left ventricular remodelling than either candesartan or enalapril alone.

Comment

This pilot study in 668 patients with NYHA-FC II–IV showed that candesartan monotherapy was similar but not superior to enalapril monotherapy in the management of patients with heart failure. The results of the main study have not yet been reported in full but the preliminary announcements indicate that candesartan has no therapeutic advantages over enalapril.

Improvement in exercise tolerance and symptoms of congestive heart failure during treatment with candesartan cilexetil.

G A J Riegger, H Bouzo, P Petr, *et al. Circulation* 1999; **100**: 2224–30.

BACKGROUND. The renin–angiotensin system plays an important part in the pathogenesis of congestive heart failure. This study evaluated the effect of an angiotensin II type I receptor antagonist on exercise tolerance and symptoms of congestive heart failure.

INTERPRETATION. In summary, treatment with candesartan cilexetil demonstrated significant improvements in exercise tolerance, cardiothoracic ratio, and symptoms and signs of congestive heart failure and was well tolerated. This was a double blind parallel group study in which patients were randomized to short-term treatment (12 weeks) with placebo ($n = 211$) or candesartan 4 mg ($n = 208$), 8 mg ($n = 212$) or 16 mg ($n = 213$). Candesartan was associated with a dose-related improvement in exercise time, whereby for the intention-to-treat analysis, all doses of candesartan were associated with improvement, although statistical significance was not always obtained.

Conclusion

There is now a considerable amount of evidence that ACE inhibitor drugs contribute positively to the management of patients with cardiac failure, left ventricular dysfunction and post-myocardial infarction. Although, on a theoretical basis, angiotensin II antagonists might be expected to provide further benefits there is no evidence so far that this is true.

Regression of left ventricular hypertrophy

There is a considerable amount of experimental evidence implicating the RAAS system in the development of left ventricular hypertrophy (LVH) and, consequently, there has been considerable interest in the effectiveness of ACE inhibitors in clinical studies. The same experimental rationale and the same experimental background has also been explored with angiotensin II receptor antagonists but with the additional expectation that, as the angiotensin II receptor antagonists block non-ACE-dependent angiotensin II generation, such as occurs within the myocardium, this class of drugs might be even more effective than the ACE inhibitor group. Unfortunately, the early studies with losartan—albeit with small numbers—totally failed to demonstrate any regression of LVH despite, in the second study, a very significant BP reduction |1,2|.

Influence of the angiotensin II antagonist valsartan on left ventricular hypertrophy in patients with essential hypertension.

P A Thürmann, P Kendi, A Schmidt, S Harder, N Rietbrock. *Circulation* 1998; **98**: 2037–42.

BACKGROUND. LVH represents an independent risk factor in patients with essential hypertension. Because reversal of LVH may be associated with an improvement of prognosis, the influence of new antihypertensive compounds, such as angiotensin II AT_1 receptor antagonists, on LVH should be determined.

INTERPRETATION. Antihypertensive treatment with the angiotensin II antagonist valsartan for 8 months produced a significant regression of LVH in predominantly previously untreated patients with essential hypertension. The drug may be safely administered in this subset of hypertensive patients; however, the long-term benefit in terms of risk reduction has still to be evaluated in further trials.

Comment

The evidence from this clinical study is consistent in showing that BP reduction leads to the regression of LVH. However, there was no evidence of any additional benefit attributable to angiotensin II antagonist activity. In this illustrative study with valsartan it is noteworthy that regression of LVH was actually achieved, whereas earlier studies with losartan had failed to confirm even this basic requirement.

Regression of left ventricular hypertrophy in human hypertension with irbesartan.
K Malmqvist, T Kahan, M Edner *et al. J Hypertens* 2001; **19**: 1167–76.

BACKGROUND. Angiotensin II induces myocardial hypertrophy. We hypothesized that blockades of angiotensin II subtype 1 (AT_1) receptor by the AT_1 receptor antagonist irbesartan would reduce the left ventricular mass (as measured by echocardiography) more than conventional treatment with beta-blocker.

INTERPRETATION. Left ventricular mass was reduced more in the irbesartan group than in the atenolol group. These results suggest that blocking the action of angiotensin II at AT_1 receptors may be an important mechanism, beyond that of lowering BP, in the regulation of left ventricular mass and geometry in patients with hypertension. This double blind trial randomized 110 hypertension patients to receive either irbesartan 150 mg daily or atenolol 50 mg daily for approximately 1 year. According to diastolic BP control, doses could be doubled and additional medications (hydrochlorothiazide and felodipine) could be prescribed as required and echocardiographic assessments were performed at 0, 12, 24 and 28 weeks. Treatments based on irbesartan and atenolol were associated with a similar reduction in BP such that the average final BP, on treatment, was closely similar at approximately 127/86 in the irbesartan group and 128/86 mmHg in the atenolol group. Baseline BP was 162/104 mmHg. Both treatments were associated with a progressive reduction in left ventricular mass index with a significantly greater reduction in the irbesartan group at 16 *vs* 9% (26 vs 14 g/m^2) ($P < 0.025$).

Comment

While there is strong experimental evidence that blockade of the RAAS should be particularly effective in promoting the regression of LVH there remains a dearth of convincing evidence when the clinical studies are evaluated. This most recent study with irbesartan similarly fails to provide definitive evidence in so far as the starting BP and the pretreatment left ventricular measurement tended to be higher in the irbesartan group compared with the atenolol group.

Pressure overload induces cardiac hypertrophy in angiotensin II type 1A receptor knockout mice.

K Harada, I Komuro, I Shiojima, *et al. Circulation* 1998; **97**: 1952–9.

BACKGROUND. Many studies have suggested that the renin–angiotensin system plays an important part in the development of pressure overload-induced cardiac hypertrophy. Moreover, it has been reported that pressure overload-induced cardiac hypertrophy is completely prevented by ACE inhibitors *in vivo* and that the stored angiotensin II is released from cardiac myocytes in response to mechanical stretch and induces cardiomyocyte hypertrophy through the angiotensin II type 1 receptor (AT$_1$) *in vitro*.

INTERPRETATION. AT$_1$-mediated angiotensin II signalling is not essential for the development of pressure overload-induced cardiac hypertrophy.

Comment

This is a very interesting and thought-provoking study concerning the role of factors other than pressure overload in the development of hypertensive LVH. The AT$_1$ receptor is the 'effector' or 'signalling' locus within the RAAS and complete or marked reduction in cardiac hypertrophy would be predicted when functional responses mediated via the AT$_1$ receptor are eliminated. In this 'knockout' animal model, elimination of the AT$_1$ receptor failed to prevent cardiac hypertrophy, thus raising considerable doubts about the proposed central role of angiotensin II and the RAAS in those non-haemodynamic processes, which are anticipated in the development of LVH.

Effects of valsartan on left ventricular diastolic function in patients with mild or moderate essential hypertension: comparison with enalapril.

A Cuocolo, G Storto, R Izzo, *et al. J Hypertens* 1999; **17**: 1759–66.

BACKGROUND. This study compares the effects of an AT$_1$ angiotensin II receptor antagonist (valsartan) with those of an ACE inhibitor (enalapril) on left ventricular diastolic function in patients with mild or moderate essential hypertension and no evidence of LVH at echocardiography.

INTERPRETATION. Valsartan-induced renin–angiotensin system blockade is able to improve left ventricular filling in patients with mild or moderate essential hypertension and impaired diastolic function. These findings support the hypothesis of a contribution of the renin–angiotensin system in the control of left ventricular diastolic function in these patients. This small scale study of 24 patients used radionuclide ambulatory monitoring to investigate left ventricular function at rest and during exercise testing. Patients received either valsartan (80–160 mg daily) and enalapril (20–40 mg daily) according to a double blind cross-over randomization scheme. Briefly, there were no significant differences between the two treatments in terms of their effects on left ventricular diastolic function. A subgroup analysis was then used to suggest that valsartan had a greater beneficial effect on left ventricular peak filling rate.

Comment

This small study is insufficiently powered to show anything other than comparability of the two different treatments that produced similar reductions in BP. The small number of patients does not justify a *post-hoc* subgroup analysis and it is not possible, in the light of a small but significant BP reduction, to draw the conclusion that the renin–angiotensin system is implicated in the control of left ventricular diastolic function in hypertensive patients. In fact, because of the reductions in BP with both active treatments it is not possible to draw any other conclusion than to suggest that BP reduction might be beneficial for left ventricular diastolic function.

Conclusion

For the clinician, the practical message from all of these studies is a reinforcement of the concept that the optimal means of preventing (or reversing) LVH is long-term BP control. While angiotensin II antagonists might usefully be incorporated into an effective antihypertensive combination regimen there is not yet clinical evidence to favour their specific use on account of any additional 'tissue' effects.

Clinical trials in renal dysfunction

The effect of selective angiotensin II blockade on renal mechanisms has been a particular feature of studies with candesartan. However, the preliminary results of outcome studies with irbesartan and losartan will be presented in 2001.

Renal haemodynamic and hormonal responses to the angiotensin II antagonist candesartan.
M C Lansang, S Y Osei, D A Prive, N D L Fisher, N K Hollenberg.
Hypertension 2000; **36**: 834–8.

BACKGROUND. The development of very specific blockers for the angiotensin II type I (AT_1) receptor made it possible to examine the contribution of angiotensin II to normal control mechanisms and disease with a specificity beyond what ACE inhibitors could provide. In this study, the contribution of angiotensin II to two renal mechanisms was explored: real haemodynamics and the short feedback loop, in which angiotensin II acts as a determinant of renin release.

INTERPRETATION. The remarkable rise in plasma renin activity after candesartan is substantially larger than that in earlier studies with ACE inhibition, providing additional evidence for non-ACE-dependent angiotensin II generation in the kidney. This was an interesting clinical pharmacological study in healthy volunteers on a very low sodium intake designed to activate the renin–angiotensin system. Candesartan was associated with a dose-related increase in renal plasma flow with the maximum vasodilator response occurring during the first 4 h post-dose. Unsurprisingly, there were dose-related increases in plasma renin activity and, on the basis of the differences with the known responses to ACE inhibitor drugs, the authors attempt to draw some mechanistic conclusions.

Comment

This is an interesting study but it constitutes only a first step in the exploration of the haemodynamic and hormonal effects in response to angiotensin II antagonism. This was a single dose study in healthy volunteers who were artificially provoked into activation of their renin–angiotensin systems. In the absence of a direct comparison in the same group of subjects with the same model it is not possible to draw a definitive conclusion about the comparative effects with ACE inhibitor drugs. Nevertheless, the conclusion that there is evidence of 'non-ACE-dependent angiotensin II generation in the kidney' appears reasonable and excites further interest in the prospects that this class of drugs may be particularly effective in the treatment of renal diseases, including hypertensive diabetic nephropathy.

Dual blockade of the renin–angiotensin–aldosterone system

There is little doubt that a more complete blockade of the RAAS can be obtained with the combination of an ACE inhibitor drug and an angiotensin II receptor antagonist. Whether or not this can translate to a more effective treatment in heart failure or in renal disorders, without compromising safety, remains to be established.

Randomized controlled trial of dual blockade of renin–angiotensin system in patients with hypertension, microalbuminuria, and non-insulin dependant diabetes: the Candesartan and Lisinopril Microalbuminuria (CALM) study.

C E Mogensen, S Neldam, I Tikkanen, et al. BMJ 2000; **321**: 1440–4.

BACKGROUND. To assess and compare the effects of candesartan or lisinopril, or both, on BP urinary albumin excretion in patients with microalbuminuria, hypertension and type 2 diabetes.

INTERPRETATION. Candesartan 16 mg, once daily, is as effective as lisinopril 20 mg, once daily, in reducing BP and microalbuminuria in hypertensive patients with type 2 diabetes. Combination treatment is well tolerated and more effective in reducing BP. This was a double blind parallel group study of 12 weeks monotherapy followed by a comparison of 12 weeks monotherapy or combination treatment. After 12 weeks of treatment there were similar reductions of about 10 mmHg in diastolic BP with both candesartan 16 mg daily and lisinopril 20 mg daily. There were correspondingly similar reductions in the urinary albumin/creatinine ratio by 30% and 46%, respectively, for candesartan and lisinopril. During the combination treatment phase after a further 12 weeks of treatment, the mean reduction in diastolic BP was 16.3 mmHg with candesartan and lisinopril combined compared with 10.4 mmHg with candesartan monotherapy and 10.7 mmHg with lisinopril monotherapy. Not surprisingly, the reductions in the urinary albumin/creatinine ratio were significantly greater with the combination treatment at 50% compared with 24% with candesartan monotherapy and 39% with lisinopril monotherapy.

Comment

This well conducted study answers some questions but, unfortunately, raises some important additional points. Reassuringly, there were additive effects in relation both to BP reduction and to improvements in urinary albumin excretion with no evidence of any adverse effect on other measures of renal function or on overall tolerability. However, some questions remain because the trends with mono-therapy favoured ACE inhibition rather than angiotensin II antagonism and the greater improvements with combination therapy were directly associated with a greater reduction in BP. Thus, this study provides no evidence to support or refute the concept that selective blockade of the RAAS through angiotensin II receptor antagonism is superior to ACE inhibition. Furthermore, it provides no definitive support for the concept that factors other than BP reduction are important.

Conclusion

There is no doubt that, as a class, angiotensin II receptor antagonists constitute a significant therapeutic advance. The good symptomatic tolerability profile and the lack of adverse metabolic effects are the principal practical advantages, and the theoretical benefits of selective blockade of the renin–angiotensin system are very attractive. Nevertheless, overall clinical effectiveness remains to be clearly estab-lished, particularly for reducing cardiovascular morbidity and mortality. Unfortun-ately, although there is a considerable amount of clinical data with the prototype drug, losartan, there remain concerns about its relative antihypertensive efficacy, ability to promote regression of LVH and its effectiveness in heart failure.

The articles cited in this chapter do not constitute a comprehensive account of every study published in the past year or so but, instead, are illustrative of the current position of this class of drugs in the setting of practical clinical issues. There is little doubt that the newer angiotensin II antagonists have generated evidence of an antihypertensive efficacy that is more directly comparable with that of other antihypertensive drug classes. However, as yet, there are no definitive outcome studies to confirm their effectiveness. Furthermore, there are no definitive dis-criminatory studies to determine which of the newer alternative agents is 'best'. Thus, selective angiotensin II receptor antagonists drugs constitute a major therapeutic advance: how much of an advance remains to be quantified and which agent(s) are the 'best buys' remains to be clarified.

References

1. Cheung B. Increased left ventricular mass (LVM) after losartan treatment. *Lancet* 1997; **349**: 1743–4.

2. Himmelmann A, Svensson A, Bergbrant A, Hansson L. *J Hum Hypertens* 1996; **10**: 729–34.

11

24-hour blood pressure measurement: current issues

Introduction

The recent guidelines from national and international authorities are consistent in their recommendations for 'tighter' blood pressure (BP) control, particularly in patients at high risk of cardiovascular disease. 'Tight' BP control applies specifically to clinic (casual or office) BP measurements—because all of the clinical trial evidence is derived from such measurements—but, increasingly, it is being recognized that BP control requires to be consistently maintained throughout the whole 24 h. However, despite the volume of evidence that adverse cardiovascular outcomes are correlated more closely with the values derived from 24-h BP assessments, rather than those derived from conventional clinic measurements, several practical considerations prevent the widespread applicability of 24-h ambulatory BP monitoring (ABPM). The following are the major areas of debate:

- guidelines for the use of the 24-h ABPM
- 24-h BP values and cardiovascular morbidity and mortality
- 24-h BP control: practical examples

Ambulatory blood pressure monitoring

The following extracts are taken from the recent guidelines to illustrate the current consensus views.

1999 World Health Organisation – International Society of Hypertension Guidelines for the Management of Hypertension.
Guidelines Committee. *J Hypertens* 1999; **17**: 151–83.

EXTRACT. Non-invasive semi-automatic and automatic devices are now available for BP measurement at home and for ABPM over periods of 24 h or more. Both of these approaches provide useful additional clinical information and have a place in the management of the hypertensive patient, but in both cases there are three important limitations.

- There are limited data available about the prognostic value of both home and ambulatory BP measurements |**1,2**|. Further prospective studies are required to determine whether such measurements offer material advantages over conventional BP measurements for the prediction of morbidity and mortality. Therefore, information obtained from these methods must be regarded as supplementary to conventional measurements, not as a substitute.
- Studies conducted in the general population and in hypertensive individuals have demonstrated that BP values obtained by home measurement or by ambulatory monitoring are several mmHg lower than those obtained by office measurements with 24-h average or home BP values of about 125/80 mmHg corresponding to clinic pressures of 140/90 mmHg |**3**|.
- The devices used should be checked for accuracy and performance over time against other well-validated BP measurement devices using standardized protocols.

ABPM also offers the advantages of providing a more realistic setting for BP measurements, and of improving patient perceptions and adherence to treatment. More important, however, is the large body of evidence indicating that the target organ damage associated with hypertension is more closely related to 24-h or daytime average BP than the clinic BP |**2,4**|, particularly if only few office values are obtained |**5**|. There is also evidence that pretreatment ambulatory BP has a prognostic value |**6,7**|, and recent prospective studies suggest that regression of target organ damage such as left ventricular hypertrophy (LVH) is more closely related to changes in the 24-h average than to changes in office BP values |**8**|. While ABPM is not a substitute for office measurement, it provides an important research tool for investigations of normal and deranged mechanisms of cardiovascular regulation, of the clinical relevance of phenomena such as BP variability and nocturnal hypotension, and of the time course and homogeneity of the antihypertensive effect of newer drugs or drug combinations |**2,9**|.

Guidelines for management of hypertension: report of the Third Working Party of the British Hypertension Society.

L E Ramsay, B Williams, G D Johnston, *et al. J Hum Hypertens* 1999; **13**: 569–92.

EXTRACT. All outcome trials on hypertension have been based on surgery or clinic BP, not ABPM, and it is therefore difficult to provide firm guidance based on evidence for use of this technique. Nevertheless, ABPM is widely used and may be valuable in special circumstances. ABPM provides numerous measurements over a short time and so reduces variability when compared with the average of a limited number of surgery or clinic readings |**5,10**|. BP by ABPM correlates more closely with target organ damage, presumably in part because of reduced variability and measurement error |**5,6**|.

ABPM may be indicated in the following circumstances:

- when BP shows unusual variability;
- in hypertension resistant to drug therapy, defined as BP > 150/90 mmHg on a regimen of three or more antihypertensive drugs;
- when symptoms suggest the possibility of hypotension;
- to diagnose white coat hypertension.

The term 'white coat hypertension' is widely used to describe consistent hypertension in the clinic with consistent normotension by ABPM. There is a systematic clinic–ABPM difference in the population that is related to the level of clinic BP and white coat hypertension is considered to be present only when the clinic–ABPM difference exceeds the population average difference [7].

It is not necessary or feasible to perform ABPM to exclude white coat hypertension in all hypertensive patients. It is not indicated in patients who are at high coronary heart disease (CHD)/cardiovascular disease risk. This includes patients who already have target organ damage or cardiovascular complications and those who have an estimated 10-year CHD risk of 15% or higher. In these patients, treatment decisions should be based on surgery or clinic pressures rather than ABPM, as was the case in outcome trials of hypertension treatment. ABPM is also unnecessary in patients with mild hypertension (140–159/90–99 mmHg) with no target organ damage, no cardiovascular complications, and an estimated 10-year CHD risk less than 15%. These patients may be left untreated without using ABPM but must be followed up.

ABPM may alter management when the average clinic BP is greater than 160/100 mmHg, there is no target organ damage or cardiovascular complications, and the estimated 10-year CHD risk is less than 15%. Here elevated BP is the only indication of high CHD/cardiovascular disease risk, and for antihypertensive treatment, and normal BP values by ABPM may alter the treatment decision.

Some important points in the interpretation of the results of ABPM records need emphasis. The average daytime BP should be used for treatment decisions, not the average 24-h BP. BP measured by ABPM is systematically lower than surgery or clinic measurements in hypertensive and normotensive people [7,8]. Because of this, treatment thresholds and targets must be adjusted downwards when making decisions based on ABPM data. Precise adjustment is complex, but the average difference between clinic and daytime mean pressures determined by ABPM is approximately 12/7 mmHg [7,8]. Thus an ABPM average daytime BP of 148/83 mmHg is approximately equivalent to a surgery BP of 160/90 mmHg, and this may require treatment in some patients. Recommended targets for ABPM measurement and for conventional clinic BP measurements are given in Table 11.1.

Comment

These extracts from the recent guidelines summarize the current recommendations concerning the use of ABPM in clinical practice. While there are some differences in points of detail, the principal practical messages are consistent:

1. Prospective (outcome) data for ABPM itself are very limited and there are no outcome studies in which drug treatment has been directed in accordance with the ABPM values.

Table 11.1 Treatment targets

	Clinic BP (mmHg)		Mean daytime ABPM (mmHg)	
	No diabetes	Diabetes	No diabetes	Diabetes
Optimal BP	< 140/85	< 140/80	< 130/80	< 130/75
Audit standard	< 150/90	< 140/85	< 140/85	< 140/80

BP = blood pressure; ABPM = ambulatory blood pressure monitoring.

Source: Ramsay *et al.* (1999)

2. ABPM is not (yet) recommended as part of the routine work-up of every hypertensive patient but instead should be reserved for those in whom there are specific management issues.

3. ABPM values are invariably lower than clinical BP readings: relative to the clinic BP, the ABPM daytime average value (which is generally preferred to the full 24-h average) will typically be lower by 10–15 mmHg systolic and 5–10 mmHg diastolic BP.

Conclusion

The overwhelming conclusion is that ABPM is important and valuable but not recommended for indiscriminate or routine use in every hypertensive patient. Instead, where major management decisions might be implicated—to withhold antihypertensive treatment in an otherwise low-risk patient, for example, or to intensify treatment in a high-risk patient with apparently 'resistant' hypertension—then the information derived from ABPM is likely to constitute an important and decisive factor.

Blood pressure measuring devices

Blood pressure measuring devices: recommendations of the European Society of Hypertension

E O'Brien, B Waeber, G Parati, J Staessen, M G Myers. *BMJ* 2001; **322**: 531–6.

BACKGROUND. There is a large market for BP measuring devices not only in clinical medicine but also among the public where the demand for self-measurement of BP is growing rapidly. For consumers, whether medical or lay, accuracy should be of prime importance when selecting a device to measure BP.

INTERPRETATION. Because most BP devices have not been independently validated, only a fraction of the many devices available have been surveyed. Devices that have

Table 11.2

Device	Mode	Protocol AAMI	BHS	Use	Recommendation
CH-DRUCK	Auscultatory	Passed	A/A	At rest	Recommended
ES-H531	Auscultatory	Passed	A/A	At rest	Recommended
QuietTrack	Auscultatory	Passed	A/A	At all times	Recommended
SpaceLabs 90217	Auscultatory	Passed	A/A	At rest	Recommended
Takeda 2430	Auscultatory	Passed	A/A	At rest	Recommended

AAMI, Association for the Advancement of Medical Instrumentation; BHS, British Hypertension Society.

Source: O'Brien et al. (2000)

been validated recently for which results have not yet been published were not included, but this shortcoming should be addressed in future. This paper describes a very important process whereby standardized criteria are applied to validate a range of different forms of sphygmomanometer, including those for self-measurement of BP and those for ambulatory BP measurement. With particular respect to ambulatory BP measurement, five devices were passed by the Association for the Advancement of Medical Instrumentation and also passed by the British Hypertension Society with a double A rating whereby both systolic and diastolic measurements showed the greatest agreement with the mercury standard with 60% of readings within 5 mmHg and 95% within 15 mmHg (Table 11.2).

Comment

With the imminent demise of the mercury sphygmomanometer and the increasing awareness and application of home or 24-h BP assessments there is a clear need for validated devices.

24-hour blood pressure and cardiovascular morbidity and mortality

The long-term consequences of uncontrolled hypertension manifest through the development of cardiovascular target organ damage. However, the predictive power of the conventional clinic BP measurement is relatively weak, whereas a number of studies have described closer relationships with the BP values derived from 24-h BP measurements [9,10]. Thus, the concept has arisen that target organ damage is more likely to occur when the BP remains elevated throughout the whole 24-h period. This concept of a BP 'load' over 24 h has typically been applied in studies assessing left ventricular mass and, generally, there are much closer relationships between measures of left ventricular mass and the values derived from 24-h BP assessments rather than those derived from conventional clinic BP measurements [11]. For example, the correlations illustrated in Fig. 11.1 show that values derived from 24-h BP assessment correlate much more closely than those obtained with a conventional clinic BP measurement. Furthermore, it can be seen that the persistence of an elevated overnight BP contributes significantly to the increase in left ventricular mass and the development of LVH.

Although many studies have focused on measurement of left ventricular mass as an index of target organ damage, similar relationships have been identified between 24-h BP measurements and other types of target organ damage (Table 11.3). Thus, it is reasonable to assume that the level of BP throughout 24-h is the principal determinant of target organ damage and this concept is entirely consistent with the results of the classical longitudinal study by Perlof *et al.* |5|, which showed that ambulatory values provided prognostic power additional to that obtained by conventional BP measurements. This seminal observation has since been confirmed

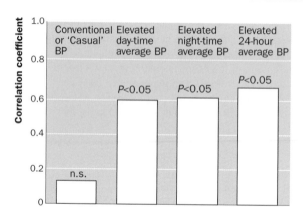

Fig. 11.1 Correlations between left ventricular mass measurements and derived ambulatory blood pressure monitoring values; ns = not significant.
Source: White *et al.* |11|.

Table 11.3 24-h average blood pressure correlates with different types of target organ damage

- Overall target organ damage score
- Left ventricular mass
- Impaired left ventricular function
- (Micro)albuminuria
- Brain damage (cerebral lacunae)
- Retinopathy
- Intima-media thickness (carotid)

by the results of several other studies, but further evidence of the predictive power of derived 24-h BP values is seen in the following studies.

Predicting cardiovascular risk using conventional *vs* ambulatory blood pressure in older patients with systolic hypertension

J A Staessen, L Thijs, R Fagard, *et al.*, for the Systolic Hypertension in Europe Trial Investigators. *JAMA* 1999; **282**: 539–46.

BACKGROUND. The clinical use of ABPM requires further validation in prospective outcome studies. To compare the prognostic significance of conventional and ambulatory BP measurement in older patients with isolated systolic hypertension.

INTERPRETATION. In untreated older patients with isolated systolic hypertension, ambulatory systolic BP was a significant predictor of cardiovascular risk over and above conventional BP.

A total of 808 untreated hypertensive patients aged more than 60 years participated in this substudy, which was part of the Systolic Hypertension in Europe (SYST-EUR) trial. The conventional BP measurement was taken as the mean of six pretreatment readings (two measurements in the sitting position at three visits each 1 month apart) and the baseline ambulatory BP assessment was also obtained prior to drug treatment. In the placebo group an increment of 10 mmHg in 24-h systolic BP average was associated with an increased relative risk rate for most outcome measurements; for example, total mortality was increased by 23% and cardiovascular mortality by 34%. Of particular interest was the finding that, statistically, the night-time systolic BP more accurately predicted end-points than the daytime level. In other words, the persistence of a (relatively) high BP overnight was an adverse prognostic feature.

Comment

This study confirms the expectation that the values derived from 24-h BP assessments, prior to treatment, are more powerful predictors of cardiovascular risk. It is noteworthy that this predictive power was apparent particularly in the placebo group but was less apparent in the active treatment group. This apparent anomaly presumably arises because the prognosis is altered by antihypertensive treatment and BP reduction such that the achieved BP during antihypertensive drug treatment becomes a more important predictor than the pretreatment value.

Reference values for 24-hour ambulatory blood pressure monitoring based on a prognostic criterion. The Ohasama study.

T Ohkubo, Y Imai, I Tsuji, *et al. Hypertension* 1998; **32**: 255–9.

BACKGROUND. Although reference values for ABPM have been investigated in several population studies, these values were derived from cross-sectional observations and were based merely on the statistical distribution of BP values. Therefore, we conducted a prospective cohort study to identify reference values for 24-h BP in relation to prognosis.

INTERPRETATION. This is the first report to propose reference values for 24-h ABP based on a prognostic criterion. This is an interesting study because it was a prospective examination attempting to identify reference values for 24-h ambulatory BP in relation to prognosis. Data were obtained from 1542 subjects (565 men) aged 40 years and over and during the follow-up period, 6.2 years on average, there were 117 deaths. The salient findings were that 24-h average BP values above 134/79 mmHg were associated with increased cardiovascular risk, whereas BPs in the range 120–133 mmHg for systolic and 65–78 mmHg for diastolic BP predicted the best prognosis. Interestingly, BP values below 119/64 mmHg were related to increased risks for non-cardiovascular mortality.

Comment

As the authors declare, this is the first report to relate 24-h ambulatory BP values to outcome information (i.e. death) rather than to an intermediate or surrogate end-point such as left ventricular mass.

Prediction of stroke by ambulatory blood pressure monitoring versus screening blood pressure measurements in a general population: the Ohasama study.

T Ohkubo, A Hozawa, K Nagai, et al. J Hypertens 2000; **18**: 847–54.

BACKGROUND. To investigate the association between 24-h, daytime and night-time ambulatory BPs and first symptomatic stroke, to compare their predictive powers for stroke with that of casual (screening) BP, and to compare the predictive power for stroke between daytime and night-time BPs, in a general population in Ohasama, Japan.

INTERPRETATION. The present study, which prospectively investigated the relation between ambulatory BP and first symptomatic stroke risk in a general population, demonstrated that: (a) ambulatory BP values were linearly related to stroke risk; (b) ambulatory BP had the stronger predictive power for stroke risk than did screening BP; and (c) daytime BP better related to stroke risk than did night-time BP. This was a prospective cohort study in 1464 subjects aged more than 40 years who were followed-up for a mean period of 6.4 years. Outcomes, in terms of first symptomatic stroke, were related to the 24-h, daytime and night-time ambulatory BP.

Comment

This is a follow-up study from the earlier Ohasama study that, arguably, is the only prospective study assessing the prognostic relevance of 24-h ambulatory BP values.

The specific focus of this follow-up study was on stroke with the identification that ambulatory BP had a stronger predictive power for stroke risk than screening (clinic or office) BP.

Prognostic value of ambulatory blood pressure monitoring in refractory hypertension: a prospective study.

J Redon, C Campos, M L Narciso, *et al. Hypertension* 1998; **31**: 712–18.

BACKGROUND. The objective of this study was to establish whether ambulatory BP offers a better estimate of cardiovascular risk than does its clinical BP counterpart in refractory hypertension.

INTERPRETATION. Higher values of ambulatory BP result in a worse prognosis in patients with refractory hypertension, supporting the recommendation that ABPM is useful in stratifying the cardiovascular risk in patients with refractory hypertension. This was a prospective study in 86 patients with essential hypertension and diastolic BP greater than 95 mmHg despite treatment with three or more antihypertensive drugs, including a thiazide diuretic. Patients were divided into tertiles of average diastolic BP according to the ABPM: the average diastolic BP was less than 88 mmHg ($n = 29$) in the lowest tertile; 88–97 mmHg ($n = 29$) in the middle tertile; and greater than 97 mmHg ($n = 28$) in the highest tertile. Interestingly, while there were significant differences in systolic and diastolic BP according to the ambulatory BP measurements there were no differences between the groups for office BP, either at the beginning or at the end of the period of observation. The incidence of cardiovascular events was significantly lower at 2.2 per 100 patient years in the lowest tertile, compared with 9.5 per 100 patient years in the middle tertile and 13.6 per 100 patient years in the upper tertile of ambulatory BP. The probability of event-free survival was also significantly different when comparing the lowest tertile with the other two groups. Thus, ambulatory BP in the highest tertile was an independent risk factor for the incidence of cardiovascular events with a relative risk of 6.2.

Comment

In one sense, this is not a novel or surprising result. However, it confirms the prognostic superiority of derived ambulatory BP measurements in a particular subgroup of patients namely those resistant to multiple antihypertensive drug treatments. Of particular interest, however, was the observation that those patients at greatest risk could not be clearly identified via the conventional clinic BP measurements. It was only in relation to their derived ambulatory BP values that the adverse prognostic significance was identified.

Conclusion

The results of these studies are entirely consistent with the guidelines from the international authorities whereby ambulatory BP measurement is advised only in those patients where it might affect the management decision and lead to a change in treatment. Following the example of the study by Redon *et al.* (1998), even greater efforts with multiple drug combination treatments might be attempted in those patients identified at the highest risk. This might even be supported by advice to the patient that adverse effects be considered acceptable (if they were relatively minor) if intensified drug treatment then led to a significant improvement in BP control and prognosis.

24-hour blood pressure control: practical issues

Recent studies from the UK and USA have clearly identified the shortcomings of current antihypertensive treatment strategies in so far as less than 50% of hypertensive patients are identified and satisfactorily treated to achieve the recommended treatment targets for clinic BP |**12,13**|. This was confirmed in a recent Italian study that was of additional and particular interest because the study design incorporated home and 24-h ambulatory measurements in addition to conventional clinic BP measurements |**14**|.

Prediction of long-term need for drug treatment

Prediction of blood pressure level and need for antihypertensive medication: 10 years of follow-up.
J M Jokiniitty, S K Majahalme, M A P Kahonen, M T Tuomisto, V M H Turjanmaa. *J Hypertens* 2001; **19**: 1193–201.

BACKGROUND. To evaluate the usefulness of BP and its variability in the prediction of future BP and need for antihypertensive medication.

INTERPRETATION. The 24-h mean BP was an excellent predictor of the future BP and the need for antihypertensive medication. Prediction of antihypertensive medication was further improved by also using BP variability. Systolic BP was more predictable than diastolic BP. At baseline, healthy untreated male volunteers were classified as normotensive ($n = 34$), borderline hypertensive ($n = 29$) or mild hypertensive ($n = 24$), according to clinic (office) measurements and the application of WHO criteria. These clinic-based measurements were supplemented by intra-arterial 24-h ABPM. After 10 years of follow-up the BP classification had deteriorated in 40% of individuals and improved in only 7%. In the borderline hypertensive group, 77% because hypertensive and the 24-h mean systolic BP was the best predictor of this outcome.

Optimal blood pressure control throughout 24 h

Although the above study identified a lack of full 24-h BP control, there is not yet any definitive evidence that BP control throughout 24 h is superior to 'intermittent' or 'incomplete' control. However, a considerable volume of indirect evidence suggests that this is likely.

Ambulatory blood pressure is superior to clinic blood pressure in predicting treatment-induced regression of left ventricular hypertrophy

G Mancia, A Zanchetti, E Agebiti-Rosei, *et al*. for the SAMPLE Study Group. *Circulation* 1997; **95**: 1464–70.

BACKGROUND. **In cross-sectional studies, ambulatory BP correlates more closely than clinic BP with the organ damage of hypertension. Whether ambulatory BP predicts development or regression of organ damage over time better than clinic BP, however, is unknown.**

INTERPRETATION. In hypertensive subjects with LVH, regression of LVH was predicted much more closely by treatment-induced changes in ambulatory BP than in clinic BP. This provides the first longitudinally controlled evidence that ambulatory BP may be clinically superior to traditional BP measurements. In this detailed study of 206 essential hypertensive patients with LVH, a number of different BP measurements were obtained before and after 1 year of treatment. BP values were obtained by 24-h ABPM, by home BP monitoring and by conventional clinic measurements. It was noted that the pretreatment left ventricular mass measurement correlated significantly with the 24-h value but not with either the clinic or home BP values. While this is confirmatory there were additional and novel findings that the improvement in BP leading to a reduction in left ventricular mass index was not related to the reduction in clinic or home BPs but was related to the reduction in the 24-h average BP.

Comment

This important study illustrates the concept that 24–h control of BP is an important requirement. Although the end-point of LVH, and its regression, is a surrogate measure for cardiovascular outcome, the findings that pretreatment left ventricular mass was related to 24-h BP and that the regression during treatment was correlated with the reduction in 24-h BP are consistent with the concept that 24-h BP control constitutes optimal BP control.

There are additional considerations that relate to an antihypertensive effect that is consistently maintained throughout 24 h. The following might be considered features of an optimal antihypertensive treatment:

- effective BP control throughout 24 h and an overall decrease in BP load;
- 'smooth' and consistent antihypertensive activity with no increase in BP variability;
- attenuation of the early morning BP surge; and
- once daily dosing (in the interests of compliance).

Conclusion

There is no doubt that 24-h BP monitoring and the BP values derived from this technique have provided additional and important insights into the relationships between hypertension and cardiovascular morbidity and mortality. Of particular practical importance is the evidence that patients at high risk, or alternatively patients at low cardiovascular risk, can be clearly identified by 24-h BP measurement but not by conventional clinic BP measurement. This observation has practical importance with respect to the need for intensified treatment in a high-risk patient and the avoidance of unnecessary treatment in a low-risk patient. This is the strategy endorsed by the guidelines from the national and international authorities, which at present do not recommend 24-h ABPM as part of the routine assessment of each individual hypertensive patient. Thus, 24-h ABPM is recommended only for selected patients and the fundamental reason for this recommendation resides in the fact that the benefits of antihypertensive drug treatment have been established through clinical trials that have used conventional clinic BP measurements and targets. As yet, there is no definitive prospective clinical outcome trial that has relied upon 24-h BP values and targets. There are also the practical considerations of expense, time and resources if 24-h BP measurements were obtained in every hypertensive patient and repeated on each occasion that a treatment change was implemented.

Accumulated evidence clearly indicates that 24-h control of BP is a desirable therapeutic goal. In turn, with the preference for once daily antihypertensive treatment, there follows the clear inference that drugs with a protracted duration of action are to be preferred. Thus, in line with the current emphasis on 'tight' BP control, there is therefore an additional practical recommendation to prescribe appropriately long-acting agents either as monotherapy or in combination therapy.

References

1. Ohkubo T, Imai Y, Tsuji I, Nagai K, Ito S, Satoh HS, Hisamichi S. Reference values for 24-hour ambulatory blood pressure monitoring based on a prognostic criterion: Ohasama study. *Hypertension* 1998; **32**: 255–9.

2. Mancia G, Zanchetti A, Agabiti-Rosei E, Benemio G, De Cesaris R, Fogari R, Pessina A, Porcellati C, Rappelli A, Salvetti A, Trimarco B, for the SAMPLE Study group. Ambulatory blood pressure is superior to clinic blood pressure in predicting treatment-induced regression of left ventricular hypertrophy. *Circulation* 1997; **95**: 1464–70.

3. Mancia G, Omboni S, Parati G. Assessment of antihypertensive treatment by ambulatory blood pressure. *J Hypertens* 1997; **15** (Suppl 2): S43–50.

4. Fagard R, Staessen J, Thijs L, Amery A. Multiple standardised clinic blood pressure may predict left ventricular mass as well as ambulatory monitoring. A meta-analysis of comparative studies. *Am J Hypertens* 1995; **8**: 533–40.

5. Perloff D, Sokolow M, Cowan R. The prognostic value of ambulatory blood pressures. *JAMA* 1983; **249**: 2792–8.

6. Verdecchia P, Porcellati C, Schillaci G, Borgioni C, Ciucci A, Battistelli M, Guerrieri M, Gatteschi C, Zampi I, Santucci A, *et al*. Ambulatory blood pressure: an independent predictor of prognosis in essential hypertension. *Hypertension* 1994; **24**: 793–801.

7. Parati G, Omboni S, Staessen J, Thijs L, Fagand R, Ulian L, Mancia G. Limitations of the difference between clinic and daytime blood pressure as a surrogate measurement of the 'white-coat hypertension' effect. *J Hypertens* 1998; **16**: 23–9.

8. Staessen JA, O'Brien ET, Atkins N, Amery AK. Ambulatory blood pressure in normotensive compared with hypertensive subjects. *J Hypertens* 1993; **11**: 1289–97.

9. Manica G. Ambulatory blood pressure monitoring: research and clinical applications. *J Hypertens* 1991; **8** (Suppl 7): S1–13.

10. Devereux RB, Pickering TG. Relationship between the level, pattern and variability of ambulatory blood pressure and target organ damage in hypertension. *J Hypertens* 1991; **9** (Suppl 8): S34–8.

11. White WB, Dey HM, Schulman P. Assessment of the daily blood pressure load as a determinant of cardiac function in patients with mild–moderate hypertension. *Am Heart J* 1989; **118**: 782–95.

12. Burt VL, Whelton P, Rocceila E, Brown C, Cutler JA, Higgins M, Horan MJ, Labarthe D. Prevalence of hypertension in the US adult population: results from the third National Health and Nutrition Examination Survey, 1988–1991. *Hypertension* 1995; **25**: 305–13.

13. Colhoun HM, Dong W, Poulter N. Blood pressure control, screening and management and control in England, results from the Health Survey for England 1994. *J Hypertens* 1998; **16**: 747–53.

14. Mancia, G, Segta R, Milesi C, Cesana G, Zanchetti A. Blood pressure control in hypertensive population. *Lancet* 1997; **349**: 454–7.

12

Surrogate measures in cardiovascular disease

Introduction

In terms of the sheer volume of evidence, the risks of uncontrolled hypertension and the benefits of antihypertensive drug treatment are indisputable. However, the association between hypertension and cardiovascular events, fatal and non-fatal, is indirect in so far as intermediate pathological processes are also implicated. Furthermore, despite the fact that blood pressure (BP) may be 'normalized', cardiovascular disease continues to account for most morbidity and mortality among treated hypertensive patients.

For the above reasons, attempts have been made to quantify alternative or additional indices that might help to identify patients at increased cardiovascular risk, thus: (a) additional haemodynamic indices, e.g. pulse wave velocity (PWV); (b) changes to the function and/or structure of the vasculature; (c) early evidence of target organ damage, e.g. microalbuminuria; (d) or the development of reversible structural changes to the heart itself [left ventricular hypertrophy (LVH)]. The following might therefore be considered to be among the most important 'intermediate' or 'surrogate' measures of hypertensive cardiovascular disease:

1. PWV (and related measurements);
2. the progressive changes to the which lead to the development of atheromatous disease of the arterial system;
3. the appearance of microalbuminuria as a marker for renal dysfunction/damage;
4. the development of LVH.

Pulse wave velocity

Systolic and diastolic BPs are the exclusive mechanical factors that predict cardiovascular risk in normotensive and hypertensive subjects. However, it has been suggested that, if hypertension is considered as a mechanical factor acting on the arterial wall with deleterious consequences, the totality of the BP curve should be considered in order to investigate the risk more accurately. The haemodynamic indices that are now considered to be of particular relevance for cardiac complications are those that originate from the pulsatile pressure and among those most widely measured are brachial pulse pressure (PP), PP amplification, early wave reflections and PWV.

Is pulse pressure useful in predicting risk for coronary heart disease?

S S Franklin, S A Khan, N D Wong, M G Larson, D Levy. *Circulation* 1999; **100**: 354–60.

BACKGROUND. Current definitions of hypertension are based on levels of systolic BP and diastolic BP, but not on PP. We examined whether PP adds useful information for predicting coronary heart disease (CHD) in the population-based Framingham Study.

INTERPRETATION. In the middle-aged and elderly, CHD risk was negative for diastolic BP at any level of systolic BP ≥ 120 mmHg, suggesting that higher PP was an important component of risk. Neither systolic BP nor diastolic BP was superior to PP in predicting CHD risk.

Comment

This analysis from the Framingham Heart Study explores the relationship between BP components and its CHD risk over a 20-year follow up in 1924 men and women aged between 50 and 79 years with no clinical evidence of CHD and not taking anti-hypertensive drug therapy. The association with CHD risk was positive for both systolic and diastolic BP, but statistically was most strongly positive for PP.

Impact of aortic stiffness attenuation on survival of patients in end-stage renal failure.

A P Guerin, J Blacher, B Pannier, *et al. Circulation* 2001; **103**: 987–92.

BACKGROUND. Aortic PWV is a predictor of mortality in patients with end-stage renal failure (ESRF). The PWV is partly dependent on BP, and a decrease in BP can attenuate the stiffness. Whether the changes in PWV in response to decreases in BP can predict mortality in ESRF patients has never been investigated.

INTERPRETATION. These results indicate that in ESRF patients, the insensitivity of PWV to decreased BP is an independent predictor of mortality and that use of angiotensin-converting enzyme (ACE) inhibitors has a favourable effect on survival that is independent of BP changes. One hundred and fifty patients with ESRF, mean age 52 years, were followed up for a mean of 51 months using ultrasonographic PWV measurements. Fifty-nine of the patients died, including 40 due to cardiovascular events. Factors predictive of mortality included absence of PWV decrease in response to BP decrease, increased left ventricular mass, age and pre-existing cardiovascular disease. Use of ACE inhibitors was predictive of improved survival, with risk ratios of 0.19 and 0.18 for all-cause and cardiovascular mortality, respectively. The risk ratios for the absence of PWV decrease were 2.59 and 2.35, for all-cause and cardiovascular mortality, respectively. In ESRF patients, therefore, the absence of a PWV change in response to a decrease in BP was strongly predictive of mortality.

Pulse pressure and aortic pulse wave are markers of cardiovascular risk in hypertensive populations.

R Asmar, A Rudnichi, J Blacher, G M London, M E Safar. *Am J Hypertens* 2001; **14**: 91–7.

BACKGROUND. PP and aortic PWV are significant markers of cardiovascular risk, but a similar role of central wave reflections has never been investigated.

INTERPRETATION. In a cross-sectional hypertensive population, PP and PWV, but not carotid amplification index (CAI), are significantly and independently associated with cardiovascular amplications.

Comment

The purpose of this cross-sectional study was to investigate whether arterial stiffness, as measured in terms of aortic PWV or CAI, is a significant risk factor for cardiovascular disease. In a cohort of 1087 subjects with essential hypertension and a mean age of 58 years, age and mean arterial pressure represented 30.4% and 5.6% of the variance of PP, PWV and CAI, respectively. After adjustment for plasma glucose, high-density lipoprotein cholesterol, plasma creatinine, tobacco consumption, age and gender, logistic regression revealed atherosclerotic alternatives to be associated with increased PP (odds ratio 1.202) and increased PWV (odds ratio 1.354), but not CAI (odds ratio 1.00). Thus, the study showed that, in a hypertensive population, PP and PWV are independently associated with cardiovascular risk, but that CAI is not.

Arterial stiffness and cardiovascular risk factor in a population-based study.

J Amar, J B Ruidavets, B Chamontin, L Drouet, J Ferriers. *J Hypertens* 2001; **19**: 381–7.

BACKGROUND. To determine the relationship between PWV, an estimate of arterial distensibility and cardiovascular risk factors.

INTERPRETATION. This study shows that, in a sample of subjects at high risk, the cumulative influence of risk factors, even treated, is an independent determinant of arterial stiffness. These results suggest that PWV may be used as a relevant tool to assess the influence of cardiovascular risk factors on aortic stiffness in high-risk patients.

Comment

This was a 3-year evaluation of the relationship between PWV and cardiovascular risk factors. The 993 subjects, aged 35-64 years, were randomly selected from the electoral roll in south-west France; 247 were being treated for hypertension, hyperlipidaemia or diabetes (mean age 54 years) and 746 were untreated (mean age 47 years).

In the untreated subjects, age, gender, systolic BP and heart rate were found to be significantly associated with PWV ($P < 0.001$). In the treated patients, age ($P < 0.01$), systolic BP ($P < 0.001$), heart rate ($P < 0.001$), apolipoprotein B ($P < 0.05$) and the number of treated cardiovascular risk factors ($P < 0.05$) had positive correlations with PWV. These authors suggested that PWV might be a useful way to quantify the impact of cardiovascular risk factors on aortic stiffness, even in patients receiving antihypertensive, hypolipidaemia and antidiabetic drugs.

Aortic stiffness is an independent predictor of all-cause and cardiovascular mortality in hypertensive patients.

S Laurent, P Boutouyrie, R Asmar, *et al. Hypertension* 2001; **37**(5): 1236–41.

BACKGROUND. Although various studies reported that PP, an indirect index of arterial stiffness, was an independent risk factor for mortality, a direct relationship between arterial stiffness and all-cause and cardiovascular mortality remained to be established in patients with essential hypertension.

INTERPRETATION. This study provides the first direct evidence that aortic stiffness is an independent predictor of all-cause and cardiovascular mortality in patients with essential hypertension.

This study set out to establish whether there is a direct link between arterial stiffness and all-cause and cardiovascular mortality. It included 1980 patients with essential hypertension who underwent measurement of arterial stiffness (as PWV) over a 16-year period at a single institution. The patients' mean age was 50 years, and the mean follow-up period was 112 months. A logistic regression model was used to estimate risk.

During follow-up, 107 fatal events occurred, of which 46 were cardiovascular. In a univariate analysis, PWV was found to be significantly associated with all-cause and cardiovascular mortality (odds ratios 2.14 and 2.35, respectively). No such relationship was found for PP. In a multivariant analysis, the significant association of PWV with all-cause and cardiovascular mortality was found to be independent of previous cardiovascular disease, age and diabetes.

The authors suggested some possible explanations for their failure to find a link between PP and mortality. They were able to conclude, however, that aortic stiffness, as measured by PWV, is significantly associated with the risk of all-cause and cardiovascular mortality in patients with essential hypertension.

Conclusion

These studies illustrate the importance of PP, PWV and related measures as predictors of adverse cardiovascular outcomes.

It is possible that the wider applicability of such techniques might refine our approaches to prevent cardiovascular events by targeting those individuals found to be at high risk even when the conventional BP measurement appears reasonably satisfactory. This needs to be established by a properly designed, prospective outcomes study. Similarly, whether or not there are specific benefits from particular drugs or drug classes also needs to be established.

Atheromatous vascular disease

Hypertension along with cigarette smoking, hypercholesterolaemia and diabetes are associated with 'premature vascular ageing' and the development of atheromatous vascular disease. This review extends the observation described for PP and PWV and further illustrates the potential role of vascular measurements as surrogate markers for the cardiovascular risk of hypertension.

Vessel wall properties and cardiovascular risk.
R Cockcroft, I B Wilkinson. *J Hum Hypertens* 1998; **12**: 343–4.

BACKGROUND. **Stiffening of the arteries, resulting in decreased compliance, is a consequence of the normal ageing process. It is accompanied by an increase in systolic and PP, and an increased risk of cardiovascular morbidity or mortality. Risk factors for the development of atherosclerosis, such as hypertension, diabetes, hypercholesterolaemia, smoking and obesity are associated with 'premature vascular ageing' and increased arterial stiffness.**

INTERPRETATION. To date both primary and secondary prevention of CHD has focused almost exclusively on modification of conventional risk factors. However, accumulating evidence suggests that increased vascular stiffness is not just a marker for atheromatous disease but may be an important additional risk factor, promoting atherogenesis and acting as a link between existing risk factors and cardiovascular disease.

Comment

This review summarizes the current thinking relating to PP, arterial stiffness or compliance, intima–media thickness and endothelial function. The following studies illustrate some of the clinical applications.

Carotid-artery intima and media thickness as a risk factor for myocardial infarction and stroke in older adults.

D H O'Leary, J F Polak, R A Kronmal, *et al.*, for the Cardiovascular Health Study Collaborative Research Group. *N Engl J Med* 1999; **340**: 14–22.

BACKGROUND. **The combined thickness of the intima and media of the carotid artery is associated with the prevalence of cardiovascular disease. We studied the associations between the thickness of the carotid artery intima and media and the incidence of new myocardial infarction (MI) or stroke in persons without clinical cardiovascular disease.**

INTERPRETATION. Increases in the thickness of the intima–media of the carotid artery, as measured non-invasively by ultrasonography, are directly associated with an increased risk of MI and stroke in older adults without a history of cardiovascular disease.

This was a large study of 5858 subject of 65 years or more in whom non-invasive measurements of the intima and media of the common and internal carotid arteries were made with high resolution ultrasonography. Correlations were then sought with a range of outcome variables over a median follow-up period of 6.2 years. The incidence of cardiovascular events correlated with measurements of carotid artery intima–media thickness. A relative risk of 3.87 for MI or stroke (adjusted for age and sex) was calculated for the quintile with the highest intima–media thickness as compared with the quintile with the lowest intima–media thickness. The association between cardiovascular events and intima–media thickness remained significant after adjustment for traditional risk factors. The results of the separate analysis for MI and stroke paralleled those for their combined end-point.

Comment

In this analysis of elderly subjects there was a clear correlation between the development of atherosclerotic vascular disease, as assessed by intima–media thickness, and adverse cardiovascular outcomes, particularly MI and stroke.

Although the volume of information is significantly less with intima–media thickness there are clear parallels with LVH in their respective roles as surrogate markers for cardiovascular disease. For example, as for echocardiographic assessment of left ventricular mass there remain methodological concerns about the reproducibility of the measurements such that specific methodological validation analyses have been undertaken.

Baseline reproducibility of B-mode ultrasonic measurement of carotid artery intima–media thickness: the European Lacidipine Study on Atherosclerosis (ELSA).

R Tang, M Hennig, B Thomasson, *et al.* for the ELSA Investigators. *J Hypertens* 2000; **18**: 197–201.

BACKGROUND. The European Lacidipine/Study of Atherosclerosis (ELSA) is a prospective, randomized, double-blind, multi-national interventional trial to determine the effect of 4-year treatment using the calcium antagonist lacidipine versus the β-blocker atenolol on the progression of carotid atherosclerosis in 2259 asymptomatic hypertensive patients.

INTERPRETATION. The results demonstrate that by implementing standardized protocols and strict quality control procedures, highly reliable ultrasonic measurements of carotid artery intima–media thickness can be achieved in large multinational trials.

Intima–media thickness was measured by B-mode ultrasound in this evaluation that sought to establish the acceptability and reproducibility of this technique. Each patient was scanned twice at baseline and scanned again at four annual visits with 80% of the replicate scans being performed by the same observer; 50% of the replicate scans were read by the same reader. The overall coefficient of the reliability was 0.859 for the maximum intima–media thickness of the carotid bifurcation (CBMmax), 0.872 for the mean maximum intima–media thickness of 12 standard sites on the common carotid artery (Mmax) and 0.794 for the overall maximum intima–media thickness (Tmax). The reliability for CBMmax was stable during the baseline period ($r = 0.848$–0.953) and was uniform among the 23 field centres ($r = 0.798$–0.926) with intra- and inter-reader reliabilities of 0.915 and 0.872, respectively.

Comment

The ELSA study is one of many that has used intima-media (intima–media) thickness of the carotid artery wall as a surrogate marker for cardiovascular morbidity and mortality. However, because of methodological shortcomings in previous studies, particular care was taken to standardize the procedures of measurement and to demonstrate the reproducibility (and, thereby, the clinical usefulness) of the techniques.

Conclusion

The first study confirms that intima–media thickness is an appropriate surrogate marker for adverse cardiovascular outcomes. The second study, the ELSA study, illustrates the methodological requirements for standardizing the procedures to make the technique sufficiently reproducible for the clinical purpose of prospective long-term evaluations. Unfortunately, previous attempts to apply these techniques in clinical studies have typically been confounded by a lack of reproducibility in the measurement techniques. It is hoped that the results of the ELSA study can clarify whether or not baseline measurements of intima–media thickness, and the changes induced by treatment are predictive of morbid and mortal cardiovascular events.

Intima–media thickness reflects structural changes in the vessel wall, but there is considerable research interest in the associated functional changes that accompany and, presumably, precede the processes involved in the structural alterations. Endothelial function/dysfunction is thought to be one of the most important early indicators of vascular disease. Whether endothelial dysfunction is a risk factor or only a risk marker, however, remains the subject of debate.

Endothelial dysfunction in cardiovascular disease: risk factor, risk marker, or surrogate end-point?

H L Elliott. *J Cardiovasc Pharmacol* 1998; **32** (Suppl 3): S67–73.

BACKGROUND. **Endothelial dysfunction is a feature of the early stages of atherosclerotic cardiovascular disease. It also is almost invariably associated with the recognized cardiovascular risk factors, including those that are irreversible (such as age and family history) and those that are reversible (such as hypertension and hypercholesterolaemia). It remains the subject of debate whether endothelial dysfunction can be considered to be an independent risk factor or, perhaps more plausibly, an intermediate or surrogate end-point.**

INTERPRETATION. While the relevance to research into cardiovascular pathophysiology is not in dispute, there remains uncertainty about its relevance as a therapeutic target. Overall, the available evidence suggests that targeting of the conventional, major risk factors remains the primary strategy, but an ancillary effect on intermediate end-points, such as an improvement or reversal of endothelial dysfunction constitute an additional potential benefit.

Comment

This short review focuses attention upon the clinical issues surrounding endothelial dysfunction. It is not yet possible to answer definitively the question that was posed but there is no doubt that endothelial dysfunction is the earliest manifestation of vascular disease albeit as a non-specific response to a range of insults, including hypertension, dyslipidaemia, diabetes mellitus and cigarette smoking. There is not yet sufficient outcome evidence to confirm whether or not endothelial function can be considered to be a surrogate end-point (in the same way as LVH or carotid intima–media thickness, for example) but there are clinical studies investigating whether or not treatment can induce beneficial changes and whether or not these changes can lead to outcome benefits beyond the obvious factors such as BP control or lipid-lowering treatment.

Nifedipine improves endothelial function in hypercholesterolaemia, independently of an effect on blood pressure or plasma lipids.

M C Verhaar, M L H Honing, T van Dam, *et al. Cardiovasc Res* 1999; **42**: 752–60.

BACKGROUND. **Dihydropyridine calcium antagonists have been shown to retard atherogenesis in animal models and to prevent the development of early angiographic lesions in human coronary arteries. Endothelial dysfunction is an early event in the pathogenesis of cardiovascular disease. We investigated whether nifedipine could**

improve endothelial function in hypercholesterolaemia, independently of changes in BP or plasma lipids.

INTERPRETATION. Our data show that nifedipine improves endothelial function in hypercholesterolaemia. It is suggested from our *in vitro* experiments that this effect is due to reduced nitric oxide degradation.

This study employed forearm venous occlusion plethysmography to assess the vasodilator responses to endothelium dependent and endothelium-independent vasodilators in 11 patients with familial hypercholesterolaemia before and after 6 weeks treatment with nifedipine gastrointestinal transport system (GITS) and in 12 matched controls. In a subgroup of six control subjects forearm vascular function was also assessed before and after 6 weeks of nifedipine GITS treatment. The salient results were that endothelium-dependent vasodilatation was impaired in hypercholesterolaemic subjects with a 47% increase in forearm blood flow compared with a 99% increase in the control subjects. Treatment with nifedipine completely restored endothelium-dependent vasodilatation whereas it had no influence on basal forearm blood flow or endothelium-independent vasodilatation. Nifedipine did not alter forearm vascular responses in the control subjects and it did not significantly alter BP or plasma lipids. These *in vivo* investigations were supported by *in vitro* investigations in which nitric oxide production was unaltered by nifedipine but production of the nitric oxide antagonist, superoxide was impaired. For this reason, the authors concluded that nifedipine improves endothelial function by a mechanism that reflects reduced nitric oxide degradation.

Effects of calcium antagonism and HMG-coenzyme reductase inhibition on endothelial function and atherosclerosis: rationale and outline of the ENCORE trials.

G Sütsch, M Büchi, A M Zeither, *et al.* on behalf of the ENCORE Trial Investigators. *Eur Heart J* 1999; **1** (Suppl M): M27–32.

BACKGROUND. In the ENCORE I trial, four groups of 100 patients each with coronary artery disease undergoing percutaneous transluminal angioplasty will be recruited. After percutaneous transluminal angioplasty, endothelial function is assessed by intracoronary methods, i.e. infusion of increasing dosages of acetylcholine in a non-obstructed coronary segment. Coronary responses to acetylcholine will be measured by quantitative coronary angiography (QCA) and Doppler flow velocity measurements. Endothelial-independent responses are tested by i.c. adenosine and nitroglycerine, respectively. Patients will then be randomly assigned in a double-blind fashion to four treatment groups: placebo, nifedipine (30–60 mg/day) or their combination. Studies will be repeated at 6 months. This trial will determine whether or not in patients with coronary artery disease calcium antagonists and/or a statin alone or in combination improve endothelial function within 6 months.

The ENCORE II trial will last 2 years, and aims at correlating endothelial function (as assessed by QCA and intravascular ultrasound; IVUS) and structural atherosclerosis in patients treated with cerivastatin, 200 receiving 200 µg/day and

200 receiving 800 μg/day, compared with 200 patients having a combination treatment with cerivastatin (800 μg/day) and nifedipine (30–60 mg). Endothelial-dependent responses of epicardial coronary arteries to acetylcholine at baseline as well as structural vascular changes as assessed by IVUS will be correlated and followed over 2 years. At the end of the 2 years another acetylcholine test, QCA and IVUS will be performed.

INTERPRETATION. The principal aim of these complementary studies is an assessment of endothelium-dependent responses in patients with known coronary artery disease. Treatment will be with a calcium channel blocker and a statin, alone or in combination, and the follow-up assessments will determine whether endothelial dysfunction and/or its improvement is associated with progression or regression of atherosclerotic coronary artery disease and possibly clinical events.

Conclusion

The first study (Verhaar *et al.*) illustrates the clinical research approach to assessing endothelial function in human subjects. The study is well designed and carefully conducted but, as the authors concede, it was not a randomized placebo-controlled assessment. Nevertheless, the conclusion that treatment with the calcium channel blocker, nifedipine, improves endothelial function in hypercholesterolaemia suggests that there may be benefit from this pharmacological intervention beyond any simple change in BP or serum cholesterol. The larger ENCORE trials seek to extend this concept of an additional and potentially protective vascular effect by investigating patients with known vascular disease. There is, however, an immediate difference in so far as these patients will already have structural vascular changes whereas these would be absent or at a much less advanced stage, in the subjects studied by Verhaar *et al.* While the results of the ENCORE trials, and particularly the results in terms of clinical events, are awaited with interest it may be that the pre-existing structural changes will compromise the identification of any functional improvement attributable to the drug treatments beyond their lipid and BP lowering.

Microalbuminuria

Microalbuminuria is defined as urinary albumin concentration of 30–200 mg/l and is thought to reflect the glomerular manifestation of a systemic capillary leak [1]. Microalbuminuria is used clinically to monitor incipient diabetic nephropathy but it is also known to be a useful predictor of outcome, including mortality, in a number of clinical situations, including mortality [2].

Microalbuminuria predicts cardiovascular events and renal insufficiency in patients with essential hypertension.

R Bigazzi, S Bianchi, D Baldari, V M Campese. *J Hypertens* 1998; **16**: 1325–33.

BACKGROUND. **Some patients with essential hypertension manifest greater than normal urinary excretion of albumin. Authors of a few retrospective studies have suggested that there is an association between microalbuminuria and cardiovascular risk.**

INTERPRETATION. This study suggests that hypertensive individuals with microalbuminuria manifest a greater incidence of cardiovascular events and a greater decline in renal function than do patients with normal urinary excretion of albumin.

This was a retrospective cohort analysis of 141 hypertensive patients who were followed up for approximately 7 years. In this study microalbuminuria was defined as an average urinary albumin excretion in the range 30–300 mg/24 h in three urine collections obtained at baseline. At baseline, 54 of these patients had microalbuminuria and 87 patients had a normal urinary albumin excretion rate. The two groups were similar in age, weight, BP and creatinine clearance rates, although the serum levels of cholesterol and uric acid were higher in those with microalbuminuria whereas high-density lipoprotein cholesterol was lower in those with microalbuminuria. During follow-up, 12 cardiovascular events occurred in the patients with microalbuminuria (an event rate of 21.3%) whereas only two such events occurred in the 87 patients with a normal urinary albumin excretion rate ($P < 0.0002$). Additionally the creatinine clearance rates decreased more rapidly in the patients with microalbuminuria at outset with a rate of decline of 12.1 ml/min versus 7.1 ml/min. A stepwise logistic regression analysis showed that urinary albumin excretion, cholesterol concentration and diastolic BP were independent predictors of adverse cardiovascular outcomes.

Treatment of diabetic nephropathy

It is a widely held view that ACE inhibitor drugs might have effects beyond BP reduction and an added ability to provide renal protection. While there is no doubt that an ACE inhibitor is the cornerstone of treatment for diabetic nephropathy there remains some doubt as to whether or not there are benefits beyond BP reduction.

Randomized placebo-controlled trial of lisinopril in normotensive patients with insulin-dependent diabetes and normoalbuminuria or microalbuminuria

The EUCLID Study Group. *Lancet* 1997; **349**: 1787–92.

BACKGROUND. **Renal disease in people with insulin-dependent diabetes (IDDM) continues to pose a major health threat. Inhibitors of ACE slow the decline of renal** function in advanced renal disease, but their effects at earlier stages are unclear, and the degree of albuminuria at which treatment should start is not yet known.

INTERPRETATION. Lisinopril slows the progression of renal disease in normotensive IDDM patients with little or no albuminuria, although greatest effect was in those with microalbuminuria (AER $>$ 20 μg/min). Our results show lisinopril does not increase the risk of hypoglycaemic events in IDDM.

This was a randomized double-blind placebo controlled trial of the ACE inhibitor lisinopril in 530 men and women with type 1 diabetes mellitus and with normoalbuminuria or microalbuminuria. All patients were considered to be normotensive with BP not more than 155/90 mmHg. On entry, the mean BP was 121/80 in the placebo group and 122/79 mmHg in the lisinopril group. The great majority of patients had normal albuminuria with only 14% in the placebo group and 19% in the lisinopril group having microalbuminuria or macroalbuminuria. For patients who completed 24 months in the trial there was a significant difference in albuminuria with a reduction by 38.5 μg/min in those with microalbuminuria at baseline (P = 0.001) and by 0.23 μg/min in those with normal albuminuria at baseline (P = 0.6). The principal conclusion from this study was that lisinopril was of clinical benefit in patients with type 1 diabetes mellitus who have early signs of renal disease without hypertension. The authors additionally recommended that the treatment of early stage renal disease, even in normotensive patients, should include an ACE inhibitor drug.

Comment

This is another paper that demonstrates the ability of an ACE inhibitor drug treatment to improve the clinical profile of diabetic patients with a significant reduction in albumin excretion rate. This adds to the volume of information that ACE inhibition is an important initial treatment in such patients. However, it should be noted that there was a small but significant difference in BP in the two groups whereby diastolic BP was 77 mmHg in the placebo group and 74 mmHg in the lisinopril group (P = 0.0001). This BP difference was maintained throughout the rest of the trial. Once again this raises the issue as to whether or not the improvements in urinary albumin excretion were attributable to ACE inhibition or, simply, to BP reduction.

Effects of intensified antihypertensive treatment in diabetic nephropathy: mortality and morbidity results of a prospective controlled 10-year study.

A K Trocha, C Schmidtke, U Didjurgeit, *et al. J Hypertens* 1999; **17**: 1497–503.

BACKGROUND. The aim of this study was to describe the effect of intensified antihypertensive therapy based on a structured teaching and treatment programme on the prognosis of hypertension type 1 (insulin-dependent) diabetic patients with kidney disease.

INTERPRETATION. We conclude that intensified antihypertensive treatment, based on a hypertension teaching and treatment programme, reduces long-term morbidity and mortality in patients with diabetic nephropathy.

This was a controlled prospective parallel group study albeit in a relatively small number of 91 hypertensive patients with type 1 diabetes mellitus. Patients were assigned to intensified antihypertensive treatment, with specialist follow-up, or to routine antihypertensive treatment as provided by family physicians, local hospitals and consultants. During the follow-up period of 10 years, there were seven deaths in the intensive treatment group and 22 deaths in the routine treatment group ($P = 0.0008$) and a cardiovascular cause was identified in three and 17 of these patients, respectively. For one of the main secondary end-points, namely renal replacement treatment, 11 patients in the intensified group reached regular dialysis treatment compared with 18 patients in the routine treatment group. Of particular interest, was the antihypertensive drug treatment regimen in the two groups. After 10 years of treatment 41% of patients in both groups were receiving an ACE inhibitor (Table 12.1). Thus, in terms of 'exposure' to ACE inhibition there was no difference between the two groups to explain the differences in outcome. However, there were significant differences in the BP values and in the number of antihypertensive drugs that averaged 2.2 after 5 years and 2.7 after 10 years in the intensified treatment group compared with corresponding number of 1.6 and 2.1 in the routine treatment group (Table 12.2).

Table 12.1 Antihypertensive treatment in diabetic nephropathy: BP control

	Intensified group	Routine group	Significance
Baseline	154/92	143/87	*$P < 0.05$ for both systolic and diastolic BP
Year 5	148/85	156/88	*$P < 0.005$ for the systolic BP difference
Year 10	151/87	150/89	

Source: Trocha *et al.* (1999).

Table 12.2 Antihypertensive treatment in diabetic nephropathy: choice of drug

	Intensified group		Routine group	
	5-year	10-year	5-year	10-year
ACE inhibitors	12	41	43	41
Beta-blockers	69	60	27	33
Calcium channel blockers	41	46	39	41
Diuretics	67	76	52	63

Source: Trocha *et al.* (1999).

Comment

This is an interesting study from which the principal message appears to be that intensified antihypertensive drug treatment and improved BP control is more important than the pharmacological characteristics of any given antihypertensive drug class. It is also important to note that multiple drug treatments were inevitably required to achieve this control and these findings are entirely consistent with the outcome benefits produced by 'tight' BP control with combinations of antihypertension drugs |3|.

Left ventricular hypertrophy

Left ventricular hypertrophy (LVH) constitutes a major independent cardio-vascular risk factor such that the cardiovascular risk of the hypertensive patient is increased beyond that associated with the level of hypertension itself. For example, in the Framingham study, the presence of the 'voltage and strain' electrocardio-graphic pattern was associated with a doubling of the risk of cardiovascular disease relative to hypertension alone. Thus, the presence of LVH is a risk factor for all the major manifestations of cardiovascular disease: for example, LVH is associated with a two- to three-fold increase in non-fatal MI and fivefold increase in sudden cardiac death.

The electrocardiogram (ECG) diagnosis of LVH has limitations particularly in relation to its sensitivity and it has now largely been superseded by echocardio-graphic assessments, which provide a more sensitive and specific method of assessing LVH. It is now well established that echocardiographic LVH is an important adverse prognostic factor. Overall, therefore, LVH can be regarded as a surrogate marker for the adverse cardiovascular consequence of uncontrolled hypertension.

Echocardiographic measurement

The Sixth Report of the Joint National Committee on prevention, detection, evaluation and treatment of high BP recommended that an extensive (optimal) preliminary investigation for risk stratification in the hypertensive patient should include assessment of the lipid profile, the status for diabetes and renal function/disease, and limited echocardiography. However, a fully quantitative echocardiographic examination is not universally recommended as part of the initial investigations for evaluation and management of arterial hypertension and this primarily reflects concerns about the ability of the technique to monitor adequately changes in left ventricular geometry in individual patients. These concerns arise because of the variability of the methodology. This issue of the reproducibility and the clinical usefulness of repeated measurements of left ventricular mass in the hypertensive patient was specifically explored in the following study.

Reliability and limitations of echocardiographic measurements of left ventricular mass for risk stratification and follow-up in single patients: the RES trial.

G de Simone, M L Muiesan, A Ganau, *et al.*, on behalf of the Working Group and Heart and Hypertension of the Italian Society of Hypertension.
J Hypertens 1999; **17**: 1955–63.

BACKGROUND. To investigate the clinical reliability of repeated measurement of left ventricular mass in a single patient.

INTERPRETATION. Measurement of left ventricular mass in single patients allows reliable risk stratification on the basis of the presence of LVH. The probability of a true change in left ventricular mass over time is maximized for a single-reader difference greater than 9% of the initial value, although differences of 10–13% might also have clinical relevance.

In this study, M-mode echocardiography was undertaken in 261 participants and repeated, on average, 5 days later. There were 131 hypertensive and 130 normotensive patients, mean age 45 years, mean body mass index 24.7 kg/m^2, with an equal sex distribution among the patients who were recruited in 16 centres in Italy. In terms of the quality of the M-mode tracings it was adjudged that 29% were optimal and 50% were sufficient. The salient result was that the categorical consistency was 87% for the identification of hypertensive patients with LVH. However, a significant but small degree of intra- and interobserver variability was noted and there also was negligible regression toward the mean.

Comment

The small but significant amount of technical variability in the M-mode measurements in this study suggests that it is not appropriate to use repeated measurement of left ventricular mass in the 'routine' or indiscriminate assessment and follow up of patients attending a hypertension clinic. Of specific technical interest was that posterior wall thickness was identified as the least reliable variable in the overall calculations used to compute left ventricular mass. However, where the measurements can be obtained systematically and according to a standardized protocol then the derived information can usefully be applied to guide the management strategy in an individual hypertensive patient. The obvious implication is that the identification of LVH should lead to intensive antihypertensive treatment and the effectiveness of that treatment can be confirmed by the evidence of regression of LVH at a subsequent echocardiographic examination.

Regression of left ventricular hypertrophy

LVH can be regarded as an adaptive or compensatory response to the increased BP and, although the focus of antihypertensive treatment should be upon BP reduction, there also should be an awareness of the potential benefits of promoting the regression of hypertension-induced structural changes. Despite the volume of evidence relating LVH to adverse cardiovascular outcomes, and despite the evidence that antihypertensive treatment may lead to the regression of LVH, the prognostic significance of the improvement in this surrogate parameter is still to be determined by an appropriate prospective study. The following study is therefore an important indicator of the potential benefits of the regression of LVH through effective antihypertensive treatment.

Prognostic significance of serial changes in left ventricular mass in essential hypertension.

P Verdecchia, G Schillaci, C Borgioni, et al. Circulation 1998; **97**: 48–54.

BACKGROUND. Increased left ventricular mass predicts an adverse outcome in patients with essential hypertension. The purpose of this study was to determine the relation between changes in left ventricular mass during antihypertensive treatment and subsequent prognosis.

INTERPRETATION. In essential hypertension, a reduction in left ventricular mass during treatment is a favourable prognostic marker that predicts a lesser risk for subsequent cardiovascular morbid events. Such an association is independent of baseline left ventricular mass, baseline clinical and ambulatory BP, and degree of BP reduction.

   This study of 430 patients with essential hypertension involved 24-h ambulatory BP measurements in addition to echocardiography before and after antihypertensive drug treatment. During the follow up, 31 patients suffered a first morbid cardiovascular event but with an event rate of 1.78 per 100 person years in the group with a decrease in left ventricular mass and a significantly greater event rate of 3.03 per 100 person years in the group with an increase in left ventricular mass ($P = 0.029$). Further statistical analysis in the group at lesser cardiovascular risk (i.e. with a decrease in left ventricular mass during treatment) identified that the benefit was independent of age and baseline LVH on the ECG. This finding was confirmed in the subset with increased left ventricular mass at baseline: thus, those who achieved regression of LVH had a lower event rate of 1.08 per 100 person years compared with those patients who did not achieve regression of LVH who had an event rate of 6.27 per 100 person years.

Comment

The most important result of this study is that the reduction of left ventricular mass in response to treatment in otherwise uncomplicated essential hypertension had a favourable impact on prognosis because it was predictive of a lesser risk for the development of subsequent cardiovascular disease. This benefit was independent of baseline left ventricular mass, baseline clinic and ambulatory BPs and the BP responses to antihypertensive drug treatment. It must be recognized, however, that this is a relatively small study in relatively young hypertensive patients with a relatively short duration of follow-up. Nevertheless, the results of other ongoing clinical trials should confirm whether or not the results of this observational study are valid. Despite these reservations, however, this is an important study because it also suggests that M mode echocardiography is a clinically valuable and cost-effective investigation because it permits the risk stratification of patients with essential hypertension. Thus, those who fail to achieve a reduction in left ventricular mass or regression of LVH should be considered at increased risk for subsequent cardiovascular disease and, accordingly, targeted for a more aggressive therapeutic approach.

Left ventricular hypertrophy: causative factors

Mechanical effects of hypertension

Hypertension leads to an increase in wall stress and this is the fundamental stimulus for the development of LVH. However, a number of other factors contribute to the increased risk of adverse cardiovascular outcomes and these include myocardial ischaemia, coexisting coronary artery disease, left ventricular dysfunction, structural myocardial changes and ventricular arrhythmias. Initially, however, hypertrophy of the left ventricular myocardium is a compensatory response attempting to restore wall stress to a normal level and thereby preserving left ventricular systolic function and reducing the possibility of myocardial perfusion abnormalities. However, this adaptive response is not limitless and eventually there is a deterioration in both cardiac function and myocardial perfusion if the BP remains elevated.

Neuroendocrine factors

In addition to the mechanical effects, 'stretching' of the myocardium promotes protein synthesis and activation of a number of important cellular signals, which also contribute to the development of cardiac hypertrophy. The adrenergic and renin–angiotensin–aldosterone systems have also been implicated in the pathogenesis of LVH and there is a wealth of experimental evidence implicating, in particular, angiotensin II and aldosterone. For example, angiotensin II has direct cardiac actions that stimulate cardiac contractility, increase protein synthesis, etc, and it also has indirect actions via the effects of aldosterone, which is implicated in myocyte hypertrophy and myocardial fibrosis. While the experimental evidence is voluminous in implicating angiotensin II as a necessary mechanistic factor there are some inconsistencies.

Pressure overload induces cardiac hypertrophy in angiotensin II type 1A receptor knockout mice.
K Harada, I Komuro, I Shiojima, *et al. Circulation* 1998; **97**: 1952–9.

B A C K G R O U N D . Many studies have suggested that the renin–angiotensin system plays an important part in the development of pressure overload-induced cardiac hypertrophy. Moreover, it has been reported that pressure overload-induced cardiac hypertrophy is completely prevented by ACE inhibitors *in vivo* and that the stored angiotensin II is released from cardiac myocytes in response to mechanical stretch and induces cardiomyocyte hypertrophy through the angiotensin II type I receptor (AT$_1$) *in vitro.*

INTERPRETATION. AT$_1$ mediated angiotensin II signaling is not essential for the development of pressure overload-induced cardiac hypertrophy.

Comment

This is an interesting experiment in which a 'knock-out' mouse model still developed LVH despite being totally deficient in angiotensin II (AT$_1$) receptors. This finding clearly raises doubts about the proposed central and causative role of the renin–angiotensin–aldosterone system in the development of LVH in humans. At a more philosophical level, the finding also sounds a cautionary note about the risk of directly and simplistically extrapolating from experimental to clinical evidence!

Regression of left ventricular hypertrophy by antihypertensive drug treatment

A question that is frequently asked is 'Which antihypertensive drug is most effective in promoting the regression of LVH?' Unfortunately, there is no individual study in which an adequate number of patients has been appropriately randomized in a double blind manner to one or two (or more) treatments and assessed after not less than 6 months of treatment with a validated measure of left ventricular mass. Accordingly, much reliance has been placed on meta-analytical techniques despite the well recognized shortcomings of this approach. In some of these meta-analyses, and in line with the experimental evidence, ACE inhibitor drugs appear to be the most effective agents for promoting regression of LVH. Correspondingly, there is an overall impression that beta-blockers are not particularly effective and there is the suggestion for thiazide diuretics that part of their measured effect is attributable to their volume depleting action leading to shrinkage of the left ventricular cavity, which is then interpreted as an overall reduction in left ventricular mass.

The shortcomings of meta-analytical techniques are considerable because they depend on the 'quality' of the studies that are included (or not included). For example, in one meta-analysis in which basic criteria were pre-defined such as the incorporation of only randomized studies comparing two or more treatments and with a blinded measurement technique, only 39 of 471 published studies fulfilled the relevant criteria |4|. In this particular analysis, ACE inhibitor drugs appeared to be associated with the greatest reduction in left ventricular mass by 13.3%, followed by calcium channel blockers at 9.3%, diuretics at 6.8% and beta-blockers at 5.5%. While this result appears to support the widely held view that ACE inhibitor drugs are the most effective agents for promoting the regression of LVH, the updated analysis by the same group gives different results.

Update of reversal of left ventricular hypertrophy in essential hypertension (a meta-analysis of all randomized double-blind studies until December 1996).

R E Schmieder, M P Schlaich, A U Klingbeil, P Martus. *Nephrol Dial Transplant* 1998; **13**: 564–9.

BACKGROUND. To provide an update on the ability of different antihypertensive drugs to reduce LVH in essential hypertension.

INTERPRETATION. Decrease in systolic BP, duration of antihypertensive therapy, degree of pretreatment LVH and antihypertensive drug class determined the reduction of LVH. ACE inhibitors and calcium channel blockers were more potent in reducing left ventricular mass than beta-blockers, with diuretics in the intermediate range.

Comment

This further meta-analysis reviewed all published articles until December 1996 and incorporated only double-blind, randomized, controlled clinical studies with parallel group designs. The data extraction was undertaken according to a predetermined protocol performed independently by two investigators. Fifty suitable studies were identified with a total of 1715 patients in 13 placebo treatments and in 89 active treatments. In summary, left ventricular mass index was reduced in relation to the decrease in systolic BP, the longer the duration of antihypertensive treatment, and the higher the pretreatment value for left ventricular mass index. With respect to the individual drug (class) effects the summarizing reductions were 12% with ACE inhibitors, 1% with calcium channel blockers, 8% with diuretics and 5% with beta-blockers (see Fig. 12.1). Subsequent testing revealed that ACE inhibitors and calcium channel blockers were significantly more effective than beta-blockers in reducing the left ventricular mass index.

Reversibility of left ventricular hypertrophy and malfunction by antihypertensive treatment.

G L Jennings, J Wong, in: L Hansson, W H Birkenhäger (eds). *Handbook of Hypertension*, Volume 18: *Assessment of Hypertensive Organ Damage*. Amsterdam: Elsevier Science 1997, p6.

BACKGROUND. Cardiac hypertrophy is a feature of many of the common cardiovascular disease, including ischaemic heart disease, cardiomyopathies, valvular disease and hypertension. For the most part, treatment has been directed towards alleviating factors contributing to cardiac load implying that hypertrophy is generally secondary to mechanical stretch. In hypertension, however, there has been considerable discussion on the strategies for optimal regression of cardiac hypertension as a goal of treatment of changes in BP.

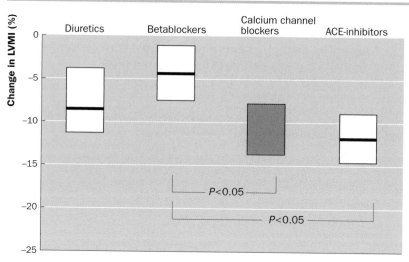

Fig 12. 1 Effectiveness of different classes of antihypertensive drug in promoting the regression of LVH. Adapted from the meta-analysis of Schmieder *et al.* (1998).

INTERPRETATION. The reasons for the recent emphasis on regression of cardiac hypertrophy in hypertension are multiple. They include the recognition from epidemiological data that LVH is a potent marker of outcome, and is particularly associated with risk of sudden death. Basic studies have shown that factors other than mechanical load can influence the development of LVH and its regression. These considerations lead to the following important questions that are the subject of this chapter: does regression of LVH occur in human hypertension, is regression beneficial when it does occur, and do different antihypertensive therapies exert selective effects on cardiac hypertrophy independent of their effects on BP?

Comment

This comprehensive review and meta-analysis calculates a closer comparability in the effectiveness of the different classes of antihypertensive drug (see Fig. 12.2). Previous indications that beta-blockers might be the least effective in promoting regression of LVH appear to be confirmed but there is no confirmation of any clear benefits attributable to ACE inhibitor drugs as the ACE inhibitor group and the calcium channel blocker group appear to be similar. Furthermore, despite insinuations about changes in internal diameter being misinterpreted as changes in left ventricular mass, the overall effectiveness of thiazide diuretics appears to be consistent with the effects of other drugs. In summary, effective BP control with treatment based upon an ACE inhibitor or a calcium channel blocker or a thiazide diuretic leads to similar reductions in left ventricular mass.

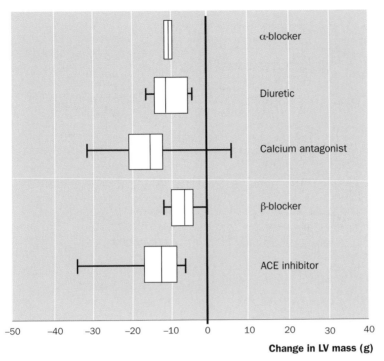

Fig. 12.2 Reversibility of LVH by antihypertensive treatment.
Source: Jennings *et al.* (1997).

Confirmation of the effectiveness of thiazide diuretics in promoting the regression of LVH is provided in the following paper.

Effect of treatment of isolated systolic hypertension on left ventricular mass.

E O Ofili, J D Cohen, J A St Vrain, *et al. JAMA* 1998; **279**: 778–80.

BACKGROUND. LVH is a common problem among elderly patients with isolated hypertension, but the effect of treatment of isolated hypertension on left ventricular mass is not known.

INTERPRETATION. Treatment of isolated hypertension with a diuretic-based regimen reduced left ventricular mass.

This was a subgroup study of 104 patients who participated in the Systolic Hypertension in the Elderly Programme (SHEP) in which it was shown conclusively that antihypertensive treatment (based upon the diuretic, chlorthalidone) was associated with significant cardiovascular benefits, particularly through a 36% reduction in stroke events.

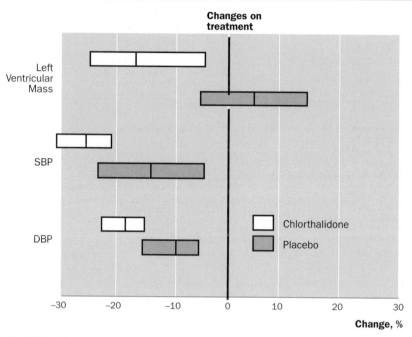

Fig. 12.3 Effect of treatment of isolated systolic hypertension on left ventricular mass. Source: Ofili *et al.* (1998).

In this substudy with a minimum follow-up of 3 years, 80% of subjects continued to receive treatment with chlorthalidone alone by the end of year 3. The left ventricular mass index declined by an average of 13% in the active group compared with a 6% increase in the placebo group (see Fig. 12.3). According to a multivariate analysis, the change in left ventricular mass was significantly correlated with the change in BP, particularly the reduction in systolic BP ($r = 0.40$; $P < 0.003$). The reduction in left ventricular mass in the active treatment group reflected an actual decrease in wall thickness as there were insignificant effects on left ventricular end diastolic dimension (5% reduction with chlorthalidone compared with a 2% reduction in the placebo group).

Conclusion

Overall, no class of drug can be clearly and consistently shown to be superior for the treatment of LVH although, alternatively, there now appears to be overall agreement that beta-blockers are the least effective group. Other antihypertensive drug classes generally have comparable effects with, on average, 12–13% reductions in left ventricular mass. While there may be differential drug effects, as identified in the experimental setting, it has not proved possible to confirm these effects in clinical studies.

Similarly, it has not proved possible to demonstrate clearly that factors other than BP reduction are important in promoting reductions in left ventricular mass in hypertensive patients. It is possible that subtle mechanistic changes are simply overwhelmed by the beneficial effects of good BP control. Thus, on the basis of the available clinical evidence, it appears that the reduction in left ventricular mass is primarily influenced by the magnitude of the BP reduction and the duration of effective antihypertensive drug treatment, rather than the class of drug itself.

Conclusion

Although BP is the most extensively studied of the cardiovascular risk factors, it must be recognized that its measurement is both indirect and relatively crude and that an elevation of BP predisposes to intermediate cardiovascular changes prior to the development of morbid and mortal events. In our attempts to refine our approaches to patient management, and also to define which patients are at greatest risk, attention had recently been focused on a number of intermediate or surrogate end-points. There are clear and important correlations between the surrogate end-points and adverse cardiovascular outcomes and there also is evidence that therapeutic intervention can exert a beneficial influence. However, the methodologies are not simple and not readily applicable in routine practice; there is only limited evidence that improvement in the surrogate measure leads to outcome benefit, i.e. a reduction in cardiovascular events; there is not yet clear evidence that ancillary properties add significantly to the benefits of BP reduction. Thus, although it is important to continue to study these intermediate factors and to try to modify them, at the present time, the balance of evidence suggests that 'tight' BP is the primary requirement. The practical message therefore remains that BP control is more important than pharmacological characteristics.

References

1. Jensen JS, Borch-Johnsen K, Jensen G, Feldt-Rasmussen B. Microalbuminuria reflects a generalised transvascular albumin leakiness in clinical healthy subjects. *Clin Sci* 1995; **88**: 629–33.

2. Damsgaard EM, Froland A, Jorgensen OD, Mogensen CE. Microalbuminuria as predictor of increased mortality in elderly people. *BMJ* 1990; **300**: 297–300.

3. UK Prospective Diabetes Study Group. Tight blood pressure control and risk of macrovascular and microvascular complications in type 2 diabetes: UKPDS 38. *Br Med J* 1998; **317**: 703–13.

4. Schmieder, RE, Martus P, Klingbeil A. Reversal of left ventricular hypertrophy in essential hypertension: A meta-analysis of randomised double-blind studies. *JAMA* 1996; 275: 1507–13.

13

Calcium channel blockers in profile

Introduction

It is well recognized that calcium channel blockers (CCBs) are effective antihypertensive drugs that can be used alone or in combination in the treatment of almost all types of hypertensive patients. Currently, in the treatment of hypertension, long-acting once daily dihydropyridine drugs (e.g. amlodipine) or modified release formulations (e.g. nifedipine GITS) are generally preferred. These agents are metabolically neutral and the only significant adverse symptomatic effect is ankle swelling (oedema), which is dose-related; is only occasionally seen at starting dose levels; and is not a harbinger of any serious pathological processes. In terms of clinical outcome studies, however, there has been considerable debate about the overall safety of CCBs and their ultimate effectiveness in reducing cardiovascular morbidity and mortality.

Unfortunately, there are not yet definitive studies that can provide clear answers to all of the questions that have been raised about antihypertensive treatment with CCBs. The available evidence is derived from disparate studies that range from case reports and retrospective case–control studies through to large-scale prospective clinical outcome trials and, recently, two summarizing meta-analyses. Useful additional information is also available from other studies in which CCBs have been used to treat patients at increased cardiovascular risk albeit not solely due to essential hypertension. It is not within the scope of this chapter to review each and every published paper but instead the focus is upon recent publications from which reasonable conclusions can be drawn about the safety and efficacy of the CCB class in general and the dihydropyridine derivatives in particular.

Prospective clinical outcome trials

The prospective double blind clinical outcome trial is generally considered to be the 'gold standard' upon which is based our concepts of evidence-based therapeutic practice. The first appropriately designed prospective trial with a dihydropyridine CCB was published in the Systolic Hypertension in Europe trial (SYST-EUR), which showed significant benefit in clinical outcomes.

Systolic Hypertension in Europe trial

Randomized double-blind comparison of placebo and active treatment for older patients with isolated systolic hypertension.
J A Staessen, R Fagard, L Thijs, *et al. Lancet* 1997; **350**: 757–64.

BACKGROUND. Isolated hypertension occurs in about 15% of people aged 60 years or older. In 1989, the European Working Party on High Blood Pressure in the Elderly investigated whether active treatment could reduce cardiovascular complications of isolated systolic hypertension. Fatal and non-fatal stroke combined was the primary end-point.

INTERPRETATION. Among elderly patients with isolated systolic hypertension, antihypertensive drug treatment starting with nitrendipine reduces the rate of cardiovascular complications. Treatment of 1000 patients for 5 years with this type of regimen may prevent 29 strokes or 53 major cardiovascular end-points.

In this study, 4695 patients were randomly assigned to nitrendipine 10–40 mg daily with the possible addition of enalapril 5–20 mg daily and hydrochlorothiazide 12.5–25 mg daily, or matching placebos. This trial was stopped prematurely by its Data and Safety Monitoring Board on account of a 43% relative reduction in stroke incidence ($P = 0.03$). This benefit was achieved after a median follow-up of 2 years. There also was a significant 31% relative reduction in cardiovascular events but, not surprisingly in such a short time period, the reduction in total mortality did not achieve statistical significance.

Comment

SYST-EUR was the first, generally accepted clinical trial to confirm the efficacy of an antihypertensive treatment regimen based upon a dihydropyridine CCB. The results, and particularly the benefits in stroke prevention, were entirely consistent with the earlier STONE study (Shanghai Trial of Nifedipine in the Elderly) |**1**|, which used a modified release form of nifedipine. However, STONE did not gain universal acceptance because of concerns about the adequacy of the randomization and 'blinding' procedures.

In addition to SYST-EUR and STONE, there is one other placebo-controlled prospective clinical outcome trial [Systolic Hypertension in China (SYST-China)], which also produced similar results in showing that antihypertensive treatment based upon a dihydropyridine CCBs significantly reduced cardiovascular morbidity and mortality.

Chinese trial on isolated systolic hypertension in the elderly.

W Ji-Guang, J A Staessen, G Lansheng, L Lisheng. *Arch Intern Med* 2000; **160**(2): 211–20.

BACKGROUND. In 1988, the SYST-China Collaborative Group initiated the placebo-controlled SYST-China trial to investigate whether antihypertensive drug treatment could reduce the incidence of fatal and non-fatal stroke in older Chinese patients with isolated systolic hypertension.

INTERPRETATION. In elderly Chinese patients with isolated systolic hypertension, stepwise antihypertensive drug treatment, starting with the dihydropyridine CCB nitrendipine, improved prognosis. The benefit was particularly evident in diabetic patients; for cardiac end-points it tended to be larger in non-smokers. Otherwise, the benefit of active treatment was not significantly influenced by the characteristics of the patients at enrolment in the trial.

Patients (1253) aged 60 years or older with a sitting systolic blood pressure (BP) of 160-219 mmHg and diastolic BP less than 95 mmHg were assigned to active treatment starting with nitrendipine (10–40 mg/day), with a possible addition of captopril (12.5–50 mg/day) and/or hydrochlorothiazide (12.5–50 mg/day). Matching placebos were administered to 1141 control patients. After 2 years of follow up BP had been reduced by 9.1/3.2 mmHg (on average) leading to significant reductions in total mortality, fatal and non-fatal stroke and all cardiovascular end-points. There were corresponding reductions in other cardiovascular events but the individual end-points failed to achieve conventional statistical significance.

Comment

Apart from the overall consistency of these results in confirming the reductions in cardiovascular morbidity and mortality achieved with dihydropyridine CCBs in STONE and SYSTEUR, a number of additional interesting observations were identified in the subgroup analyses. For example, the benefits of treatment were particularly apparent when nitrendipine monotherapy was administered on a twice-daily basis. In this group there were significant reductions in total mortality by 50%, in cardiovascular mortality by 49%, in cardiovascular end-points by 52% and in cardiac events by 74% (Table 13.1). For the study as a whole, the benefits of active treatment in high-risk patients were again apparent, including those with diabetes mellitus.

Conclusion

Through 'gold standard' prospective clinical outcome trials there is clear evidence of cardiovascular outcome benefits with CCBs. By way of comparison, the reductions in cardiovascular morbidity and mortality in SYST-EUR were closely similar to those obtained with thiazide diuretics in the SHEP study |2| (Table 13.2). An

Table 13.1 Nitrendipine: once *vs* twice daily

	Adjusted relative hazard rate	
	Once daily (n = 735)	Twice daily (n = 518)
Mortality	0.73	0.50*
Cardiovascular mortality	0.75	0.51*
Cardiovascular end-points	0.73	0.52*
Stroke events	0.62	0.71
Cardiac events	0.94	0.36**

*$P < 0.05$ compared with placebo; **$P < 0.05$ compared with placebo and once daily nitrendipine.
Source: Ji-Guang *et al.* (2000).

Table 13.2 Isolated systolic hypertension in the elderly: comparison of SYST-EUR and SHEP

	SYSTEUR	SHEP	P<
Relative risk reduction			
Stroke	42%	36%	0.01
MI	30%	27%	0.05
CV events	31%	32%	0.01
All cause mortality	14%	13%	
Absolute benefit (5 year NNT)			
Stroke	34	33	
CV events	19	17	

incidental and additionally reassuring observation was that there was no increase in mortality from any other cause in any of these three trials.

Comparative clinical outcome trials

 Morbidity and mortality in patients randomized to double-blind treatment with long-acting calcium channel blocker or diuretic in the international nifedipine GITS study: intervention as a goal in hypertension treatment.
M J Brown, C R Palmer, A Castaigne, *et al. Lancet* 2000; **356**: 366–72.

BACKGROUND. The efficacy of antihypertensive drugs newer than diuretics and β-blockers has not yet been established. We compared the effects of the CCB nifedipine once daily with the diuretic combination co-amilozide on cardiovascular mortality and morbidity in high-risk patients with hypertension.

INTERPRETATION. Nifedipine once daily and co-amilozide were equally effective in preventing overall cardiovascular or cerebrovascular complications. The choice of drug can be decided by tolerability and BP responses rather than long-term safety or efficacy.

This was a prospective randomized double blind trial in 6321 patients aged 55–80 years with BP greater than 150/95 mmHg, or with a systolic BP greater than 160 mmHg, and at least one additional cardiovascular risk factor. Patients were randomly assigned to nifedipine GITS in a starting dose of 30 mg or to co-amilozide (hydrochlorothiazide 25 mg plus amiloride 2.5 mg) and the achieved BPs were closely similar in the two groups at about 138/82 mmHg sitting.

The results of this comparative clinical trial, against an established or reference antihypertensive agent (thiazide diuretic) are consistent with, and complementary to, the results of the earlier placebo-controlled clinical trials. Although the withdrawal rates were relatively high in both treatment groups—on account mainly of symptomatic and metabolic adverse effects (about 40% with nifedipine GITS and 33% with co-amilozide)—the intention-to-treat analysis confirmed a remarkable similarity for primary end-points and all-cause mortality (Fig. 13.1). Thus, 6.3% and 5.8% of patients with treatment based upon nifedipine GITS and co-amilozide, respectively, sustained a primary cardiovascular end-point, which comprised combined fatal and non-fatal stroke, myocardial infarction (MI) and heart failure. Other major predetermined subgroups are shown in Table 13.3.

Table 13.3 INSIGHT: primary outcome results

	Nifedipine	Co-amilozide	
Major cardiovascular events	6.3%	5.8%	
Myocardial infarction			
Non-fatal	1.9%	1.8%	
Fatal	0.5%	0.2%	*$P < 0.05$
Sudden death	0.5%	0.7%	
Stroke			
Non-fatal	1.7%	2.0%	
Fatal	0.3%	0.3%	
Heart failure			
Non-fatal	0.8%	0.3%	
Fatal	0.1%	0.1%	*$P < 0.05$
Other cardiovascular death	0.4%	0.4%	

Source: Brown *et al.* (2000).

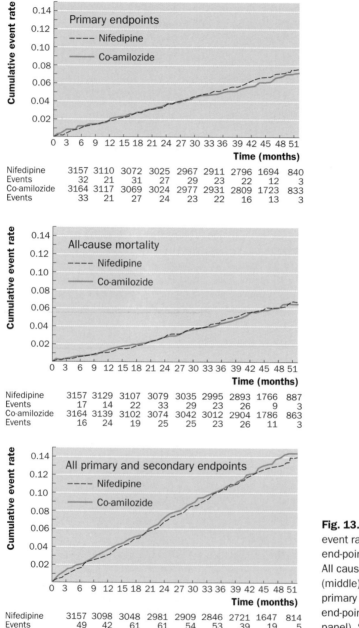

Fig. 13.1 Cumulative event rates for primary end-points (upper), All cause mortality (middle) and all primary and secondary end-points (lower panel). Source: Brown *et al.* (2000).

Comment

Further subdivision of the results into 18 possible outcome categories has led some authors to fuel the speculation that there may be less coronary heart disease (CHD) protection with CCBs. For example, MI and cardiac failure, when further sub-divided into fatal and non-fatal events, were less effectively prevented with CCBs and statistical benefits were found in favour of diuretic-based treatment. However, with small numbers and multiple statistical comparisons these findings obviously require cautious interpretation and this is well illustrated for fatal MI and sudden cardiac death. There were 16 fatal MIs in the nifedipine group and five in the co-amilozide group but there were 23 sudden deaths in the co-amilozide group compared with 17 in the nifedipine group. Clearly, the Intervention as a Goal in Hypertension Treatment (INSIGHT) trial was not intended to nor statistically empowered to address these particular subdivisions.

Retrospective (*post hoc*) analyses

It is noteworthy that adverse publicity for CCBs has generally arisen from retro-spective analyses (typically case–control studies) and from studies that have often involved relatively small patient numbers. Arguably the most rigorous of these retrospective analyses, with substantial patient numbers studied over a protracted time period, has produced reassuring but non-definitive results.

Do inhibitors of angiotensin-I-converting enzyme protect against risk of cancer?

A F Lever, D J Hole, C R Gillis, *et al. Lancet* 1998; **352**: 179–84.

BACKGROUND. Previous studies have reported an increased risk of cancer with CCBs in humans. Other work in animals suggests that inhibitors of angiotensin-converting enzyme (ACE) protect against cancer. We aimed to assess the risk of cancer in hypertensive patients receiving ACE inhibitors or other antihypertensive drugs.

INTERPRETATION. Long-term use of ACE inhibitors may protect against cancer. The status of this finding is more that of hypothesis generation than hypothesis testing; randomized controlled trials are needed.

In 5020 patients registered with the Glasgow Blood Pressure Clinic between 1980 and 1995 there were 134 cases of cancer in patients receiving CCBs and this translated to a clearly non-significant relative risk of 1.02 in comparison with patients receiving other types of antihypertensive drug. This interpretation was reinforced by further comparisons that showed no association between CCBs and cancer in two other control groups from the same geographical location.

Comment

This *post hoc* analysis has clearly demonstrated that, over a protracted period of observation, CCBs are not associated with any increased risk of cancer. It remains to be established whether or not the apparently protective effect of ACE inhibitors is a real effect.

Meta-analyses

Two major meta-analyses have been recently published in the *Lancet*.

Health outcomes associated with calcium antagonists compared with other first-line antihypertensive therapies: a meta-analysis of randomized controlled trials.

M Pahor, B M Psaty, M H Alderman, *et al. Lancet* 2000; **356**: 1949–54.

BACKGROUND. **Several observational and individual randomized trials in hypertension have suggested that, compared with other drugs, calcium antagonists may be associated with a higher risk of coronary events, despite similar BP control. The aim of this meta-analysis was to compare the effects of calcium antagonists and other antihypertensive drugs on major cardiovascular events.**

INTERPRETATION. In randomized controlled trials, the large available database suggests that calcium antagonists are inferior to other types of antihypertensive drugs as first-line agents in reducing the risk of several major complications of hypertension. On the basis of these data, the longer-acting calcium antagonists cannot be recommended as first-line therapy for hypertension.

Effects of ACE Inhibitors, calcium antagonists, and other blood-pressure-lowering drugs: results of prospectively designed overviews of randomized trials.

Blood Pressure Lowering Treatment Trialists' Collaboration. *Lancet* 2000; **355**: 1955–64.

BACKGROUND. **The programme of overviews of randomized trials was established to investigate the effects of ACE inhibitors, calcium antagonists and other BP-lowering drugs on mortality and major cardiovascular morbidity in several populations of patients. We separated overviews of trials comparing more intensive and less intensive BP-lowering strategies, and trials comparing treatment regimens based on different drug classes.**

INTERPRETATION. Strong evidence of benefits of ACE inhibitors and calcium antagonists is provided by the overviews of placebo-controlled trials. There is weaker evidence of differences between treatment regimens of differing intensities and of differences between treatment regimens based on different drug classes. Data from continuing trials of BP-lowering drugs will substantially increase the evidence available about any real differences that might exist between regimens.

Comment

It is remarkable that these two analyses, which contained essentially the same data, involved closely similar methodologies and derived closely similar summarizing figures and percentages, should have derived almost diametrically opposing conclusions. Thus, one meta-analysis determined that CCBs had an adverse effect on outcome, whereas the other analysis showed that there were no statistically significant outcome differences for CCBs relative to other types of antihypertensive drug. In my opinion, the analysis by the Blood Pressure Lowering Treatment Trialists' Collaboration is the more rigorous and this showed no statistically significant differences. The summarizing results for major end-points are shown in Table 13.4.

Conclusion

The available data from the individual 'robust', appropriately designed, prospective clinical trials and, in essence, the two meta-analyses shows no significant differences between CCBs and 'conventional' antihypertensive drug treatments in terms of the impact on all-cause mortality and cardiovascular events.

The only remaining contentious issue appears to be the 'pattern' of cardiovascular events prevented. The benefits of CCBs in stroke prevention have been demonstrated repeatedly but the reduction in CHD events (including cardiac failure) appears to be less than that associated with, for example, ACE inhibitor treatment. However, CHD events are remarkably under-represented in the clinical outcome trials contained within these meta-analyses. In fact, if individual studies are to be considered there is no completed clinical outcome study with sufficient statistical power to address the treatment effect on CHD events. Only the ongoing Antihypertensive and Lipid Lowering to prevent Heart Attack Trial (ALLHAT) and

Table 13.4 Major end-points: summarizing meta-analytical results of 'conventional' antihypertensive drugs *vs* ACE inhibitors and CCBs

	'Conventional'	ACE inhibitors	CCB
BP reduction (mmHg)	16/6.5	3/1	9/5
CHD	−16%	−20%	−21%
Stroke	−38%	−30%	−39%
Cardiovascular death	−21%	−26%	−28%
Total mortality	−13%	−16%	−13%
Heart failure	NA	−13% (NS)	−28%

Source: Blood Pressure Lowering Treatment Trialists' Collaboration (2000).

Anglo Scandinavian Cardiac Outcomes Trial (ASCOT) (both with amlodipine) have sufficient statistical power to independently assess the impact of different antihypertensive treatments on CHD outcomes |3,4|. In the fullness of time, the ALLHAT and ASCOT data are proscribed to be incorporated into the meta-analysis of the Blood Pressure Lowering Treatment Trialists' Collaboration.

Are calcium channel blockers homogeneous?

It is interesting to note in the meta-analytical methodology that steps are taken to confirm homogeneity of the data derived from disparate clinical trials. However, it is remarkable that no corresponding consideration is given to the CCBs themselves and, generally, the CCBs are considered as a homogeneous class despite the fact that there are clear, clinically relevant differences between different agents. Verapamil (a phenylalkylamine), diltiazem (a benzothiazepine) and the dihydropyridine derivatives (e.g. nifedipine, amlodipine and felodipine) are chemically, pharmacologically and therapeutically different from each other: of equal importance (but less well recognized) are the clinically relevant differences within the dihydropyridine class in relation to intrinsically long-acting drugs, or modified-release formulator, and then in therapeutic features such as rapidity of onset, frequency of dosing, duration of action, etc.

With the overall preference in current antihypertensive practice for long-acting once daily dihydropyridine CCBs it can be argued that there are only three studies to be assessed: nifedipine GITS in the INSIGHT study, felodipine ER in the Hypertension Optimal Treatment (HOT) study, and amlodipine in the Prospective Randomized Evaluation of the Vascular Effects of Norvasc Trial (PREVENT) (although this was not a hypertension study). The PREVENT study assessed the impact of amlodipine on the progression of atherosclerosis in 825 patients with angiographically proven CHD |5|. If there was a harmful effect in provoking MI or CCF then it might have been expected in these high-risk CHD patients . In terms of clinical events (albeit not a primary end-point) there was evidence of a beneficial effect from CCB treatment rather than a harmful effect (Table 13.5). For example, one

Table 13.5 PREVENT: summary of major clinical events

	No. of patients		
	Amlodipine	Placebo	
Any death	6	8	
Fatal/non-fatal MI	19	20	
Major vascular event	23	28	
Documented angina/CCF	61	88	$P < 0.01$
Major vascular procedure	52	88	$P < 0.001$

case of heart failure compared with five cases, and significantly fewer cases of unstable angina.

Other studies with long-acting calcium channel blockers

Effects of intensive blood-pressure lowering and low-dose aspirin in patients with hypertension: principal results of the Hypertension Optimal Treatment (HOT) randomised trial.
L Hansson, A Zanchetti, S G Carruthers, *et al. Lancet* 1998; **351**: 1755–62.

BACKGROUND. Despite treatment, there is often a higher incidence of cardiovascular complications in patients with hypertension than in normotensive individuals. Inadequate reduction of their BP is a likely cause, but the optimum target BP is not yet known. The impact of acetylsalicylic acid (aspirin) has never been investigated in patients with hypertension. We aimed to assess the optimum target diastolic BP and the potential benefit of a low dose of acetylsalicylic acid in the treatment of hypertension.

INTERPRETATION. Intensive lowering of BP in patients with hypertension was associated with a low rate of cardiovascular events. The HOT study shows the benefits of lowering the diastolic BP down to 82.6 mmHg. Acetylsalicylic acid significantly reduced major cardiovascular events with the greatest benefit seen in all MI. There was no effect on the incidence of stroke or fatal bleeds, but non-fatal major bleeds were twice as common.
   Patients (18 790) aged 50–80 years with a diastolic BP between 100 and 150 mmHg were randomly assigned to three different targets for diastolic BP. Patients were targeted to a diastolic BP < 90 mmHg, < 85 mmHg and < 80 mmHg, and felodipine (ER) was administered as the baseline treatment with the addition of other agents, according to a five-step regimen, to achieve the target BP. The salient results are summarized in Table 13.6.

Comment

In many respects, one of the most important pieces of supportive evidence for the antihypertensive effectiveness of CCBs appears in the HOT study involving the dihydropyridine CCB, felodipine in a modified release formulation. For example, in the diabetic subgroup in this study, who were obviously at high risk of cardio-vascular disease in general and CHD in particular, there were important outcome differences in the three different treatment cohorts in association with very small differences in BP. Thus, for an achieved BP difference of 2/2 mmHg there was a

Table 13.6 High-risk (diabetic) patients in the HOT study

Diastolic group	Cardiovascular events per 1000 patient years		
	<90	**<85**	**<80 mmHg**
Patients (*n*)	6264	6264	6264
Major cardiovascular events	24.4	18.6	11.9
Cardiovascular mortality	15.9	15.5	9.0

Source: Hansson *et al.* (1998).

further 33% relative reduction in major cardiovascular events in the lowest BP group compared with the middle group. The HOT study was not a placebo or positively controlled clinical trial but was an assessment of the benefits of intensive antihypertensive drug treatment to relatively low BP targets (co-administration of aspirin was also shown to be beneficial).

Relevant parallels can be drawn between the HOT study (based on a CCB) and the Heart Outcomes Prevention Evaluation (HOPE) study based upon an ACE inhibitor (ramipril) in which high-risk cardiac and diabetic patients were treated either with placebo or with the ACE inhibitor |6|. Thus, a 2/2 mmHg difference was associated with a 33% reduction in major cardiovascular events in HOT and a similarly modest BP reduction of 3/2 mmHg in the HOPE study was associated with 20–30% relative reductions in cardiovascular events.

Conclusion

Aggressive antihypertensive treatment in high-risk patients produced significant cardiovascular benefits irrespective of whether the treatment was based upon a dihydropyridine CCB or an ACE inhibitor.

Discussion

In summary, there are no definitive answers about the safety and efficacy of CCBs because these are no definitive studies. The following appear to be the main conclusions that can reasonably be drawn from the available evidence.

1. Although not discussed specifically in this chapter, there is no place for short-acting CCBs for which there is no outcome evidence and for which there is evidence of inferior efficacy. The positive prospective clinical studies involving a relatively large number of patients have been derived from studies with medium- and long-acting CCBs.

2. The overall effectiveness of antihypertensive treatment with dihydropyridine CCBs has now been incontrovertibly established with a significant reduction in

cardiovascular events. This has been a recurring feature of all of the prospective clinical outcome trials.

3. As a side issue, it is interesting to note that twice daily nitrendipine was associated with significant reductions in cardiovascular events, whereas there were non-significant reductions with once daily dosing. While this may be a dose-dependent phenomenon (although doses were adjusted according to achieved BP) it might also be argued that the better result reflected more protracted and better sustained pharmacological activity, i.e. the benefits of long-lasting calcium channel blockade.

4. There has been no evidence in the prospective trials of problems with increased bleeding risk or increased cancer risk. Furthermore, one of the most robust of the retrospective analyses also failed to find evidence of any association between cancer and CCBs. Stroke prevention is clearly established but there are insufficient data to draw clear conclusions regarding specific effects on acute MI, CCF, etc. Unfortunately, none of the prospective clinical outcome studies has been appropriately powered and the summarizing meta-analyses contain relatively small numbers of such patients. In due course, it is hoped that the results from the appropriately powered ALLHAT and ASCOT studies might shed light on the effectiveness of long acting CCBs in the prevention of CHD events.

5. For the moment, therefore, the emphasis should remain upon the identification of hypertensive patients at increased cardiovascular risk; drug treatment should be targeted to achieve BP control at the recommended levels of 140/85 mmHg or less; and antihypertensive drug treatment regimens should incorporate long-acting CCBs because their well recognized antihypertensive efficacy has been shown to translate to outcome benefits and reduced cardiovascular morbidity and mortality.

References

1. Gong L, Zhang W, Zhu Y, Zhu J, Kong D, Page V, Ghadirian P, LeLorier J, Hamet P. Shanghai trials of nifedipine in the elderly (STONE). *J Hypertens* 1996; 15 (Suppl 2): S123–8.

2. SHEP Cooperative Research Group. Prevention of stoke by antihypertensive drug treatment in older persons with isolated systolic hypertension: final results of the Systolic Hypertension in the Elderly Program (SHEP). *JAMA* 1991; 265: 3255–64.

3. Davis BR, Cutler JA, Gordon DJ, Furberg D, Wright JT, Cushman WC, Grimm RH, LaRosa J, Whelton PK, Perry HM, Alderman MH, Ford CE, Oparil S, Francis C, Proschan M, Pressel S, Black HR, Hawkins CM, for the ALLHAT Research Group.

Rationale and design for the antihypertensive and lipid lowering treatment to prevent heart attack trial (ALLHAT). *Am J Hypertens* 1996; **9:** 342–60.

4. Sever PS, Dahlof B, Poulter NR, Wedel H, Beevers G, Caulfield M, Collins R, Kjeldsen SE, McInnes GT, Mehlsen J, Nieminen M, O'Brien E, Ostergren J, for the ASCOT investigators. Rationale, design, methods and baseline demography of participants of the Anglo-Scandinavian Cardiac Outcomes Trial. *J Hypertens* 2001; **19:** 1139–47.

5. Pitt B, Byington RP, Furberg CD, Hunninghake DB, Mancini J, Miller ME, Riley W, for the PREVENT Investigators. Effect of amlodipine on the progression of atherosclerosis and the occurrence of clinical events. *Circulation* 2000; **102:** 1503–10.

6. HOPE (Heart Outcomes Prevention Evaluation) Study Investigators. Effects of an angiotensin-converting enzyme inhibitor, ramipril, on cardiovascular events in high-risk patients. *N Engl J Med* 2000; **342:** 145–53.

Abbreviations

AB	alpha blocker	BP	blood pressure
ABCD	Appropriate Blood Pressure Control in Diabetes	BPLT	Blood Pressure Lowering Treatment
ABP	ambulatory BP	BS	blood sugar
ABPM	ambulatory blood pressure monitoring	CAD	coronary artery disease
		CAI	carotid amplification index
ACC	associated clinical conditions	CALM	Candesartan and Lisinopril Microalbuminuria
ACC	American College of Cardiology	CAPPP	Captopril Prevention Project
ACE	angiotensin-converting enzyme	CARE	Cholesterol and Recurrent Events
ACEI	angiotensin-converting enzyme inhibitor	CASTEL	Cardiovascular Study in the Elderly
ADVANCE	Action in Diabetes and Vascular Disease—PreterAx AND DiamicroN MR Controlled Evaluation	CCB	calcium channel blocker
		CHD	coronary heart disease
		CHF	congestive heart failure
		CI	confidence interval
AFCAPS/ TexCAPS	Air Force/Texas Coronary Atherosclerosis Prevention Study	COPD	chronic obstructive pulmonary disease
		CT	computed tomography
AGT	angiotensinogen	CV	cardiovascular
AHA	American Heart Association	CVD	cardiovascular disease
ALLHAT	Antihypertensive and Lipid Lowering to prevent Heart Attack Trial	CVS	cardiova
		CXR	chest X-ray
		DAIS	Diabetes Atherosclerosis Intervention Study
aLVH	appropriate LVH		
ANBP2	Australian National Blood Pressure study 2	DBP	diastolic blood pressure
APA	aldosterone producing adenomas	DCCT	Diabetes Control and Complications Trial
ARB	angiotensin receptor blocker	DHP	dihydropyrindine
ARR	aldosterone renin ratio	DM	diabetes mellitus
ASCOT	Anglo Scandinavian Cardiac Outcomes Trial	ECG	electrocardiogram
		ECTIM	Etude Cas-Témoins sur l'Infarctus du Myocarde
AT	angiotensin		
AVS	arterial venous sampling	EF	ejection fraction
BHS	British Hypertension Society	ELITE	Evaluation of Losartan in the Elderly Study
BMI	body mass index		

ELSA	European Lacidipine/Study of Atherosclerosis	ISA	intrinsic sympathomimetic activity
ENCORE	Evaluation of Nifedipine and Cerivastatin on Recovery of Endothelial function	ISH	International Society of Hypertension
		ISH	isolated systolic hypertension
ENOS	endothelial nitric oxide syn-thase	IVRT	isovolumetric relaxation time
		IVUS	intravascular ultrasound
ERT	estrogen replacement therapy	JNC	Joint National Committee
ESRF	end-stage renal failure	LDL	low-density lipoprotein
ET1	Endothelin-1	LIFE	Losartan Intervention For End-point reduction
ETA	endothelin A		
ETB	endothelin B	LIPID	Long-term Intervention with Pravastatin in Ischaemic Disease Study
EWPHE	European Working Party on High Blood Pressure in the Elderly		
		LOD	Logorphanetic odds
FACET	Fosinopril vs Amlodipine Cardiovascular Events Trial	LVH	left ventricular hypertrophy
		MAP	mitogen-activated protein
FFA	free fatty acids	MCE	major cardiovascular events
FH	family history	MI	myocardial infarction
FSS	fluid shear stress	MICRO-	Microalbuminuria and
GITS	gastrointestinal therapeutic system	HOPE	Renal Outcomes Heart Outcomes Prevention Evaluation trial
GOALLS	Getting to Appropriate LDL cholesterol Levels with Simvastatin	MIDAS	Multicenter Isradipine Diuretic Atherosclerosis Study
GRA	Glucocorticoid remediable hyperaldosteronism	MIRACL	Myocardial Ischaemia Reduction with Aggressive Cholesterol Lowering
HCTZ	hydrochlorothiazide		
HDL	high-density lipoprotein	MMSE	Mini Mental State Examination
HEP	Hypertension in Elderly Patients in Primary Care		
		MONICA	Monitoring Trends and Determinants of Cardiovascular Disease
HERS	Heart and Estrogen/progestin Replacement Study		
HF	heart failure	MRC1	Medical Research Council trials in mild hypertension and (MRC2) in older adults
HMG	hydroxy-methylglutaryl		
HOPE	Heart Outcomes Prevention Evaluation		
		MRI	magnetic resonance imaging
HOT	Hypertension Optimal Treatment	NHANES	National Heart and Nutrition Examination Surveys
HRT	hormone replacement therapy	NICS-EH	National Intervention Cooperative Study in Elderly Hypertensives study
HYVET	HYpertension in the Very Elderly Trial		
IC	intronic conversion	NIDDM	non-insulin dependent diabetes mellitus
IDDM	insulin-dependent diabetes		
IGT	impaired glucose tolerance	NO	nitric oxide
iLVH	inappropriate LVH	NORDIL	Nordic Diltiazem
INSIGHT	Intervention as a Goal in Hypertension Treatment	NSAID	non-steriodal anti-inflammatory drug

NT	no treatment	SHEP	Systolic Hypertension in the Elderly Programme
NYHA	New York Heart Association		
PA	primary aldosteronism	SIGN	Scottish Intercollegiate Guidelines Network
PAC	plasma aldosterone concentration		
		SMAC	Standing Medical Advisory Committee
PGWB	Psychological General Well-Being		
		SRIF	infusion of somatostatin
PKB	protein kinase B	STONE	Shanghai Trial of Nifedipine in the Elderly
PP	pulse pressure		
PPAR	peroxisome proliferator-activated receptor	STOP-2	Swedish Trial of Old Patients with Hypertension-2
PRA	plasma renin activity	SYST-CHINA	Systolic Hypertension in China trial
PREVENT	Prospective Randomized Evaluation of the Vascular Effects of Norvasc Trial		
		SYST-EUR	Systolic Hypertension in Europe trial
PROBE	Prospective, Randomized, Open, Blinded End-point	TC	total serum cholesterol
		TC:HDL-C	total serum cholesterol: HDL cholesterol
PROGRESS	Perindopril Protection against Recurrent Stroke Study		
		TDT	transmission disequilibrium testing
pt-years	patient treatment years		
PWV	pulse wave velocity	THALDO	tetrahydroaldosterone
QCA	quantitative coronary angiography	TIA	transient ischaemic attack
		TNA	tumour necrosis factor
QTL	Quantitative Trait Locus	TOD	target organ damage
RAAS	renin–angiotensin–aldosterone system	U and E	serum urea and electrolytes
		UK	United Kingdom
RESOLVD	Randomised Evaluation of Strategies for Left Ventricular Dysfunction	UKPDS	UK Prospective Diabetes Study
		US	ultrasound
RI	renal insufficiency	USA	United States of America
RF	risk factor	VALUE	Valsartan Anithypertensive Long-term Use Evaluation
RR	relative risk		
SBP	systolic blood pressure	VHAS	Verapamil in Hypertension and Atherosclerosis Study
SCOPE	Study on COgnition and Prognosis in Elderly patients with hypertension		
		vs	*versus*
		WHIMS	Women's Health Initiative Memory Study
SECRET	Study on Evaluation of Candesartan cilexetil after REnal Transplantation		
		WHO	World Health Organization
Ser cr	serum creatinine	WOSCOPS	West of Scotland Coronary Prevention Study

Index of Papers Reviewed

Guidelines

Part II Interface: hypertension and other cardiovascular risk factors

D Curb, SL Pressel, JA Cutler, PJ Savage, WB Applegate, H Black, G Camel, BR Davis, PH Frost, N Gonzalez, G Guthrie, A Oberman, GH Rutan, J Stamler; Systolic Hypertension in the Elderly Program Cooperative Research Group. Effect of diuretic-based antihypertensive treatment on cardiovascular disease risk in older diabetic patients with isolated systolic hypertension. *JAMA* 1996; 276: 1886–92. **142**

Diabetes Atherosclerosis Intervention Study Investigators. Effects of fenofibrate on progression of coronary artery disease in type 2 diabetes: the Diabetes Atherosclerosis Intervention Study, a randomized study. *Lancet* 2001; 357: 905–10. **146**

JR Downs, M Clearfield, S Weis, E Whitney, DR Shapiro, PA Beere, A Langendorfer, EA Stein, W Kruyer, AM Gotto Jr. Primary prevention of acute coronary events with lovastatin in men and women with average cholesterol levels : results of AFCAPS/TexCAPS, Air Force/Texas Coronary Atherosclerosis Prevention Study. *JAMA* 1998; 279: 1615–22. **157**

D Einhorn, M Rendell, J Rosenzweig, JW Egan, AL Mathisen, RL Schneider; the Pioglitazone 027 Study Group. Pioglitazone hydrochloride in combination with metformin in the treatment of type 2 diabetes mellitus: a randomized, placebo-controlled study. *Clin Ther* 2000; 22: 1395–409.

RO Estacio, BW Jeffers, WR Hiatt, SL Biggerstaff, N Gifford, RW Schrier. The effect of nisoldipine as compared with enalapril on cardiovascular outcomes in patients with non-insulin-dependent diabetes and hypertension. *N Engl J Med.* 1998; 338: 645–52. **152**

EUROASPIRE I and II Group. Clinical reality of coronary prevention guidelines: a comparison of EUROASPIRE I and II in nine countries. *Lancet* 2001; 357: 995–1001. **162**

M Farnier, J-J Portal, P Maigret. Efficacy of atorvastatin compared with simvastatin in patients with hypercholesterolaemia. *J Cardiovasc Pharmacol Ther* 2000; 5: 27–32. **173**

DJ Freeman, J Norrie, N Sattar, RD Neely, SM Cobbe, I Ford, C Isles, AR Lorimer, PW Macfarlane, JH McKillop, CJ Packard, J Shepherd, A Gaw. Pravastatin and the development of diabetes mellitus: evidence for a protective treatment effect in the West of Scotland Coronary Prevention Study. *Circulation* 2001; 103: 357–62. **147**

P Gaede, P Vvedel, H-H Parving, O Pederson. Intensified multifactorial intervention in patients with type 2 diabetes mellitus and microalbuminuria: The Steno type 2 randomized study. *Lancet* 1999; 353: 617–22. **148**

F Garmendia, AS Brown, I Reiber, PC Adams. Attaining United States and European guideline LDL-cholesterol levels with simvastatin in patients with coronary heart disease (the GOALLS study). *Curr Med Res Opin* 2000; 16: 208–19. **169**

RB Goldberg, MJ Mellies, FM Sacks, LA Moye, BV Howard, WJ Howard, BR Davis, TG Cole, MA Pfeffer, E Braunwald; the Care Investigators. Cardiovascular events and their reduction with pravastatin in diabetic and glucose-intolerant myocardial infarction survivors with average cholesterol levels: subgroup analyses in the Cholesterol and Recurrent Events (CARE) trial. *Circulation* 1998; 98: 2513–19. **145**

L Hansson, LH Lindholm, L Niskanen, J Lanke, T Hedner, A Niklason, K Luomanmaki, B Dahlöf, U de Faire, C Morlin, BE Karlberg, PO Wester, JE Bjorck. Effect of angiotensin-converting-enzyme inhibition compared with conventional therapy on cardiovascular morbidity and mortality in hypertension:

the Captopril Prevention Project (CAPPP) randomized trial. *Lancet* 1999; 353: 611–16. **138**

L Hansson, A Zanchetti, SG Carruthers, B Dahlöf, D Elmfeldt, S Julius, J Menard, KH Rahn, H Wedel, S Westerling; HOT Study Group. Effects of intensive blood pressure lowering and low-dose aspirin in patients with hypertension: principal results of the Hypertension Optimal Treatment (HOT) randomized trial. *Lancet* 1998; 351: 1755–62. **140**

PJ Harvey, LM Wing, J Savage, D Molloy. The effects of different types and doses of oestrogen replacement therapy on clinic and ambulatory blood pressure and the renin–angiotensin system in normotensive postmenopausal women. *J Hypertens* 1999, 17: 405–14. **179**

TJ Harris, DG Cook, PD Wicks, FP Cappuccio. Ethnic differences in use of hormone replacement therapy: community based survey. *Br Med J* 2000; 319: 610–11. **189**

Heart Outcomes Prevention Evaluations (HOPE) Study Investigators. Effects of ramipril on cardiovascular and microvascular outcomes in people with diabetes mellitus; results of the HOPE study and MICRO-HOPE substudy. *Lancet* 2000; 355: 253–9. **143**

DM Herrington, DM Reboussin, KB Brosnihan, PC Sharp, SA Shumaker, TE Snyder, CD Furberg, GJ Kowalchuk, TD Stuckey, WJ Rogers, DH Givens, D Waters. Effects of estrogen replacement on the regression of coronary artery atherosclerosis. *N Engl J Med* 2000; 343: 522–9. **185**

L Hooper, CD Summerbell, JPT Higgins, RL Thompson, NE Capps, GD Smith, RA Riemersma, S Ebrahim. Dietary fat intake and prevention of cardiovascular disease: systematic review. *BMJ* 2001; 322: 757–63. **166**

FB Hu, MJ Stampfer, JE Manson, F Grodstein, GA Colditz, FE Speizer, WC Willett. Trends in the incidence of coronary heart disease and changes in diet and lifestyle in women. *N Engl J Med* 2000; 343: 530–7. **187**

S Hulley, D Grady, T Bush, C Furberg, D Herrington, B Riggs, E Vittinghoff, for the Heart and Estrogen/progestin Replacement Study (HERS) Research Group. Randomized trial of estrogen plus progestin for secondary prevention of coronary heart disease in postmenopausal women. *JAMA* 1998; 280: 605–13. **184**

P Jones, S Kafonek, I Laurora, D Hunninghake. Comparative dose efficacy study of atorvastatin, lovastatin, and fluvastatin ion patients with hypercholesterolaemia (the CURVES study). *Am J Cardiol* 1998; 81: 582–7. **171**

S Kim-Schulze, WL Lowe, W Schnaper. Estrogen stimulates delayed mitogen-activated protein kinase activity in human endothelial cells via an autocrine loop that involves basic fibroblast growth factor. *Circulation* 1998; 98: 413–21. **183**

RH Knopp. Drug treatment of lipid disorders. *N Engl J Med* 1999; 341: 498–510. **169**

KC Light, AL Hinderliter, SG West, KM Grewen, JF Steege, A Sherwood, SS Girdler. Hormone replacement improves haemodynamic profile and left ventricular geometry in hypertensive and normotensive postmenopausal women. *J Hypertens* 2001; 19: 269–78. **182**

LH Lindholm, L Hansson, T Ekbom, B Dahlöf, J Lanke, E Linjer, B Schersten, PO Wester, T Hedner, U de Faire, for the STOP Hypertension-2 Study Group. Comparison of antihypertensive treatments in preventing cardiovascular events in elderly diabetic patients: results from the Swedish Trial in Old Patients with Hypertension-2. *J Hypertens* 2000; 18:1671–5. **144**

W März, H Wollschläger, G Kleinm, A Neiß, M Wehling. Safety of low-density lipoprotein cholesterol reduction with atorvastatin versus simvastatin in a coronary heart disease population (the TARGET TANGIBLE trial). *Am J Cardiol* 1999; 84: 7–13. **173**

ER Mathieson, E Hommel, HP Hansen, UM Smidt, H-H Parving. Randomized control trial of long-term efficacy of captopril on preservation of kidney function in normotensive patients with insulin-dependent diabetes and microalbuminuria. *BMJ* 1999; 319: 24–5. **150**

H Neil, G Fowler, H Patel, Z Eminton, S Maton. An assessment of the efficacy of atorvastatin in achieving LDL cholesterol target levels in patients with coronary heart disease: a general practice study. *IJCP* 1999; 53: 422–6. **170**

B Pitt, D Waters, WV Brown, AJ van Boven, L Schwartz, LM Title, D Eisenberg, L Shurzinske, LS McCormick. Aggressive lipid-lowering therapy compared with angioplasty in stable coronary artery disease. *N Engl J Med* 1999; 341: 70–6. **174**

P Primatesta, NR Poulter. Lipid concentrations and the use of lipid lowering drugs: evidence from a national cross sectional survey. *BMJ* 2000; 321: 1322–5. **164**

U Pripp, G Hall, G Csemiczky, S Eksborg, BM Landgren, K Schenck-Gustafsson. A randomized trial on effects of hormone therapy on ambulatory blood pressure and lipoprotein levels in women with coronary artery disease. *J Hypertens* 1999; 17: 1379–86. **179**

HB Rubins, SJ Robins, D Collins, CL Fye, JW Anderson, MB Elam, FH Faas, E Linares, EJ Schaefer, G Schectman, TJ Wilt, J Wittes. Gemfibrozil for the secondary prevention of coronary heart disease in men with low levels of high-density lipoprotein cholesterol. *N Engl J Med* 1999; 341: 410–18. **167**

S Shumaker, BA Reboussin, MA Espeland, SR Rapp, WL McBee, M Dailey, D Bowen, T Terrell, BN Jones. The Women's Health Initiative Memory Study (WHIMS): a trial of the effect of estrogen therapy in preventing and slowing the progression of dementia. *Control Clin Trials* 1998; 19: 604–21. **191**

GG Schwartz, AG Olsson, MD Ezekowitz, P Ganz, MF Oliver, D Waters, A Zeiher, BR Chaitman, S Leslie, T Stern; Myocardial Ischemia Reduction with Aggressive Cholesterol Lowering (MIRACL) Study Investigators. Effects of atorvastatin on early recurrent ischemic events in acute coronary syndromes. The MIRACL study: a randomized controlled trial. *JAMA* 2001; 285: 1711–18. **160**

S Seshadri, GL Zornberg, LE Derby, MW Myers, H Jick, DA Drachman. Postmenopausal estrogen replacement therapy and the risk of Alzheimer's disease. *Arch Neurol* 2001; 58: 435–40. **188**

JA Simon, J Hsia, JA Cauley, C Richards, F Harris, J Fong, E Barrett-Connor, SB Hulley. Postmenopausal hormone therapy and risk of stroke. *Circulation* 2001; 103: 638. **186**

L Sourander, T Rajala, I Räihä, J Makinen, R Erkkola, H Helenius. Cardiovascular and cancer morbidity and mortality and sudden cardiac death in postmenopausal women on oestrogen replacement therapy (ERT). *Lancet* 1998; 352: 1965–9. **177**

MJ Stampfer, FB Hu, JE Manson, EB Rimm, WC Willett. Primary prevention of coronary heart disease in women through diet and lifestyle. *N Engl J Med* 2000; 3436: 16–22. **186**

U Stenestrand, L Wallentin, for the Swedish Register of Cardiac Intensive Care. Early statin treatment following acute myocardial infarction and 1-year survival. *JAMA* 2001; 285: 430–6. **160**

IM Stratton, AI Adler, HA Neil, DR Matthews, SE Manley, CA Cull, D Hadden, RC Turner, RR Holman, on behalf of the UK prospective Diabetes Study Group. Association of glycaemia with macrovascular and microvascular complications of type 2 diabetes (UKPDS 35): prospective observational study. *BMJ* 2000; 321:405–12. **136**

BH Sung, M Ching, JL Izzo Jr, P Dandona, MF Wilson. Estrogen improves abnormal norepinephrine-induced vasoconstriction in postmenopausal women. *J Hypertens* 1999, 17: 523–8. **181**

JL Tang, JM Armitage, T Lancaster, CA Silagy, GH Fowler, HA Neil. Systematic review of dietary intervention trials to lower blood total cholesterol in free-living subjects. *BMJ* 1998; 316: 1213–20. **165**

P Tatti, M Pahor, RP Byington, P Di Mauro, R Guarisco, G Strollo, F Strollo. Outcome results of the Fosinopril versus Amlodipine Cardiovascular Events randomized Trial (FACET) in patients with hypertension and NIDDM. *Diabetes Care* 1999; 21: 597–603. **151**

J Tuomilehto, D Rastenyte, WH Berkenhager, L Thijs, R Antikainen, CJ Bulpitt, AE Fletcher, F Forette, A Goldhaber, P Palatini, C Sarti, R Fagard; Systolic Hypertension in Europe Trial Investigators. Effects of calcium channel blockade in older patients with diabetes and systolic hypertension. *N Engl J Med* 1999; 340: 677–84. **139**

United Kingdom Prospective Diabetes Study Group. Effect of intensive blood glucose control with metformin on complications in overweight patients with type 2 diabetes: UKPDS 34. *Lancet* 1998; 352: 854–65. **131**

United Kingdom Prospective Diabetes Study Group. Efficacy of atenolol and captopril in reducing risk of macrovascular and microvascular complications in type 2 diabetes: UKPDS 39. *BMJ* 1998; 317: 713–20. **133**

United Kingdom Prospective Diabetes Study Group. Intensive blood-glucose control with sulphonylureas or insulin compared with conventional treatment and risk of complications in patients with type 2 diabetes: UKPDS 33. *Lancet* 1998; 352: 837–53. **130**

United Kingdom Prospective Diabetes Study Group. Tight blood pressure control and risk of macrovascular and microvascular complications in type 2 diabetes: UKPDS 38. *BMJ* 1998; 317: 703–13. **132**

TK Waddell, C Rajkumar, JD Cameron, GL Jennings, AM Dart, BA Kingwell. Withdrawal of hormone therapy for 4 weeks decreases arterial compliance in postmenopausal women. *J Hypertens* 1999; 17: 413–18. **181**

HD White, J Simes, NE Anderson, GJ Hankey, JD Watson, D Hunt, DM Colquhoun, P Glasziou, S MacMahon, AC Kirby, MJ West, AM Tonkin. Pravastatin therapy and the risk of stroke. *N Engl J Med* 2000; 343: 317–26. **161**

AS Wierzbicki, PJ Lumb, Y Semra, G Chik, ER Christ, MA Crook. Atorvastatin compared with simvastatin-based therapies in the management of severe familial hyperlipidaemias. *Q J Med* 1999; 92: 387–94. **171**

MI Wiggam, SJ Hunter, AB Atkinson, CN Ennis, JS Henry, JN Browne, B Sheridan, PM Bell. Captopril does not improve insulin action in essential hypertension: a double-blind placebo-controlled study. *J Hypertens* 1998; 16: 1651–7. **153**

K Yaffe, L Lui, D Grady, J Cauley, J Kramer, SR Cummings. Cognitive decline in women relation to non-protein-bound oestradiol concentrations. *Lancet* 2000; 356: 708–12. **188**

K Yaffe, K Krueger, S Sarkar, D Grady, E Barrett-Connor, DA Cox, T Nickelsen; Multiple Outcomes of Raloxifene

Evaluation Investigators. Cognitive function in postmenopausal women treated with raloxifene. *N Engl J Med* 2001: 344(16): 1207–13. **188**

Part III Hypertension: emerging concepts

H Abriel, J Loffig, JF Rebhun, JH Pratt, L Schild, JD Horisberger, D Rotin, O Staub. Defective regulation of the epithelial Na+ channel by Nedd4 in Liddle's syndrome. *J Clin Invest* 1999; 103: 667–73. **239**

EH Baker, YB Dong, GA Sagnella, M Rothwell, AK Onipinla, ND Markandu, FP Cappuccio, DG Cook, A Persu, P Corvol, X Jeunemaitre, ND Carter, GA MacGregor. Association of hypertension with T594M mutation in β subunit of epithelial sodium channels in black people resident in London. *Lancet* 1998: 351: 1388–92. **240**

I Barroso, M Gurnell, VE Crowley, M Agostini, JW Schwabe, MA Soos, GL Maslen, TD Williams, H Lewis, AJ Schafer, VK Chatterjee, S O'Rahilly. Dominant negative mutations in human PPAR associated with severe insulin resistance, diabetes mellitus and hypertension. *Nature* 1999: 402(6764): 880–3. **224**

AV Benjafield, BJ Morris. Association analyses of endothelial nitric oxide synthase gene polymorphisms in essential hypertension. *Am J Hypertens* 2000; 13: 994–8. **206**

E Brand, N Chatelain, B Keavney, M Caulfield, L Citterio, J Connell, D Grobbee, S Schmidt, H Schunkert, H Schuster, AM Sharma, F Soubrier. Evaluation of the angiotensinogen locus in human essential hypertension: a European study. *Hypertension* 1998; 31: 725–9. **198/233**

E Brand, N Chatelain, P Mulatero, I Fery, K Curnew, X Jeunemaître, P Corvol, L Pascoe, F Soubrier. Structural analysis and evaluation of the aldosterone synthase gene in hypertension. *Hypertension* 1998; 32: 198–204. **234**

G Candy, N Samani, G Norton, A Woodiwiss, I Radevski, A Wheatley, J Cockcroft, IP Hall. Association analysis of β₂ adrenoceptor polymorphisms with hypertension in a black African population. *J Hypertens* 2000, 18: 167–72. **208**

CJ Clark, E Davies, NH Anderson, R Farmer, EC Friel, R Fraser, JM Connell. α-adducin and angiotensin 1-converting enzyme polymorphisms in essential hypertension. *Hypertension* 2000; 36: 990–4. **203**

SJ Cleland, JR Petrie, M Small, HL Elliott, JM Connell. Insulin action is associated with endothelial function in hypertension and type 2 diabetes. *Hypertension* 2000; 35(1 Pt 2): 507–11. **218**

E Davies, CD Holloway, MC Ingram, GC Inglis, EC Friel, C Morrison, NH Anderson, R Fraser, JM Connell. Aldosterone excretion rate and blood pressure in essential hypertension are related to polymorphic differences in the aldosterone synthase gene (*CYP11B2*). *Hypertension* 1999; 33: 703–7. **201/235**

JA Ellis, M Stebbing, SB Harrap. Association of the Human Y chromosome with high blood pressure in the general population. *Hypertension* 2000; 36: 731–3. **211**

CE Fardella, L Mosso, C Gomez-Sanchez, P Cortes, J Soto, L Gomez, M Pinto, A Huete, E Oestreicher, A Foradori, J Montero. Primary hyperaldosteronism in essential hypertensives: prevalence, biochemical profile and molecular biology. *J Clin Endocrinol Metab* 2000; 85: 1863–7. **249**

E Ferrannini, A Natali, B Capaldo, M Lohtovirta, S Jacob, H Yki-Jarvinen. Insulin resistance, hyperinsulinemia, and blood pressure: role of age and obesity. *Hypertension* 1997; 30: 1144–9. **214**

T Heise, K Magnusson, L Heinemann, PT Sawicki. Insulin resistance and the effect of insulin on blood pressure in essential hypertension. *Hypertension* 1998; 32: 243–8. **215**

V Herrmann, R Buscher, MM Go, KM Ring, JK Hofer, MT Kailasam, DT O'Connor, RJ Parmer, PA Insel. β_2 adrenergic receptor polymorphisms at codon 16, cardiovascular phenotypes and essential hypertension in whites and African Americans. *Am J Hypertens* 2000; 13: 1021–6. **208**

ZY Jiang, YW Lin, A Clemont, EP Feener, KD Hein, M Igarashi, T Yamauchi, MF White, GL King. Characterization of selective resistance to insulin signaling in the vasculature of obese Zucker (fa/fa) rats. *J Clin Invest* 1999; 104: 447–57. **219**

A Kamitani, ZYH Wong, R Fraser, DL Davies, JM Connor, CJ Foy, GC Watt, SB Harrap. Human α-adducin gene, blood pressure, and sodium metabolism. *Hypertension* 1998; 32: 138–43. **203**

N Kato, T Sugiyama, H Morita, T Nabika, H Kurihara, Y Yamori, Y Yazaki. Lack of evidence for association between the endothelial nitric oxide synthase gene and hypertension. *Hypertension* 1999; 33: 933–6. **205**

F Kim, B Gallis, MA Corson. TNF-α inhibits flow and insulin signaling leading to NO production in aortic endothelial cells. *Am J Physiol Cell Physiol* 2001; 280(5): C1057–65. **223**

K Kuboki ZY Jiang, N Takahara, SW Ha, M Igarashi, T Yamauchi, EP Feener, TP Herbert, CJ Rhodes, GL King. Regulation of endothelial constitutive nitric oxide synthase gene expression in endothelial cells and in vivo : a specific vascular action of insulin. *Circulation* 2000; 101(6): 676–81. **220**

H Laine, MJ Knuuti, U Ruotsalainen, M Raitakiari, H Iida, J Kapanen, O Kirvela, M Haaparanta, H Yki-Jarvinen, P Nuutila. Insulin resistance in essential hypertension is characterized by impaired insulin stimulation of blood flow in skeletal muscle. *Hypertension* 1998: 16: 211–9. **217**

D Levy, AL DeStefano, MG Larson, CJ O'Donnell, RP Lifton, H Gavras, LA Cupples, RH Myers. Genome scan linkage results for longitudinal blood pressure phenotypes in subjects from the Framingham Heart Study. *Hypertension* 2000; 36(4): 469–70. **209**

PO Lim, E Dow, G Brennan, RT Jung, TM MacDonald. High prevalence of primary hyperaldosteronism in the Tayside hypertension clinic population. *J Hum Hypertens* 2000; 14: 311–15. **250**

PO Lim, RT Jung, TM MacDonald. Raised aldosterone to renin ratio predicts antihypertensive efficacy of spironolactone: a prospective cohort follow-up study. *Br J Clin Pharmacol* 1999; 48: 756–60. **254**

WR Litchfield, BF Anderson, RJ Weiss, RP Lifton, RG Dluhy. Intracranial aneurysm and hemorrhagic stroke in glucocorticoid remediable aldosterone. *Hypertension* 1998: 31: 445–50. **244**

K-C Loh, ES Koay, M-C Khaw, SC Emmanuel, WF Young Jr. Prevalence of primary aldosteronism among Asian hypertensive patients in Singapore. *J Clin Endocrinol Metab* 2000; 85(8): 2854–9. **248**

AA MacConnachie, KF Kelly, A McNamara, S Loughlin, IJ Gates, GC Inglis, A Jamieson, JM Connell, NE Haites. Rapid diagnosis and identification of cross-over sites in patients with glucocorticoid remediable aldosteronism. *J Clin Endocrinol Metal* 1998; 83: 4328–31. **246**

SB Magill, H Raff, JL Shaker, RC Brickner, TE Knechtges, ME Kehoe, JW Findling. Comparison of adrenal vein sampling and computed tomography in the differentiation of primary aldosteronism. *J Clin Endocrinol Metab* 2001; 86(3): 1066–71. **258**

AP Guerin, J Blacher, B Pannier, SJ Marchais, ME Safar, GM London. Impact of aortic stiffness attenuation on survival of patients in end-stage renal failure. *Circulation* 2001; 103: 987–92. **300**

L Hansson, A Zanchetti, SG Carruthers, B Dahlöf, D Elmfeldt, S Julius, J Menard, KH Rahn, H Wedel, S Westerling; HOT Study Group. Effects of intensive blood-pressure lowering and low-dose aspirin in patients with hypertension: principle results of the Hypertension Optimal Treatment (HOT) randomized trial. *Lancet* 1998; 351: 1755–62. **333**

K Harada, I Komuro, I Shiojima, D Hayashi, S Kudoh, T Mizuno, K Kijima, H Matsubara, T Sugaya, K Murakami, Y Yazaki. Pressure overload induces cardiac hypertrophy in angiotensin II type 1A receptor knockout mice. *Circulation* 1998; 97: 1952–9. **279/315**

GL Jennings, J Wong, in: L Hansson, WH Birkenhäger (eds). Reversibility of left ventricular hypertrophy and malfunction by antihypertensive treatment. *Handbook of Hypertension*, Volume 18: *Assessment of Hypertensive Organ Damage*. Amsterdam: Elsevier Science 1997, p6. **317**

W Ji-Guang, JA Staessen, G Lansheng, L Lisheng. Chinese trial on isolated systolic hypertension in the elderly. *Arch Intern Med* 2000; 160(2): 211–20. **325**

JM Jokiniitty, SK Majahalme, MAP Kahonen, MT Tuomisto, VMH Turjanmaa. Prediction of blood pressure level and need for antihypertensive medication: 10 years of follow-up. *J Hypertens* 2001; 19: 1193–201. **294**

BE Karlberg, L-E Lins, K Hermansson for the TEES Group. Efficacy and safety of telmisartan, a selective AT$_1$ receptor antagonist, compared with enalapril in elderly patients with primary hypertension. *J Hypertens* 1999, 17: 293–302. **271**

MC Lansang, SY Osei, DA Prive, NDL Fisher, NK Hollenberg. Renal haemodynamic and hormonal responses to the angiotensin II antagonist candesartan. *Hypertension* 2000; 36: 834–8. **280**

S Laurent, P Boutouyrie, R Asmar, I Gautier, B Laloux, L Guize, P Ducimetiere, A Benetos. Aortic stiffness is an independent predictor of all-cause and cardiovascular mortality in hypertensive patients. *Hypertension* 2001; 37(5): 1236–41. **302**

AF Lever, DJ Hole, CR Gillis, IR McCallum, GT McInnes, PL MacKinnon, PA Meredith, LS Murray, JL Reid, JW Robertson. Do inhibitors of angiotensin-I-converting enzyme protect against risk of cancer. *Lancet* 1998; 352: 179–84. **329**

JM Mallion, JP Siche, Y Lacourcière, and the Telmisartan Blood Pressure Monitoring Group. ABPM comparison of the antihypertensive profiles of the selective angiotensin II receptor antagonists telmisartan and losartan in patients with mild to moderate hypertension. *J Hum Hypertens* 1999, 13: 657–64. **269**

K Malmqvist, T Kahan, M Dahl. Angiotensin II type 1 (AT$_1$) in hypertensive women: candesartan cilexetil versus enalapril or hydrochlorothiazide. *Am J Hypertens* 2000; 13: 504–11. **272**

K Malmqvist, T Kahan, M Edner, C Held, A Hagg, L Lind, R Muller-Brunotte, F Nystrom, KP Ohman, MD Osbakken, J Ostergern. Regression of left ventricular hypertrophy in human hypertension with irbesartan. *J Hypertens* 2001; 19: 1167–76. **278**

G Mancia, A Zanchetti, E Agabiti-Rosei, G Benemio, R De Cesaris, R Fogari, A Pessina, C Porcellati, A Rappelli, A Salvetti, B Trimarco, for the SAMPLE Study Group. Ambulatory blood pressure is superior to clinic blood pressure in predicting treatment-induced regression of left ventricular hypertrophy. *Circulation* 1997; 95: 1464–70. **295**

L Mazzolai, M Maillard, J Rossat, J Nussberger, HR Brunner, M Burnier. Angiotensin II receptor blockade in normotensive subjects: a direct comparison of three AT_1 receptor antagonists. *Hypertension* 1999; 33: 850–5. **267**

RS McKelvie, S Yusuf, D Pericak, A Avezum, RJ Burns, J Probstfield, RT Tsuyuki, M White, J Rouleau, R Latini, A Maggioni, J Young, J Pogue; the RESOLVD Pilot Study Investigators. Comparison of candesartan, enalapril, and their combination in congestive heart failure. Randomized Evaluation of Strategies for Left Ventricular Dysfunction (RESOLVD) Pilot Study. *Circulation* 1999; 100: 1056–64. **276**

CE Mogensen, S Neldam, I Tikkanen, S Oren, R Viskoper, RW Watts, ME Cooper. Randomized controlled trial of dual blockade of renin–angiotensin system in patients with hypertension, microalbuminuria, and non-insulin dependant diabetes: the Candesartan and Lisinopril Microalbuminuria (CALM) study. *BMJ* 2000; 321: 1440–4. **281**

E O'Brien, B Waeber, G Parati, J Staessen, MG Myers. Blood pressure measuring devices: recommendations of the European Society of Hypertension. *BMJ* 2001; 322: 531–6. **288**

EO Ofili, JD Cohen, JA St Vrain, A Pearson, TJ Martin, ND Uy, R Castello, AJ Labovitz. Effect of treatment of isolated systolic hypertension on left ventricular mass. *JAMA* 1998; 279: 778–80. **319**

T Ohkubo, A Hozawa, K Nagai, M Kikuya, I Tsuji, S Ito, H Satoh, S Hisamichi, Y Imai. Prediction of stroke by ambulatory blood pressure monitoring versus screening blood pressure measurements in a general population: the Ohasama study. *J Hypertens* 2000; 18: 847–54. **292**

T Ohkubo, Y Imai, I Tsuji, K Nagai, S Ito, H Satoh, S Hisamichi. Reference values for 24-hour ambulatory blood pressure monitoring based on a prognostic criterion. The Ohasama study. *Hypertension* 1998; 32: 255–9. **291**

DH O'Leary, JF Polak, RA Kronmal, TA Manolio, GL Burke, SK Wolfson Jr, for the Cardiovascular Health Study Collaborative Research Group. Carotid-artery intima and media thickness as a risk factor for myocardial infarction and stroke in older adults. *N Engl J Med* 1999; 340: 14–22. **304**

M Pahor, BM Psaty, MH Alderman, WB Applegate, JD Williamson, C Cavazzini, CD Furberg. Health outcomes associated with calcium antagonists compared with other first-line antihypertensive therapies: a meta-analysis of randomized controlled trials. *Lancet* 2000; 356: 1949–54. **330**

B Pitt, P Poole-Wilson, R Segal, FA Martinez, K Dickstein, AJ Camm, MA Konstam, G Riegger, GH Klinger, J Neaton, D Sharma, B Thiyagarajan. Effects of losartan compared with captopril on mortality in patients with symptomatic heart failure: randomized trial—the Losartan Heart Failure Survival Study ELITE II. *Lancet* 2000; 355: 1582–7. **275**

B Pitt, R Segal, FA Martinez, G Meurers, AJ Cowley, I Thomas, PC Deedwania, DE Ney, DB Snavely, PI Chang. Randomized trial of losartan versus captopril in patients over 65 with heart failure (Evaluation of Losartan in the Elderly Study, ELITE). *Lancet* 1997; 349: 747–52. **274**

LE Ramsay, B Williams, GD Johnston, G MacGregor, L Poston, J Potter, N Poulter, G Russell. Guidelines for management of hypertension: report of the Third Working Party of the British Hypertension Society. *J Hum Hypertens* 1999; 13: 569–92. **286**

J Redon, C Campos, ML Narciso, G MacGregor, L Poston, J Potter, N Poulter, G Russell. Prognostic value of ambulatory blood pressure monitoring in refractory hypertension: a prospective study. *Hypertension* 1998; 31: 712–18. **293**

GAJ Riegger, H Bouzo, P Petr, J Munz, R Spacek, H Pethig, V von Behren, M George, H Arens; Symptom, Tolerability, Response to Exercise Trial of Candesartan Cilexetil in Heart Failure (STRETCH) Investigators. Improvement in exercise tolerance and symptoms of congestive heart failure during treatment with candesartan cilexetil. *Circulation* 1999; 100: 2224–30. **276**

RE Schmieder, MP Schlaich, AU Klingbeil, P Martus. Update of reversal of left ventricular hypertrophy in essential hypertension (a meta-analysis of all randomized double-blind studies until December 1996). *Nephrol Dial Transplant* 1998; 13: 564–9. **317**

JA Staessen, R Fagard, L Thijs, H Celis, GG Arabidze, WH Birkenhager, CJ Bulpitt, PW de Leeuw, CT Dollery, AE Fletcher, F Forette, G Leonetti, C Nachev, ET O'Brien, J Rosenfeld, JL Rodicio, J Tuomilehto, A Zanchetti; the Systolic Hypertension in Europe (Syst-Eur) Trial Investigators. Randomized double-blind comparison of placebo and active treatment for older patients with isolated systolic hypertension. *Lancet* 1997; 350: 757–64. **324**

JA Staessen, L Thijs, R Fagard, ET O'Brien, D Clement, PW de Leeuw, G Mancia, C Nachev, P Palatini, G Parati, J Tuomilehto, J Webster, for the Systolic Hypertension in Europe Trial Investigators. Predicting cardiovascular risk using conventional vs ambulatory blood pressure in older patients with systolic hypertension. *JAMA* 1999; 282: 539–46. **291**

KO Stumpe, D Haworth, C Hoglund, L Kerwin, A Martin, T Simon, C Masson, K Kassler-Taub, M Osbakken. Comparison of the angiotensin II receptor antagonists irbesartan with atenolol for treatment of hypertension. *Blood Pressure* 1998; 7: 31–7. **271**

G Sütsch, M Büchi, AM Zeither, *et al.* on behalf of the ENCORE Trial Investigators. Effects of calcium antagonism and HMG-coenzyme reductase inhibition on endothelial function and atherosclerosis: rationale and outline of the ENCORE trials. *Eur Heart J* 1999; 1 (Suppl M): M27–32. **307**

R Tang, M Hennig, B Thomasson, R Scherz, R Ravinetto, R Catalini, P Rubba, A Zanchetti, MG Bond, for the ELSA Investigators. Baseline reproducibility of B-mode ultrasonic measurement of carotid artery intima–media thickness: the European Lacidipine Study on Atherosclerosis (ELSA). *J Hypertens* 2000, 18: 197–201. **304**

P A Thürmann, P Kendi, A Schmidt, S Harder, N Rietbrock. Influence of the angiotensin II antagonist valsartan on left ventricular hypertrophy in patients with essential hypertension. *Circulation* 1998; 98: 2037–42. **277**

A K Trocha, C Schmidtke, U Didjurgeit, I Muhlhauser, R Bender, M Berger, PT Sawicki. Effects of intensified antihypertensive treatment in diabetic nephropathy: mortality and morbidity results of a prospective controlled 10-year study. *J Hypertens* 1999; 17: 1497–503. **310**

P Verdecchia, G Schillaci, C Borgioni, A Ciucci, R Gattobigio, I Zampi, G Reboldi, C Porcellati. Prognostic significance of serial changes in left ventricular mass in essential hypertension. *Circulation* 1998; 97: 48–54. **314**

General Index